IgE Regulation

MOLECULAR MECHANISMS

IgE Regulation

MOLECULAR MECHANISMS

Edited by

DONATA VERCELLI

Istituto di Ricovero e Cura
a Carattere Scientifico,
Milan, Italy

JOHN WILEY & SONS

Chichester · New York · Weinheim · Brisbane · Singapore · Toronto

Other Wiley Editorial Offices

John Wiley & Sons, Inc., 605 Third Avenue,
New York, NY 10158-0012, USA

WILEY-VCH Verlag GmbH, Pappelallee 3,
D-69469 Weinheim, Germany

Jacaranda Wiley Ltd, 33 Park Road, Milton,
Queensland 4064, Australia

John Wiley & Sons (Asia) Pte Ltd, 2 Clementi Loop #02-01,
Jin Xing Distripark, Singapore 129809

John Wiley & Sons (Canada) Ltd, 22 Worcester Road,
Rexdale, Ontario M9W 1L1, Canada

Library of Congress Cataloging-in-Publication Data

IgE regulation : molecular mechanisms / edited by Donata Vercelli.
 p. cm.
 Includes bibliographical references and index.
 ISBN 0-471-97138-3 (cased)
 1. Immunoglobulin E.   2. Immune response—Regulation.   3. Immune
response—molecular aspects. I. Vercelli, Donata.
QR186.8.E2I45   1997   97–15134
616.07'98—dc21   CIP

British Library Cataloguing in Publication Data

A catalogue record for this book is available from the British Library

ISBN 0-471-97138-3

Typeset in 10/12pt Times from the author's disks by Techset Composition Ltd, Salisbury
Printed and bound in great Britain by Biddles Ltd, Guildford and King's Lynn
This book is printed on acid-free paper responsibly manufactured from sustainable forestation, for which at least two trees are planted for each one used for paper production.

Contents

Contributors

Alessandra A. Agresti
Molecular Immunoregulation Unit, DIBIT, San Raffaele Scientific Institute, Via Olgettina, 58, 20132 Milano, Italy

Dr Frederick W. Alt
Howard Hughes Medical Institute, Children's Hospital, 300 Longwood Avenue, Boston MA 02115, USA

Dr Tanya Ball
Experimentelle Pathologie, Universität Wien, Wahringer Gurtel 18-20, 1090 Wien, Austria

Dr Rebecca L. Beavil
The Randall Institute, King's College London, 26–29 Drury Lane, London WC2B 5RL, UK

Dr Eugene R. Bleecker
University of Maryland School of Medicine, Baltimore, MD, USA

Dr Andrea Bottaro
Howard Hughes Medical Institute, Children's Hospital, 300 Longwood Avenue, Boston MA 02115, USA

Dr Volker Brinkmann
Novastis Pharma Inc., Research Department, Therapeutic Area Respiratory Diseases, CH-4002 Basel, Switzerland

Dr Melissa A. Brown
Department of Experimental Pathology, Emory University School of Medicine, 1639 Pierce Drive, Atlanta GA 30322, USA

Dr Sylvia K. Chai
Department of Medicine and Microbiology, Columbia University, Morningside Heights, New York, NY 10027, USA

Dr Gianfranco Del Prete
Istituto di Clinica Medica III, Universitá di Firenze – Policlinico di Careggi, Viale Morgagni, 85, 50134 Firenze, Italy

Dr Stephen R. Durham
Imperial College School of Medicine, National Heart and Lung Institute, Dovehouse Street, London SW3 6LY, UK

Dr Rodolfo Ghirlando
Centre de Biochemie Structurale, Faculte de Pharmacie, CNRS UMR 9955-UM1-INSERM U414, 15, 34060 Montpellier, France

Professor Hannah J. Gould
The Randall Institute, King's College London, 26–29 Drury Lane, London WC2B 5RL, UK

Dr Qutayba A. Hamid
McGill University, Meakins-Christie Laboratories, Montreal, Quebec H2X 2P2, Canada

Dr Bernd Kinzel
Novastis Pharma Inc., Research Department, Therapeutic Area Respiratory Diseases, CH-4002 Basel, Switzerland

Dr Check W. Ma
The Randall Institute, King's College London, 26–29 Drury Lane, London WC2B 5RL, UK

Dr Deborah A. Meyers
Professor of Pediatrics, University of Maryland at Baltimore, 108 N. Greene Street, Baltimore, MD21201, USA

Professor Dr Andreas Radbruch
Deutsches Rheumaforschungszentrum Berlin, Monbijouhaus, Monbijoustr. 2A, D-10117 Berlin, Germany

Dr Rajko Reljić
The Randall Institute, King's College London, 26–29 Drury Lane, London WC2B 5RL, UK

Professor Sergio Romagnani
Istituto di Clinica Medica III, Universitá di Firenze – Policlinico di Careggi, Viale Morgagni, 85, 50134 Firenze, Italy

Dr Paul B. Rothman
Department of Medicine and Microbiology, Columbia University, New York, NY 10027, USA

Dr Andrew Saxon
Division of Clinical Immunology and Allergy, University of Los Angeles, California School of Medicine, 10833 Le Conte Avenue, Los Angeles, CA 90024-1680, USA

Dr Jianguo Shi
The Randall Institute, King's College London, 26–29 Drury Lane, London WC2B 5RL, UK

Dr Gregor Siebenkotten
Miltenyi Biotec GmBh, Friedrich-Ebert-Str. 68, D-51429 Bergisch Gladbach, Germany

Dr Brian J. Sutton
The Randall Institute, King's College London, 26–29 Drury Lane, London WC2B 5RL, UK

Dr Rudolf Valenta
Experimentelle Pathologie, Universität Wien, Wahringer Gurtel 18-20, 1090 Wien, Austria

Dr Donata Vercelli
Molecular Immunoregulation Unit, DIBIT, San Raffaele Scientific Institute, Via Olgettina, 58, 20132 Milano, Italy

Dr Ke Zhang
Division of Clinical Immunology and Allergy, University of Los Angeles, California School of Medicine, 10833 Le Conte Avenue, Los Angeles, CA 90024-1680, USA

Preface

It all started in Stockholm, although at the time I didn't know it. The Pharmacia Allergy Research Foundation, an institution that has the commendable habit of keeping close track of what its members are up to, had assembled a nice meeting within the meeting, a symposium on the latest developments in allergy research held during the 1994 ICACI. Thus, I flew from Milano on a warm day in late June and presented the most recent developments of our work on the molecular mechanisms of IgE regulation in front of a pleasantly packed room.

The meeting was lively and enjoyable, the bright summer nights astonishing and exhilarating. I went back home perfectly satisfied with the trip. Later, however, I realized that in a way the best was yet to be. One day, not very long after the Stockholm meeting, I received a letter from Dr Farouk Shakib, who first expressed interest in the field of IgE regulation and IgE switching (how could I, of all people, disagree?), then kindly acknowledged the contribution of my lab – as highlighted in my Stockholm talk – as substantial (who wouldn't be flattered?), and finally proceeded to tempt me (any resemblance between Dr Shakib and Mephistopheles is purely accidental). John Wiley & Sons might, he wrote, be interested in a book on IgE regulation with you as the editor. The time is right, the field is blooming, there isn't much around about the molecular work (molecular was going to become the code word from the very start), would you like to do it? I was intrigued and pleased, but deep down I was also scared. Editing a book was something I had sworn to myself never to do, having seen so many of my friends and colleagues engage in this task only to live to repent. On the other hand, I instantly saw a chance of doing something different and possibly novel, a tight, 'vertical' account of a field that is technically complex, and perhaps even a bit arcane, but also truly fascinating. To understand how and why a B lymphocyte makes the choice of the immunoglobulin isotype it will produce has always seemed to me an exciting intellectual challenge, something that can take us right into the heart of the decision-making process of immune cells. These are, to wit, fateful decisions, so fateful in fact that they involve subtle tuning and tight regulatory mechanisms. To understand how and why a B lymphocyte picks IgE as the isotype to produce is even more challenging, because in the highly regulated world of switching this is the most unlikely, hence the most demanding, choice. On top of everything else, the topic isn't an easy one to study. The experimental models one can choose are not as amenable to manipulation and as transparent as we would like them to be. Even with the most recent, technically powerful approaches (knock-out mice, for instance) often more questions have been raised than answers given – not to mention the ever-pervasive difficulty of extrapolating to humans results obtained in animal models. For quite some time I did not know how to answer, and I struggled to find a way to bring order to my own decision making. Finally, I realized that in my heart of hearts I wanted to do this book, and I knew how I wanted to do it. Yet, I was reluctant to stick my neck out because I was afraid that my views might be too uncompromising and therefore unpalatable. *À la guerre comme à la guerre*: I wrote back, and I simply said what I thought, i.e. that I would do this IgE book if and only if the outcome was going to be something I myself would like to read. That meant having a free hand in picking authors and topics. Most of all, it meant dispensing with issues that, although very popular in certain quarters, are in my own view somewhat trivial. IgE switching is a topic of compelling interest for any articulate biologically-orientated mind. It certainly requires explanations, but can do without cheap simplifications. When the experiments are well presented, the relevance of this work to general issues in biology and medicine comes out loud and clear.

The outline of the book that I sent to England was short, dry and did not make much of an effort to be eloquent. But as it turned out, I was indeed very fortunate because I had an enlightened counterpart who gave me a green light and never flinched. In no time contracts were signed, and it all got moving. Right from the beginning and all the way through, the support from the people at Wiley has been unswerving. Michael Osuch in particular has been invaluable in steering me, using the carrot much more than the stick.

Now that I am sitting in my cozy New England hide-out surrounded by snow and I finally have the complete manuscript in front of me, I can say that all promises have been kept. Working on this book was hard, but was also fun. I am proud, very proud, of all my authors, of what they told, of how they told it. They all graciously accepted, they all graciously complied. I asked for something different, no party line, no 'scientific correctness', say what you think, and say why you think it. Be focussed and not unnecessarily user friendly. No need to be smooth, if there are differences in opinions and views, stress them. Discuss only your own work, don't write a review, other people will have a chance to speak for themselves. All my authors gave me what I asked for, even though writing something of this kind is unusual and therefore more time-consuming, more demanding. I am deeply grateful to all of them. I feel that what these scientists have contributed amounts to a lucid, very often provocative, always compelling account of a unique biological process: a model system for how a highly specialized immune cell makes a lifetime choice. Even though (or perhaps because) it is up to date, this book won't last forever. In fact, at the risk of making our publisher unhappy, one should hope for progress so fast as to make it quickly obsolete. It will not matter. If this book convinces one, just one, bright young researcher that this is the kind of problem she wants to tackle, my authors and I will feel that it was worth the effort.

Donata Vercelli
Marblehead, MA, USA

1 How T Cells Direct IgE Switching

SERGIO ROMAGNANI and GIANFRANCO DEL PRETE
Institute of Internal Medicine and Immunoallergology, University of Florence, Florence, Italy

1.1 INTRODUCTION

Atopic allergy is a genetically determined disorder affecting a considerable proportion of the population, whose main pathophysiological feature is an enhanced ability of B cells to produce immunoglobulin (Ig)E antibodies in response to certain ubiquitous antigens (allergens) able to activate the immune system after inhalation, ingestion, and perhaps diffusion through the skin. Evidence for the importance of the IgE antibody response in atopic diseases comes from both epidemiology and experimental models (1). IgE antibodies bind to high affinity (type I) Fcε receptors (FcεRI) expressed on mast cells and basophils. Allergen-induced FcεRI cross-linking triggers the release of powerful vasoactive mediators, chemotactic factors and cytokines, which are responsible for several pathophysiological changes, known as 'the allergic cascade' (2). In addition to IgE-producing B cells and IgE-binding mast cells/basophils, eosinophils are also consistently involved in allergic reactions, inasmuch as these cells tend to accumulate at the sites of allergic inflammation where their toxic products significantly contribute to tissue damage (3).

In recent years, the cellular basis of IgE regulation has been actively investigated. The studies of molecular events underlying IgE synthesis have provided an interesting model to identify and characterize the signals involved in isotype-specific regulation of Ig synthesis in humans. More importantly, the intense study of the functional properties of T helper (Th) cells that help B cells in antibody production has clarified the mechanisms accounting for the joint involvement of IgE-producing B cells, mast cells/basophils and eosinophils in the pathogenesis of allergic disorders.

This chapter mainly focuses on the regulatory mechanisms of IgE synthesis in humans and the mechanisms which regulate the development of type 2 T helper cells (Th2), which are responsible for both IgE synthesis and the recruitment and activation of the other cell types involved in allergic reactions.

1.2 SIGNALS INVOLVED IN IGE PRODUCTION

For many years, studies performed in rodents suggested that IgE production could be regulated by antigen-specific helper and suppressor T cells, as well as by isotype-

IgE Regulation: Molecular Mechanisms. Edited by D. Vercelli. © 1997 John Wiley & Sons Ltd.

specific factors showing affinity for IgE (IgE-binding factors) (1). Since 1986, a completely different pathway of murine IgE regulation has emerged that is based on the reciprocal activity of interleukin (IL)-4 (at that time still termed B cell stimulatory factor-1; BSF-1) and interferon (IFN)-γ (4).

1.2.1 The IgE Switching Cytokines: IL-4 and IL-13

Murine B cells stimulated *in vitro* with lipopolysaccharide (LPS) could be induced by BSF-1/IL-4 to produce IgE and IgG1, and this activity was strongly inhibited by IFN-γ (4). The crucial role of IL-4 in the induction of murine IgE synthesis has also been confirmed *in vivo*. Suppression of *in vivo* polyclonal IgE responses could be achieved by injection of an anti-IL-4 antibody, and no IgE synthesis could be detected in IL-4-deficient mouse mutants obtained by IL-4 gene targeting (5). Stimulation of murine B cells with IL-4 and LPS induced the appearance of 1.7–1.9 kb ε germline transcripts. Such transcripts contain an Iε exon, located 2 kb upstream of the ε switch region, spliced to the Cε 1–4 exons (6) (see also Chapters 7–10).

In 1988, the crucial role of IL-4 in the induction of human IgE synthesis could be demonstrated in an *in vitro* model based on the use of T-cell clones (7, 8). Phytohemagglutinin (PHA)—or anti-CD3 antibody-stimulated—T-cell clones, as well as their supernatants, were able to provide substantial help for IgE synthesis by normal B cells. When the ability of PHA-induced T-cell clones (or their supernatants) to induce IgE synthesis was compared with their ability to produce (or their content of) IL-2, IL-4 and IFN-γ, a significant positive correlation was found between the helper function for IgE synthesis and the production of IL-4. Conversely, a significant inverse relationship was found between the IgE helper activity of T-cell clones (or their supernatants) and their ability to produce (or their content of) IFN-γ (7). This opposite regulatory role for IL-4 and IFN-γ in human IgE synthesis *in vitro* was further supported by the observation that, (i) addition of human recombinant IL-4 resulted in IgE synthesis by peripheral blood mononuclear cells (PBMC) (7, 8), and, (ii) this effect was dose-dependently inhibited by the addition of recombinant IFN-γ (7, 8). Furthermore, a neutralizing anti-IL-4 antibody markedly suppressed IgE synthesis induced in B cells by all the active T-cell clones tested (or their supernatants), whereas it had little, if any, inhibitory activity on the synthesis of IgM and IgG. Besides inducing IgE, IL-4 was also found to induce *in vitro* production of IgG4, the human counterpart of murine IgG1 (8).

More recently IL-13, a cytokine showing about 30% homology with IL-4 but sharing similar IgE switching activity, was discovered (9). Mouse and human IL-13 are not active on T cells, exert similar effects on macrophages, but differ in their effects on B cells. Mouse IL-13 is inactive on B cells, whereas human IL-13 has IL-4-like effects, being able to induce both B cell proliferation and isotype switching to IgE and IgG4. Like IL-4, IL-13 induces ε germline mRNA expression in highly purified B cells, and this accounts for its ability to drive B-cell switching to the IgE isotype. IL-13, which seems to be about two- to five-fold less potent than IL-4 in inducing IgE production, has neither additive nor synergistic effects with IL-4 in the induction of IgE or IgG4 isotypes. This is in favor of the possibility that IL-4 and IL-13 use a common signaling pathway for the induction of these Ig isotypes. Indeed, it has recently been shown that receptors for IL-4 and IL-13 are distinct, but share a common subunit (10). Like human IL-4, human IL-13 is produced by activated T cells, but the kinetics of IL-13 production is markedly different from that of IL-4. Although IL-13 mRNA expression peaks approximately 2 hours after activation, considerable steady levels of IL-13 mRNA are still observed after 72 hours. In contrast, IL-4 mRNA peaks after 4–6 hours, but becomes minimal or undetectable after 24 hours. Based on these observations, it was inferred that IL-13 may also play a role in the regulation of enhanced IgE synthesis in atopy (10) (see also Chapter 5).

1.2.2 T-B Cell-to-cell Contact-mediated Signals

Although both IL-4 and IL-13 are sufficient for the initiation of ε germline transcription, additional signals are required for the expression of mature ε mRNA transcripts and IgE protein production. Both IL-4 and IL-13 failed to induce IgE synthesis in highly purified B cells, but IL-4-dependent IgE synthesis could be restored by the addition of appropriate concentrations of autologous or allogeneic activated T cells. Addition of monocytes further potentiated this effect (11). In contrast, IgE synthesis by highly purified B cells was not restored by using mixtures of different concentrations of T cell- (and/or monocyte-) derived cytokines, suggesting that a physical interaction between T and B cells is required for IL-4- (and IL-13-) dependent IgE synthesis. Direct evidence in support of this hypothesis was provided by assessing IgE synthesis in a double-compartment culture system. When T and B cells were cultured in different chambers separated by microporous membranes permeable to molecules but not to cells, IL-4 failed to induce IgE synthesis by purified B cells. Indeed, IL-4-induced IgE synthesis occurred only when T and B cells were co-cultured in the same compartment (12, 13). This observation led to the proposition of a two-signal model for the induction of human IgE synthesis (11, 14). The hypothesis was that cognate T-B cell-to-cell interaction was required to induce the release of IL-4 (and/or IL-13) by activated T cells, but the molecules involved in contact-mediated signaling were independent of the T cell receptor (TCR)–CD3/ major histocompatibility complex (MHC) class II (11). Indeed, both CD4$^+$ and CD8$^+$ PHA-induced T-cell clones were able to induce IgE synthesis by B cells from randomly selected donors if exogenous IL-4 was added in culture. Further evidence for the role of a 'non-cognate' interaction in the induction of IgE synthesis was provided by assessing the activity of an alloreactive Th2-like T-cell clone (TR46). This clone could induce IgE synthesis when co-cultured with B cells possessing the appropriate alloantigen (DR4). When DR4$^+$ B cells were irradiated, IgE synthesis did not occur, but their presence in culture enabled DR4^A unirradiated B cells to produce IgE. More importantly, in the presence of exogenous IL-4, the TR46 clone enabled B cells from all donors tested to produce IgE, regardless of their DR haplotype (13). Finally, mouse EL-4 thymoma cells potently induced IgE synthesis by human B cells provided that both phorbol ester and exogenous IL-4 were added (11).

The nature of the molecule(s) involved in the contact-mediated non-cognate signaling required for IgE production has been investigated. Different couples of molecules may be involved in T-B cell-to-cell interaction; however, a critical signal seems to be provided by the interaction of CD40 expressed on B cells with its natural ligand (CD40L) expressed by activated T cells (15). CD40 is a member of the tumor necrosis factor receptor (TNF-R) superfamily that includes both type I and type II TNF-R, the nerve growth factor receptor, CD27, CD30, and Fas antigen (16). CD40 is a 50 kDa glycoprotein expressed on all human B cells, but not by resting T cells. Interestingly, anti-CD40 monoclonal antibodies (mAbs) could replace activated T cells in induction of IgE synthesis driven by IL-4 (15). The ability of anti-CD40 mAbs to replace T cells in the induction of IgE synthesis suggested the presence of a ligand for CD40 on activated T cells. CD40L, a 33 kDa type II glycoprotein with significant homology to TNF-α and TNF-β, has indeed been cloned from cDNA libraries derived from activated T cells (15). Transfectants expressing CD40L induced B-cell proliferation and differentiation into IgE-secreting cells in the presence of IL-4, indicating that all signals required for IgE switching could be delivered by CD40L and IL-4 (17). More importantly, the gene encoding CD40L was mapped on the X-chromosome (q26.3–q27.1), in the same region where a gene defect in patients with X-linked hyper-IgM syndrome was identified. Patients with hyper-IgM syndrome, who have minimal levels of IgG, IgA and IgE in their sera, have mutations in their CD40L gene that result in defective expression of CD40L and impaired isotype switching *in vivo* (18). In addition, T cells from a subset of patients suffering from common variable immunodeficiency were found to express suboptimal levels of CD40L, further supporting an essential role for CD40/CD40L interactions in productive T/B cell collaboration (19).

T/B cell contact-mediated signals, other than CD40/CD40L interactions, may also be involved in the events leading to B-cell activation, proliferation and differentiation. Indeed, when B cells are stimulated with anti-CD40 mAbs in the presence of activated CD4$^+$ T cells and optimal concentrations of IL-4, a synergistic effect on IgE synthesis is observed. The 26 kDa membrane form of TNF-α (mTNF-α) expressed on CD4$^+$ T cells after activation is another molecule associated with productive T cell/B cell interactions. Anti-TNF-α mAbs strongly inhibit IgE synthesis induced by activated CD4$^+$ T-cell clones or their membranes (20), as well as Ig production induced by human immunodeficiency virus- or herpesvirus saimiri-infected CD4$^+$ T-cell clones (21, 22). Likewise, the ligation of B cell CD58 (leukocyte function-associated antigen-3; LFA-3) by CD2 (its natural ligand expressed on T cells) or anti-CD58 mAb, in concert with IL-4-stimulated ε germline transcription induced the appearance of productive ε transcripts and IgE production (23). Interestingly, anti-CD58 mAbs also inhibited Ig production induced in B cells by herpesvirus saimiri-infected CD4$^+$ T-cell clones (22). Recently, the ligand for CD30 (CD30L) was cloned (24) and found to be active in inducing CD40L-independent IgE secretion (25). Thus, although CD40/CD40L interactions seem to be essential for B-cell differentiation and

Ig isotype switching, other molecules—including mTNF-α, CD2 and CD30L—can modulate the isotype switching events during T/B cell interactions.

1.2.3 T-Cell Independent Models of IL-4-dependent IgE Synthesis

Apart from the above mentioned model of IgE synthesis induced by stimulation with IL-4 and anti-CD40 mAb (that mimics the activity of CD40L expressed on activated T cells), other T-cell independent systems of IgE synthesis have been described (26). Stimulation with IL-4 and Epstein–Barr virus (EBV) induces T-cell independent IgE synthesis in human B cells (27). The nature of the EBV-mediated signal favoring the transcription of mature Cε transcripts is presently unknown. However, it does not simply result from engagement of the EBV receptor/CD21/complement receptor 2 (CR2). Indeed, mAbs to different CD21 epitopes could not synergize with IL-4 in IgE induction. EBV infection results in the expression of a variety of viral genes in B cells, one of which may facilitate recombination indirectly, through effects on transcription or cell proliferation (26).

IgE synthesis has also been induced in human CD5$^+$ leukemic B cells by a combination of IL-4 and hydrocortisone (28). Normal polyclonal IgE$^-$ B cells isolated by cell sorting are also inducible to IgE synthesis by hydrocortisone and IL-4, in the absence of both T cells and monocytes. The nature of the hydrocortisone-derived signal is unknown. Analysis of the effects of hydrocortisone on ε] germline transcription showed that hydrocortisone by itself did not induce ε germline transcripts, but modestly enhanced their accumulation. Since both hydrocortisone and CD40 engagement induced vigorous IgE synthesis in the presence of IL-4, it is likely that IgE synthesis induced by hydrocortisone also reflects effect(s) on step(s) other than ε germline transcription (29).

It has recently been reported that mast cell and basophilic cell lines are able to increase IgG and to induce IgE synthesis in purified B cells stimulated with IL-4 in the absence of T cells. Both effects were inhibited by competition with a chimeric recombinant fusion protein consisting of the extracellular domain of human CD40 fused to a murine IgG constant region (CD40-Fc) (30). These results suggest that mast cell or basophilic cell lines can replace T cells in providing the contact-mediated signal required (together with IL-4) for the induction of IgE synthesis *in vitro*. Inhibition by CD40-Fc indicates the involvement of CD40L. Accordingly, purified normal lung mast cells and blood basophils were found to support IgE production by B cells in the absence of T cells (30). Basophils, but not mast cells, were able to induce IgE synthesis even in the absence of exogenous IL-4. This would be consistent with the observation that basophils are able to release IL-4 (31), whereas the ability of normal mast cells to release IL-4 (32) is more controversial. Based on these findings, it has been suggested that mast cells and basophils may play a role in the regulation of IgE synthesis *in vivo* and that Ig isotype switching may occur also outside the germinal centers, in peripheral organs such as lung or skin (30) (see also Chapter 2). However, the *in vivo* relevance of this *in vitro* model is unclear.

1.3 MODULATION OF IGE SYNTHESIS

1.3.1 IgE Enhancing Factors

T cell- and IL-4-dependent IgE synthesis can be modulated by cytokines other than IL-4. IL-2, IL-5, IL-6, TNF-α (33) and IL-9 (34) enhance IL-4-induced IgE synthesis. IL-5 and IL-6 have been shown to upregulate IgE production induced by IL-4 in unfractionated peripheral blood mononuclear cells (PBMC). However, upregulation of IgE by IL-5 could be observed only when suboptimal IL-4 concentrations were used (35), whereas IL-6 could enhance IgE synthesis even in the presence of high concentrations of IL-4 (36). IL-6 is known to act at a late stage in B-cell differentiation with no isotype preference. IL-6 induces the secretion of IgG1 by coordinated transcriptional activation, selective accumulation of mRNA for the secreted form of IgG, and possibly differential mRNA stabilization. Even though no direct evidence is available, IL-6 might amplify IgE secretion by similar mechanisms (33). The mechanisms responsible for the enhancement of IgE synthesis by IL-2 and TNF-α are not completely clear. Both cytokines influence the proliferation of both T and B lymphocytes, as well as the differentiation of B cells into antibody-producing cells. However, the effects of IL-2 and TNF-α on IgE production induced in the presence of T cells or in their absence (stimulation of purified B cells with anti-CD40 antibody or soluble CD40L) have not been compared. Interestingly, in the T-cell dependent model, IL-2 was found to exert opposite effects on IgE helper activity by naive or memory T cells. IgE helper activity by naive T cells was inhibited, whereas in the presence of IL-2 the IgE helper activity of memory T cells was enhanced (37). However, the finding that IL-2 was able to potentiate T-cell/IL-4-dependent IgE synthesis even when T cells had been treated with mitomycin C suggested that the enhancing effect of IL-2 on IgE synthesis was not merely due to its T-cell growth factor activity (38).

1.3.2 IgE Inhibitory Factors

Cytokines or mediators such as IFN-α, IFN-γ (7, 8), transforming growth factor (TGF)-β (39), IL-8 (40), IL-10 (41), IL-12 (42), PAF-acether (43), and prostaglandin E2 (8) have been shown to downregulate IgE synthesis *in vitro* (33). IFN-α and IFN-γ inhibit IL-4-dependent IgE synthesis in both mice and humans (4, 7, 8), but the mechanisms by which they inhibit IgE synthesis are not well understood. IFN-γ was found to suppress the expression of ε germline transcripts in murine B cells stimulated with LPS and IL-4. By contrast, no inhibition was observed when IFN-γ was added to highly purified human B cells stimulated with IL-4, suggesting that activation of ε germline transcription and switch recombination may not be necessarily coupled. TGF-β and PAF-acether suppress both ε germline transcription and IgE synthesis in human B cells stimulated with IL-4. IL-8 also suppresses IgE synthesis by purified B cells stimulated with IL-4 and anti-CD40 mAb, but the mechanism has not been investigated. IL-8 was found to block spontaneous IgE synthesis, and this effect was apparently mediated by its ability to decrease the production of IL-6 and TNF-α (44). IL-10 blocks IgE synthesis by PBMC by inhibiting the accessory cell function of monocytes (41). However, IL-10 also directly stimulates B cells cultured in the presence of IL-4 and anti-CD40 mAbs cross-linked to CD32 (FcγRII) on murine L cells (45). The mechanism responsible for the inhibitory activity of IL-12 on IgE synthesis is still unknown. However, inhibition by this cytokine may well be mediated by IFN-γ, since IL-12 is a powerful inducer of IFN-γ release by both T cells and natural killer (NK) cells (46).

1.3.3 CD23

The effects on human IgE production *in vitro* of signals delivered via CD23 deserve a separate discussion. CD23 is the low-affinity receptor for IgE. Two forms of CD23, FcεRIIa and FcεRIIb, which differ only in their N-terminal cytoplasmic portion, are generated through the use of different transcription sites and alternative RNA splicing (47). FcεRIIa is expressed by B cells, whereas FcεRIIb is expressed by monocytes and Langerhansí cells upon activation by IL-4. CD23 is a labile protein, since a soluble fragment (sCD23) is released from the carboxy-terminal extracellular portion of the molecule. The studies on the role of sCD23 in the regulation of IgE synthesis have resulted in somewhat contradictory results. Supernatants of CD23$^+$ B cell lines or purified sCD23 were shown to enhance IgE synthesis (48, 49), and mAbs specific for CD23 inhibited B-cell proliferation and differentiation (50). By contrast, other studies suggested that recombinant sCD23 had no B-cell growth promoting activity *in vitro* (51). Administration to mice of anti-CD23 mAbs strongly inhibited antigen-specific IgE synthesis (52), suggesting a role for CD23 in the regulation of IgE production *in vivo*. In addition, CD21, another ligand for CD23, was apparently able to modulate IgE production (53). More recent experiments performed in both CD23 gene-targeted and CD23 transgenic mice suggest that membrane CD23 is involved in a feedback regulatory circuit active on IgE synthesis (54–56). Such a regulatory effect is probably mediated by a negative signal delivered by the interaction of IgE-containing immune complexes with CD23 expressed on the B cell surface (56). However, at least in these very reliable experimental models, the role for sCD23 in the regulation of IgE synthesis does not seem to be noteworthy (see also Chapter 3 in this book).

1.4 TH2 CELLS: FUNCTIONAL ASPECTS AND MODULATION OF DEVELOPMENT

The role of Th cells and Th cell-derived cytokines in the induction of IgE synthesis was further clarified by the demonstration that functionally distinct subsets of CD4$^+$ Th cells, reminiscent of those already described in mice (57), do also exist in humans (58).

1.4.1 The Th1/Th2 Dichotomy

Two very polarized forms of the specific Th cell-mediated response have been described, based on their distinct and mutually exclusive patterns of cytokine secretion. Th1, but not Th2, cells produce IFN-γ and TNF-β; whereas Th2, but not Th1, cells produce IL-4 and IL-5. In humans, the production of other cytokines, such as IL-2, IL-10 and IL-13, is less restricted than in mice (59), although IL-2 is mainly released by Th1 cells, whereas IL-10 and IL-13 are mainly released by Th2 cells. Different cytokine patterns also imply distinct effector functions. Th1 cells, which trigger both cell-mediated immunity and production of opsonizing antibodies, are involved in phagocyte-dependent defense in response to intracellular pathogens (60). In contrast, Th2 cells are responsible for IgE and IgG4 antibody production, differentiation and activation of mast cells and eosinophils, inhibition of some macrophage functions, and are mainly involved in the phagocyte-independent defense against extracellular parasites (60). Human Th1 and Th2 cells also differ in their cytolytic potential and mode of providing B cells with help for Ig synthesis *in vitro*. Th2 clones, which usually lack cytolytic potential, were found to induce IgM, IgG, IgA, and IgE synthesis by autologous B cells that bear the specific antigen, with a response which was proportional to the number of Th2 cells added to B cells. In contrast, Th1 clones (most of which are cytolytic) provided B cell help for the synthesis of IgM, IgG and IgA, but not IgE, at low T/B cell ratios. At ratios higher than 1:1, a decline in Ig production was observed, due to a concomitant Th1-mediated lysis of antigen-presenting autologous B cells (61). Another functional difference between human Th1 and Th2 clones was found in their ability to induce monocyte procoagulant activity (PCA) and tissue factor (TF) production. Th1, but not Th2, clones induced both PCA and TF in monocytes by both physical cell-to-cell interaction and release of soluble factors. Antigen-dependent induction of TF synthesis in monocytes was at least partially mediated by IFN-γ released by Th1 clones, whereas IL-4, IL-13 and IL-10 released by Th2 clones were strongly inhibitory (62) (Table 1.1).

In addition to cells that fit into the Th1 or Th2 polarized phenotypes, CD4$^+$ Th0 cells have been identified that show a composite profile, with production of both Th1- and Th2-type cytokines and effects that depend on the ratio of cytokines produced (60). More recently, human T cell clones producing Th2-type cytokines were found to differ from those producing Th1-type cytokines in their ability to express membrane CD30 (63), a member of the TNF-R superfamily (16), and to release CD30 in soluble form (sCD30) (63).

1.4.2 Preferential Development of Allergen-specific Th2 Cells in Atopic Subjects, and Their Role in the Pathogenesis of Allergy

Because of their ability to produce IL-3, granulocyte–macrophage colony-stimulating factor (GM-CSF), IL-4, IL-5 and IL-10, Th2 cells represent an excellent candidate to explain why the mast cell/eosinophil/IgE-producing B cell triad is

Table 1.1. Main properties of human CD4$^+$ T helper (Th) cells

Functions	Th1	Th2	Th0
Cytokine secretion			
IFN-γ	++	−	++
TNF-β	++	−	++
IL-2	++	+/−	++
IL-3	+/−	++	+
IL-6	+/−	++	+
GM-CSF	+/−	++	+
LIF	+	++	++
TNF-α	++	+	++
IL-10	+/−	++	+
IL-13	+/−	++	+
IL-4	−	++	+
IL-5	−	++	+
Cytotoxic activity	++	−	+
Induction of monocyte procoagulant activity	++	−	+
Help for Ig synthesis			
IgE	−	++	+/−
IgM, IgG, IgA			
(low T : B ratio)	+	+	+
(high T : B ratio)	−	++	+
Expression and release			
CD30	−/+	++	+
LAG-3	++	−/+	+

involved in the pathogenesis of allergy. Cytokines such as IL-3, IL-4 and IL-10 are growth factors for mast cells; IL-3, GM-CSF and IL-5 promote eosinophil differentiation, activation and survival in tissues (64).

The analysis of cytokine production by T-cell clones specific for different antigens has clearly shown that, in contrast to clones specific for bacterial antigens which generally show a prevalent Th1/Th0 phenotype, the great majority of allergen-specific T cell clones generated from peripheral blood lymphocytes of atopic donors express a Th0/Th2 phenotype, with high production of IL-4 and IL-5 and no or low production of IFN-γ (65, 66). Evidence suggesting that Th2-like cells accumulate in target organs of different allergic disorders has been provided by using either cloning techniques or *in situ* hybridization. The majority of T-cell clones generated from the conjunctival infiltrates of patients with vernal conjunctivitis was found to preferentially express the Th2 cytokine profile (67). *In situ* hybridization showed mRNA for Th2, but not Th1, cytokines at the site of late phase skin reactions in skin biopsies from atopic patients, in mucosal bronchial biopsies or bronchoalveolar lavage (BAL) from patients with allergic asthma (68–70), and in the nasal mucosa of patients with allergen-induced rhinitis following local allergen challenge (71) (see also Chapter 2 in this book). Likewise, increased levels of IL-4 and IL-5 were measured in BAL of allergic asthmatics, whereas in non-allergic asthmatics IL-2 and IL-5 were predominant (72). Finally, 14–22% of T-cell clones generated from the airway mucosa of grass-allergic patients following inhalation challenge with grass pollen appeared to be specific for grass allergens, and most of them exhibited a definite Th2 profile (73). Accordingly, high proportions of *Dermatophagoides pteronyssinus* (DP)-specific Th2-like CD4$^+$ T-cell clones were generated from intact skin of patients with atopic dermatitis obtained after contact challenge with DP (74). Recently, CD30 expression was evaluated in circulating CD4$^+$ T cells from six grass-pollen sensitive patients and six non-atopic controls, before and during the seasonal exposure to grass pollens. Virtually no CD4$^+$ CD30$^+$ cells were detected in any of the non-atopic donors or the atopic patients examined before the pollen season, whereas four out of six grass-sensitive donors examined during the season, when they were suffering from allergic symptoms, showed small but consistent proportions of circulating CD4$^+$ CD30$^+$ cells (up to 0.3%). Circulating CD4$^+$ T cells from these patients were fractionated into CD30$^+$ and CD30$^-$ cells by sorting with an anti-CD30 mAb, the two cell fractions were expanded in IL-2-conditioned medium, and then assessed for their ability to produce type 1 (IFN-γ and TNF-β) or type 2 (IL-4 and IL-5) cytokines, and to proliferate in response to *Lolium perenne* group I (Lol p I). Only CD30$^+$ cells proliferated in response to Lol p I and produced IL-4 and IL-5, whereas production of IFN-γ and TNF-β was prevalent in the CD30$^-$ cell fraction (63). These findings clearly demonstrate that grass allergen-reactive CD4$^+$ CD30$^+$ T cells inducible to produce Th2 cytokines can circulate in the peripheral blood of allergic patients during the *in vivo* natural exposure to allergen.

Recent studies devoted to investigating the effect of allergen-specific immunotherapy on the cytokine profile of allergen-specific T cells have provided further evidence for the role of Th2-like cells in the pathogenesis of IgE-mediated allergic disorders. Immunotherapy did not affect the expression of Th2-type cytokines in response to grass pollen exposure at the level of late-phase cutaneous reactions, but the expression of mRNA for Th1-type cytokines was enhanced in many patients showing clinical improvement (75). Successful immunotherapy was also found to reduce IL-4 production by allergen-specific CD4$^+$ T cells to levels observed in T cells from non-allergic subjects, whereas IFN-γ production was not affected (76). Finally, both decreased production of IL-4 and increased production of IFN-γ was observed in bee venom-sensitized patients treated with specific immunotherapy (77, 78). Although these reports are partially discordant, probably due to the different experimental approaches, they all support the concept that cytokine profiles of allergen-specific memory CD4$^+$ T cells can be therapeutically manipulated *in vivo*. This possibility is also supported by studies in mice injected with chemically modified allergen (79) or infected with *Leishmania major* and treated with IL-12 and pentostam (80) (see also Chapters 2 and 5).

1.4.3 Regulatory Mechanisms of Th2 Development

The mechanisms responsible for the preferential development of allergen-reactive T cells into Th2 effectors in atopics have not yet been fully elucidated. Attention has focused on the possible role of antigen-presenting cells (APC), the T cell repertoire, and soluble factors present in the microenvironment at the time of allergen presentation.

It is possible that skin Langerhans' cells and mucosal dendritic cells represent the primary cells of the immune system which come in contact with allergens, and are probably involved in allergen transport to regional lymph nodes, where allergen presentation to allergen-specific CD4$^+$ T cells does occur. However, the actual role of APC in driving the preferential development of allergen-reactive T cells into Th2 cells is still unclear. It will be of interest to establish whether alterations of the expression and/or activity of CD30L (24) may play some role in the development of allergen-specific Th2 responses in atopic individuals. We have recently shown that co-stimulation through CD30 at the time of allergen presentation favors the development of Th2 responses, whereas blocking of CD30L on APC (by soluble CD30 or anti-CD30L mAbs) shifts the *in vitro* differentiation of allergen-specific T cells from the Th0/Th2 to the Th0/Th1 phenotype (81).

The role of the T-cell repertoire in determining the development of Th1- or Th2-type responses is still controversial (82, 83). A role of hormones in promoting the differentiation of Th cells or in favoring the shift of already differentiated Th cells to a different cytokine profile has also been suggested. Glucocorticoids enhance Th2 activity and synergize with IL-4, whereas dehydroepiandrosterone sulfate enhances Th1 activity (84). Another major pro-hormone, 25-hydroxy-cholecalciferol (25-OH vitamin D3) may have an opposite effect on the Th1/Th2 balance (84). Finally, progesterone favors the *in vitro* development of human Th0/Th2 cells and promotes both IL-4 production and membrane CD30 expression in established human Th1 clones (64). This may represent one of the mechanisms involved in the Th1/Th2 switch which has been hypothesized to occur at the maternal–fetal interface in order to guarantee fetal survival and promote successful pregnancy (85).

The clearest example of factors able to substantially affect the differentiation pathways of Th cells in both mice and humans are the cytokines released by APC and/or other cell types present in the microenvironment at the time of antigen presentation. IFN-α, IL-12 and TGF-β produced by macrophages and B cells play an important role in the induction of Th1 expansion in various systems (86). IFN-γ produced by T cells and natural killer (NK) cells also promotes the differentiation of Th1 cells (87). Likewise IL-12, a powerful IFN-γ inducer (46), appears to be the most important natural initiator of Th1 responses by acting either directly or indirectly via the induction of IFN-γ secretion (88, 89).

The effect of cytokines produced by macrophages and/or B cells on the development of Th2 cells seems to be less critical. IL-10 has been shown to favor the development of Th2 cells both in mouse and man. IL-1 is a selective co-factor for the growth of some murine Th2 clones and can favor the *in vitro* development of human Th2-like clones (64). However, recent data indicate that IL-4 is an essential requirement for the maturation of Th cells into Th2 cells. In both mice and humans, IL-4 is indeed the dominant factor in determining the likelihood of Th2 polarization in cultured T cells (87, 90). Accordingly, IL-4 gene-targeted mice fail to generate mature Th2 cells *in vivo* and to produce IgE antibodies (91), suggesting that early

IL-4 production by another cell type must be involved. Possible candidates include a peculiar CD1-restricted CD4$^+$ NK1.1$^+$ T-cell subset (92), as well as mast cells and basophils, which have been shown to release stored IL-4 in response to FcεRI triggering (31, 32). However, it is not clear how parasites or allergens might activate CD4$^+$ NK1.1$^+$ T cells nor how they would cross-link FcεRI on mast cells/basophils prior to a primary specific immune response resulting in the production of allergen (or parasite)-specific IgG and IgE. On the other hand, Th2 responses in mast cell-deficient mice were not substantially affected (93). More importantly, only recon-stitution with IL-4-producing T cells, but not with IL-4-producing non-T cells (i.e. mast cells/basophils) resulted in the production of antigen-specific IgE in IL-4-deficient mice (94). Thus, IL-4 production by mast cells triggered by antigen-IgE immune complexes may play a role in amplifying secondary responses, but cannot account for Th2 development in primary immune responses. An alternative expla-nation is that some proteolytic enzymes produced by helminths, or anaphylotoxins formed via the alternative complement pathway, trigger mast cells to release IL-4 and other cytokines that induce Th2 differentiation during primary responses. In this regard, it is of note that some environmental allergens are proteases. Injection of papain in BALB/c mice resulted in 10–30-fold increases in IL-4 and IL-5 in draining lymph nodes, whereas inactivated papain was much less potent (95). Recent studies suggest that naive Th cells themselves may represent the primary source of IL-4 in primary responses. Low intensity signaling of TCR, such as that mediated by low peptide doses or by mutant peptides, led to the secretion of small amounts of IL-4 by naive murine T cells (96). Moreover, human CD45RA$^+$ (naive) adult or neonatal peripheral blood T cells were found to develop into IL-4-producing cells in the absence of any pre-existing source of IL-4 and in spite of the presence of anti-IL-4 antibodies (97, 98). Recently, high proportions of T-cell clones showing a definite Th2 profile could be generated from individual CD4$^+$ T cells isolated from the thymus of newborns (99). Thus, evidence is accumulating to suggest that the maturation of naive T cells into the Th2 pathway mainly depends on the levels and the kinetics of IL-4 production by naive T cells themselves at the time of antigen priming. These are likely determined by: (i) the genetic background of the indivi-dual, and (ii) the nature and the intensity of TCR signaling. The fact that allergens induce Th2-type responses only in selected individuals suggests that atopic subjects may have a genetic dysregulation in the production of IL-4 (and/or of cytokines exerting regulatory effects on the development and/or function of Th2 cells) at level of T cells (100) (see also Chapter 4). This possibility is supported by several observations. A remarkable proportion of CD4$^+$ T-cell clones generated from atopics produce IL-4 and IL-5 in response to bacterial antigens, such as purified protein derivative (PPD) and streptokinase (101), which usually evoke Th1-type responses in non-atopic individuals (58). In addition, T-cell clones generated from cord blood lymphocytes of newborns whose parents were atopic produced higher amounts of IL-4 than clones derived from T cells of newborns with non-atopic parents (102). Moreover, large series of T cell clones specific for *Parietaria officinalis* group I (Par O 1) were generated from atopic subjects with low or high serum IgE levels and assessed for their cytokine secretion profile and reactivity to p92 and p96 immu-nodominant Par O 1 peptides. In general, both p92- and p96-specific clones gen-erated from [å]high IgEí donors were able to produce high amounts of IL-4 and low amounts of IFN-γ. In contrast, among the T cell clones derived from 'low IgE' donors, those specific for p96 produced high amounts of both IL-4 and IFN-γ whereas most of the clones reactive against p92 showed a Th1-like profile (102). Taken together, these data support the concept that the type of allergen peptide may influence the cytokine profile of responding Th cells, even though the mechanisms underlying non-cognate regulation of IgE responsiveness seem to be largely pre-dominant.

Recently, it has been suggested that IFN-γ released by MHC class I-restricted CD8$^+$ T cells plays a role in preventing the development of Th2-like cells in response to non-replicating antigens presented at mucosal surfaces (103, 104). Furthermore, inhaled, but not parenteral, IFN-γ decreased IgE production and nor-malized airway functions in a murine model of allergen sensitization (105), sug-gesting that the immediate allergic response to allergen sensitization through the airways may be modulated by locally produced cytokines (see also Chapter 2).

1.5 CONCLUSIONS

The mechanisms accounting for the joint involvement of IgE-producing B cells, mast cells/basophils and eosinophils in the pathogenesis of allergic disorders remained unclear until the existence of functional subsets of CD4$^+$ Th cells with distinct profiles of cytokine secretion was discovered. At least three different subsets of Th cells have been described in both mice and humans: Th1 cells that produce IL-2, IFN-γ and TNF-β; Th2 cells that produce IL-4, IL-5 and IL-10; and Th0 cells that produce both Th1- and Th2-type cytokines. Other cytokines such as IL-3, GM-CSF and TNF-α are variably produced by all Th subsets. It is of note that IL-3, IL-4 and IL-10 are growth factors for mast cells, and IL-5 is a selective activation and dif-ferentiation factor for eosinophils. Finally, it has clearly been shown that IgE synthesis results from a collaboration between Th2 cells producing IL-4 (and IL-13) and B cells. Th2 cells provide B cells with at least two signals: the soluble one is delivered by IL-4/1L-13; the other signal is represented by a T-B cell-to-cell physical interaction occurring between the CD40 molecule constitutively expressed on the B cell and CD40L expressed by Th cells upon activation. Th2 cell-derived IL-4 induces ε germline expression in B cells, whereas the CD40L/CD40 interaction is required for both expression of productive ε mRNA and IgE protein synthesis. Another cytokine, IL-13, is also able to induce ε germline expression, but its role in the pathogenesis of allergic disorders has not been fully elucidated. On the other hand Th1 cells, which produce IFN-γ but not IL-4, as well as those Th0 cells which produce high concentrations of IFN-γ in addition to IL-4 and/or IL-13 (low IL-4/IFN-γ ratio), are unable to support, or rather they suppress, IL-4-dependent IgE synthesis. Other soluble factors produced by either T cells or 'non-T' cells have been found to exert positive (IL-5, IL-6, TNF-α) or negative (IFN-α, TGF-β, IL-8, IL-10, IL-12) regulatory effects on human IgE synthesis, at least *in vitro*.

The question of how and why common environmental allergens preferentially evoke Th2 responses, even though only in a minority of subjects, is still obscure. The recent demonstration that one or more polymorphisms exist in a coding or, more probably, in a regulatory region of the IL-4 gene points to an alteration of the molecular mechanisms involved in the regulation of IL-4 gene expression. Over-expression of other cytokine genes, such as IL-13 and IL-5, located with IL-4 within the cluster on chromosome 5 (5q31.1) may also occur (see also Chapter 4). Of note is that IL-4 not only acts as an IgE switching cytokine, but also represents the critical factor required for the differentiation of both naive and memory Th cells into the Th2-type functional subset. On the other hand, the possible role of a deficient regulatory activity of cytokines (IL-12, IFN-α and IFN-γ) which are inhibitory on both IgE synthesis and development of Th2 cells, cannot be excluded.

1.6 REFERENCES

1. Ishizaka K and Ishizaka T (1978) Mechanisms of reaginic hypersensitivity and IgE antibody response. *Immunol Rev* **41:**122–148.
2. Siraganian RP (1993) Mechanism of IgE-mediated hypersensitivity. In: Middleton E *et al* (eds) *Allergy. Principles and Practice*, pp 105–134. Mosby, St. Louis.
3. Sur S, Adolphson CR and Gleich GJ (1993) Eosinophils. Biochemical and cellular aspects. In: Middleton E *et al* (eds) *Allergy. Principles and Practice*, pp. 169–200. Mosby, St. Louis.
4. Coffman RL and Carty J (1986) A T cell activity that enhances polyclonal IgE production and its inhibition by interferon-γ. *J Immunol* **136:**949–954.
5. Kuhn R, Rajewski K and Muller W (1991) Generation and analysis of IL-4-deficient mice. *Science* **254:**707–710.
6. Rothman P, Li SC, Gorham B, Glimcher L, Alt F and Boothby M (1991) Identification of a conserved lipopolysaccharide-plus-interleukin-4 responsive element located at the promoter of germ line ε transcripts. *Mol Cell Biol* **11:**5551–5561.
7. Del Prete G, Maggi E, Parronchi P *et al* (1988) IL-4 is an essential factor for the IgE synthesis induced *in vitro* by human T cell clones and their supernatants. *J Immunol* **140:**4193–4198.
8. Pene J, Rousset F, Briere F *et al* (1988) IgE production by normal human B cells is induced by interleukin 4 and suppressed by interferon γ and α and prostaglandin E2. *Proc Nat Acad Sci USA* **85:**6880–6884.
9. Punnonen J, Aversa G, Cocks BG *et al* (1993) Interleukin 13 induces interleukin 4-independent IgG4 and IgE synthesis and CD23 expression by human B cells. *Proc Natl Acad Sci USA* **90:**3730–3734.
10. Zurawski G and de Vries JE (1994) Interleukin 13, an interleukin 4-like cytokine that acts on monocytes and B cells, but not on T cells. *Immunol Today* **15:**19–26.
11. Romagnani S (1990) Regulation and deregulation of human IgE synthesis. *Immunol Today* **11:**316–321.
12. Vercelli D, Jabara HH, Arai K and Geha RS (1989) Induction of human IgE synthesis requires interleukin-4 and T/B cell interactions involving the T cell receptor/CD3 complex and MHC class II antigens. *J Exp Med* **169:**1295–1307.

13. Parronchi P, Tiri A, Macchia D *et al* (1990) Noncognate contact-dependent B cell activation can promote IL-4-dependent *in vitro* human IgE synthesis. *J Immunol* **44**:2102–2108.
14. Vercelli D and Geha RS (1991) Regulation of IgE synthesis in humans: a tale of two signals. *J Allergy Clin Immunol* **8**:285–295.
15. Armitage R, Fanslow W, Strockbine L *et al* (1992) Molecular and biological characterization of a murine ligand for CD40. *Nature* **357**:80–82.
16. Smith CA, Davis T, Anderson D *et al* (1990) A receptor for tumor necrosis factor defines an unusual family of cellular and viral proteins. *Science* **248**:1019–1023.
17. Spriggs MK, Armitage RJ, Strockbine L *et al* (1992) Recombinant human CD40 ligand stimulates B cell proliferation and immunoglobulin E secretion. *J Exp Med* **176**:1543–1550.
18. Aruffo A, Farrington M, Hollenbaugh D *et al* (1993) The CD40 ligand, gp39, is defective in activated T cells from patients with X-linked hyper IgM syndrome. *Cell* **72**:291–300.
19. Farrington M, Grosmaire LS, Nonoyama S *et al* (1994) CD40 ligand is defective in a subset of patients with common variable immunodeficiency. *Proc Natl Acad Sci USA* **91**:1099–1103.
20. Aversa G, Punnonen J and de Vries JE (1993) The 26-kD transmembrane form of tumor necrosis factor α on activated CD4$^+$ T cell clones provides a co-stimulatory signal for human B cell activation. *J Exp Med* **177**:1575–1585.
21. Macchia D, Almerigogna F, Parronchi P, Ravina A, Maggi E and Romagnani S (1993) Membrane tumor necrosis factor-α is involved in the polyclonal B cell activation induced by HIV-infected human T cells. *Nature* **363**:464–466.
22. Del Prete G, De Carli M, D'Elios MM *et al* (1994) Polyclonal B cell activation induced by Herpesvirus saimiri-transformed human CD4$^+$ T cell clones: role for membrane TNF-α/TNF-α receptors and CD2/CD58 interactions. *J Immunol* **152**:4872–4879.
23. Diaz-Sanchez D, Chegini S, Zhang K and Saxon A (1994) CD58 (LFA-3) stimulation provides a signal for human isotype switching and IgE production distinct from CD40. *J Immunol* **153**:10–20.
24. Smith CA, Gruss H-J, Davis T *et al* (1993) CD30 antigen, a marker for Hodgkin's lymphoma, is a receptor whose ligand defines an emerging family of cytokines with homology to TNF. *Cell* **273**:1349–1360.
25. Shanebeck KD, Maliszewski CR, Kennedy MK *et al* (1995) Regulation of murine B cell growth and differentiation by CD30 ligand. *Eur J Immunol* **25**:2147–2153.
26. Vercelli D and Geha RS (1995) Regulation of immunoglobulin E synthesis. In: Busse WW and Holgate ST (eds) *Asthma and Rhinitis*, pp. 437–449. Blackwell Scientific Publications, Oxford.
27. Thyphronitis G, Tsokos GC, June CH, Levine AD and Finkelman FD (1989) IgE secretion by Epstein–Barr virus-infected purified human B lymphocytes is stimulated by interleukin 4 and suppressed by interferon γ. *Proc Natl Acad Sci USA* **86**:5580–5584.
28. Sarfati M, Luo H and Delespesse G (1989) IgE synthesis by chronic lymphocytic leukemia cells. *J Exp Med* **170**:1775–1780.
29. Jabara HH, Ahern DJ, Vercelli D and Geha RS (1991) Hydrocortisone and IL-4 induce IgE isotype switching in human B cells. *J Immunol* **147**:1557–1560.
30. Gauchat J-F, Henchoz S, Mazzei G *et al* (1993) Induction of human IgE synthesis in B cells by mast cells and basophils. *Nature* **365**:340–343.
31. Brunner T, Heusser CH and Dahinden CA (1993) Human peripheral blood basophils primed by interleukin 3 (IL-3) produce IL-4 in response to immunoglobulin E receptor stimulation. *J Exp Med* **177**: 605–611.
32. Bradding P, Feather IH, Howarth PH *et al* (1992) Interleukin 4 is localized and released by human mast cells. *J Exp Med* **76**:1381–1386.

33. Punnonen J, Aversa G, Cocks BG and de Vries JE (1994) Role of interleukin-4 and interleukin-13 in the synthesis of IgE and expression of CD23 by human B cells. *Allergy* **49**:576–586.
34. Dugas B, Renauld JC, Pene J *et al* (1993) Interleukin-9 potentiates the interleukin-4-induced immunoglobulin (IgG, IgM and IgE) production by normal human B lymphocytes. *Eur J Immunol* **23**:1687–1692.
35. Pene J, Rousset F, Briere F *et al* (1988) Interleukin 5 enhances interleukin-4-induced IgE production by normal human B cells. The role of soluble CD23 antigen. *Eur J Immunol* **18**:929–935.
36. Vercelli D, Jabara HH, Arai K, Yokota T and Geha RS (1989) Endogenous IL-6 plays an obligatory role in IL-4-induced human IgE synthesis. *Eur J Immunol* **19**:1419–1424.
37. van Kooten C, van der Pouw Kraan T, Resnink I, van Oers R and Aarden L (1992) Both naive and memory T cells can provide help for human IgE production, but with different cytokine requirements. *Eur Cytokine Network* **3**:289–297.
38. Maggi E, Del Prete G, Parronchi P *et al* (1989) Role for T cells, IL-2 and IL-6 in the IL-4-dependent *in vitro* human IgE synthesis. *Immunology* **68**:300–306.
39. Gauchat J-F, Aversa GC, Gascan H and de Vries JE (1992) Modulation of IL-4-induced germline ε RNA synthesis in human B cells by tumor necrosis factor-α, anti-CD40 monoclonal antibodies or transforming growth factor-β correlates with levels of IgE production. *Int Immunol* **4**:397–406.
40. Kimata H, Yoshida A, Ishioka C, Lindley I and Mikawa H. (1992) Interleukin 8 selectively inhibits immunoglobulin E production induced by IL-4 in human B cells. *J Exp Med* **176**:1227–1231.
41. Punnonen J, de Waal Malefyt R, van Vlasselaer P, Gauchat J-F and de Vries JE (1993) IL-10 and viral IL-10 prevent IL-4-induced IgE synthesis by inhibiting the accessory cell function of monocytes. *J Immunol* **151**:1280–1289.
42. Kiniwa M, Gately M, Gubler U, Chizzonite R, Fargeas C and Delespesse G (1992) Recombinant interleukin-12 suppresses the synthesis of immunoglobulin E by interleukin-4 stimulated human lymphocytes. *J Clin Invest* **90**:262–266.
43. Deryckx S, de Waal Malefyt R, Gauchat J-F, Vivier E, Thomas Y and de Vries JE (1992) Immunoregulatory functions of paf-acether. VIII. Inhibition of IL-4-induced human IgE synthesis. *J Immunol* **148**:1465–1470.
44. Kimata H, Lindley I and Furusho K (1995) Selective inhibition of spontaneous IgE and IgG4 production by interleukin-8 in atopic patients. *Blood* **85**:3191–3198.
45. Rousset F, Garcia E, DeFrance T *et al* (1992) Interleukin-10 is a potent growth and differentiation factor for activated human B lymphocytes. *Proc Natl Acad Sci USA* **89**:1890–1894.
46. Chehimi J and Trinchieri G (1994) Interleukin-12: a bridge between innate resistance and adaptive immunity with a role in infection and acquired immunodeficiency. *J Clin Immunol* **14**:149–161.
47. Yokota A, Kikutani H, Tanaka T *et al* (1988) Two species of human Fcε receptor II (Fcε RII/CD23): tissue-specific and IL-4-specific regulation of gene expression. *Cell* **55**:611–618.
48. Sarfati M and Delespesse G (1988) Possible role of human lymphocyte receptor for IgE (CD23) or its soluble fragments in the *in vitro* synthesis of human IgE. *J Immunol* **141**:2195–2199.
49. Sherr E, Macy E, Kimata H, Gilly M and Saxon A (1989) Binding the low affinity FcεR on B cells suppresses ongoing human IgE synthesis. *J Immunol* **142**:481–489.
50. Luo H, Hofstetter H, Banchereau J and Delespesse G (1991) Cross-linking of CD23 antigen by its natural ligand (IgE) or by anti-CD23 antibody prevents B lymphocyte proliferation and differentiation. *J Immunol* **146**:2122–2129.

51. Uchibayashi N, Kikutani H, Barsumian E *et al* (1989) Recombinant soluble Fcε receptor II (FcεRII/CD23) has IgE binding activity but no B cell growth promoting activity. *J Immunol* **142**:3901–3908.

52. Bonnefoy J-Y, Shields J and Mermod J-J (1990) Inhibition of human interleukin-4-induced IgE synthesis by a subset of anti-CD23/FceRII monoclonal antibodies. *Eur J Immunol* **20**:139–144.

53. Aubry J-P, Pochon S, Graber P, Jansen K and Bonnefoy J-Y (1992) CD21 is a ligand for CD23 and regulates IgE production. *Nature* **358**:505–507.

54. Texido G, Eibel H, Le Gros G and van der Putten H (1994) Transgene CD23 expression on lymphoid cells modulates IgE and IgG1 responses. *J Immunol* **153**:3028–3042.

55. Fujiwara H, Kikutani H, Suematsu S *et al* (1994) The absence of IgE antibody-mediated augmentation of immune responses in CD23-deficient mice. *Proc Natl Acad Sci USA* **91**:6835–6839.

56. Yu P, Kosco-Vilbois M, Richards M, Kohler G and MC Lamers (1994) Negative feedback regulation of IgE synthesis by murine CD23. *Nature* **369**:753–756.

57. Mosmann TR, Cherwinski H, Bond MW, Giedlin MA and Coffman RL (1986) Two types of murine helper T cell clone. I. Definition according to profiles of lymphokine activities and secreted proteins. *J Immunol* **136**:2348–2356.

58. Del Prete G, De Carli M, Mastromauro C *et al* (1991) Purified protein derivative of *Mycobacterium tuberculosis* and excretory–secretory antigen(s) of *Toxocara canis* expand *in vitro* human T cells with stable and opposite (type 1 T helper or type 2 T helper) profile of cytokine production. *J Clin Invest* **88**:346–350.

59. Del Prete G, De Carli M, Almerigogna F, Giudizi MG, Biagiotti R and Romagnani S (1993) Human IL-10 is produced by both type 1 helper (Th1) and type 2 helper (Th2) T cell clones and inhibits their antigen-specific proliferation and cytokine production. *J Immunol* **150**: 353–360.

60. Romagnani S (1994) Lymphokine production by human T cells in disease states. *Annu Rev Immunol* **12**:227–257.

61. Del Prete G, De Carli M, Ricci M and Romagnani S (1991) Helper activity for immunoglobulin synthesis of T helper type 1 (Th1) and Th2 human T cell clones: the help of Th1 clones is limited by their cytolytic capacity. *J Exp Med* **174**:809–813.

62. Del Prete G, De Carli M, Lammel R *et al* (1995) Th1 and Th2 T helper cells exert opposite regulatory effects on procoagulant activity and tissue factor production by human monocytes. *Blood* **86**:250–257.

63. Del Prete G, De Carli M, Almerigogna F *et al* (1995) Preferential expression of CD30 by human CD4$^+$ T cells producing Th2-type cytokines. *FASEB J* **9**:81–86.

64. Romagnani S (1994) Regulation of Th2 development in allergy. *Curr Opin Immunol* **6**:838–846.

65. Wierenga EA, Snoek M, de Groot C *et al* (1990) Evidence for compartmentalisation of functional subsets of CD4$^+$ T lymphocytes in atopic patients. *J Immunol* **144**:4651–4656.

66. Parronchi P, Macchia D, Piccinni M-P *et al* (1991) Allergen- and bacterial antigen-specific T cell clones established from atopic donors show a different profile of cytokine production. *Proc Natl Acad Sci USA* **88**:4538–4542.

67. Maggi E, Biswas P, Del Prete G *et al* (1991) Accumulation of Th2-like helper T cells in the conjunctiva of patients with vernal conjunctivitis. *J Immunol* **146**:1169–1174.

68. Kay AB, Ying S, Varney V *et al* (1991) Messenger RNA expression of the cytokine gene cluster, interleukin 3 (IL-3), IL-4, IL-5, and granulocyte/macrophage colony-stimulating factor, in allergen-induced late-phase cutaneous reactions in atopic subjects. *J Exp Med* **173**:775–778.

69. Hamid Q, Azzawi M, Ying S *et al* (1991) Expression of mRNA for interleukin-5 in mucosal bronchial biopsies from asthma. *J Clin Invest* **87**:1541–1546.

70. Robinson DS, Hamid Q, Ying S *et al* (1992) Predominant Th2-like bronchoalveolar T-lymphocyte population in atopic asthma. *N Engl J Med* **326**:295–304.
71. Bradding P, Feather IH, Wilson S *et al* (1993) Immunolocalization of cytokines in nasal mucosa of normal and perennial rhinitic subjects. *J Immunol* **151**:3853–3865.
72. Walker C, Bode E, Boer L, Hansel TT, Blaser K and Virchow J-C (1992) Allergic and non-allergic asthmatics have distinct patterns of T cell activation and cytokine production in peripheral blood and bronchoalveolar lavage. *Am Rev Resp Dis* **146**:109–115.
73. Del Prete G, De Carli M, D'Elios MM *et al* (1993) Allergen exposure induces the activation of allergen-specific Th2 cells in the airway mucosa of patients with allergic respiratory disorders. *Eur J Immunol* **23**:1445–1449.
74. van Reijsen FC, Bruijnzeel-Koomen CAFM, Kalthoff FS *et al* (1992) Skin-derived aeroallergen-specific T cell clones of Th2 phenotype in patients with atopic dermatitis. *J Allergy Clin Immunol* **90**:184–192.
75. Varney VA, Hamid Q, Gaga M *et al* (1993) Influence of grass pollen immunotherapy on cellular infiltration and cytokine mRNA expression during allergen-induced late-phase cutaneous responses. *J Clin Invest* **92**:644–651.
76. Secrist H, Chelen CJ, Wen Y, Marshall JD and Umetsu DT (1993) Allergen immunotherapy decreases interleukin 4 production in CD4$^+$ T cells from allergic individuals. *J Exp Med* **178**:2123–2130.
77. Jutel M, Pichler WJ, Skrbic D, Urwyler A, Dahinden C and Muller UR (1995) Bee venom immunotherapy results in decrease of IL-4 and IL-5 and increase of IFN-γ secretion in specific allergen-stimulated T cell cultures. *J Immunol* **154**:4187–4194.
78. McHugh SM, Deighton J, Stewart AG, Lachmann PJ and Ewan PW (1995) Bee venom immunotherapy induces a shift in cytokine responses from a Th2 to a Th1 dominant pattern: comparison of rush and conventional immunotherapy. *Clin Exp Allergy* **25**:828–838.
79. Gieni RS, Yang X and Hay Glass KT (1993) Allergen-specific modulation of cytokine synthesis pattern and IgE responses *in vivo* with chemically modified allergen. *J Immunol* **150**:302–310.
80. Nabors GS, Afonso LCC, Farell JP and Scott P (1995) Switch from a type 2 to a type 1 T helper cell response and cure of established *Leishmania major* infection in mice is induced by combined therapy with interleukin 12 and pentostam. *Proc Natl Acad Sci USA* **92**:3142–3146.
81. Del Prete G, De Carli M, D'Elios MM *et al* (1995) CD30-mediated signaling promotes the development of human T helper type 2-like T cells. *J Exp Med* **182**:1655–1661.
82. Reiner SL, Wang Z-E, Hatam F, Scott P and Locksley RM (1993) Th1 and Th2 cell antigen receptors in experimental leishmaniasis. *Science* **259**:1457–1460.
83. Renz H, Saloga J, Bradley KL *et al* (1993) Specific Vβ T cell subsets mediate the immediate hypersensitivity response to ragweed allergen. *J Immunol* **151**:1907–1917.
84. Rook GAW, Hernandez-Pando R and Lightman SL (1994) Hormones, peripherally activated prohormones and regulation of the Th1/Th2 balance. *Immunol Today* **15**:301–303.
85. Wegmann TG, Lin H, Guilbert L and Mosmann TR (1993) Bidirectional cytokine interactions in the maternal–fetal relationship: is successful pregnancy a Th2 phenomenon? *Immunol Today* **14**:353–356.
86. Romagnani S (1992) Induction of Th1 and Th2 responses: a key role for the 'natural' immune response? *Immunol Today* **13**:379–380.
87. Maggi E, Parronchi P, Manetti R *et al* (1992) Reciprocal regulatory role of IFN-γ and IL-4 on the *in vitro* development of human Th1 and Th2 clones. *J Immunol* **148**:2142–2148.

88. Manetti R, Parronchi P, Giudizi M-G *et al* (1993) Natural killer cell stimulatory factor (interleukin 12) induces T helper type 1 (Th1)-specific immune responses and inhibits the development of IL-4-producing Th cells. *J Exp Med* **177**:1199–1204.
89. Hsieh C-S, Macatonia SE, Tripp CS, Wolf SF, O'Garra A and Murphy KM (1993) Development of Th1 CD4$^+$ T cells through IL-12 produced by *Listeria*-induced macrophages. *Science* **260**:547–549.
90. Swain SL (1993) IL-4 dictates T cell differentiation. *Res Immunol* **144**:616–620.
91. Kopf M, Le Gros G, Bachmann M, Lamers MC, Bluthmann H and Kohler G (1993) Disruption of the murine IL-4 gene blocks Th2 cytokine responses. *Nature* **362**:245–248.
92. Yoshimoto T and Paul WE (1994) CD4^{pos}, NK1.1^{pos} T cells promptly produce interleukin 4 in response to *in vivo* challenge with anti-CD3. *J Exp Med* **179**:1285–1295.
93. Wershil BK, Theodos CM, Galli SJ and Titus RG (1994) Mast cells augment lesion size and persistence during experimental *Leishmania major* infection in the mouse. *J Immunol* **152**:4563–4571.
94. Schmitz J, Thiel A, Kuhn R *et al* (1994) Induction of interleukin-4 (IL-4) expression in T helper (Th) cells is not dependent on IL-4 from non-T cells. *J Exp Med* **179**:1349–1353.
95. Finkelman FD and Urban JF (1992) Cytokines: making the right choice. *Parasitol Today* **8**:311–314.
96. Pfeiffer C, Stein J, Southwood S, Ketelaar H, Sette A and Bottomly K (1995) Altered peptide ligands can control CD4 T lymphocyte differentiation *in vivo*. *J Exp Med* **181**:1569–1574.
97. Kalinski P, Hilkens GMU, Wierenga EA *et al* (1995) Functional maturation of human naive T helper cells in the absence of accessory cells. Generation of IL-4-producing T helper cells does not require exogenous IL-4. *J Immunol* **154**:3753–3760.
98. Yang L-P, Byun D-G, Demeure CE, Vezzio N and Delespesse G (1995) Default development of cloned human naive CD4 T cells into interleukin-4- and interleukin 5-producing effector cells. *Eur J Immunol* **25**: 3517–3520.
99. Mingari MC, Maggi E, Cambiaggi A *et al* (1996) Development *in vitro* of human CD4 thymocytes into functionally mature Th2 cells. Exogenous interleukin-12 is required for priming thymocytes to produce both Th1 cytokines and interleukin-10. *Eur J Immunol* **26**: 1083–1087.
100. Marsh DG, Neely JD, Breazeale DR *et al* (1994) Linkage analysis of IL-4 and other chromosome 5q31.1 markers and total serum immunoglobulin E concentration. *Science* **264**:1152–1156.
101. Parronchi P, De Carli M, Manetti R *et al* (1992) Aberrant interleukin (IL)-4 and IL-5 production *in vitro* by CD4$^+$ helper T cells from atopic subjects. *Eur J Immunol* **22**:1615–1620.
102. Romagnani S (1995) Atopic allergy and other hypersensitivities. *Curr Opin Immunol* **7**:745–750.
103. McMenamin C and Holt PG (1993) The natural immune response to inhaled soluble protein antigens involves major histocompatibility complex (MHC) class I-restricted CD8+ T cell-dependent immune deviation resulting in selective suppression of immunoglobulin E production. *J Exp Med* **178**:889–899.
104. Kemeny DM and Diaz-Sanchez D (1993) The role of CD8$^+$ T cells in the regulation of IgE. *Clin Exp Allergy* **23**:466–470.
105. Lack G, Renz H, Saloga J *et al* (1993) Nebulized but not parenteral IFN-γ decreases IgE production and normalizes airways function in a murine model of allergen sensitization. *J Immunol* **152**:2546–2554.

2 IgE Regulation in Tissues

STEPHEN R. DURHAM*, HANNAH J. GOULD[†] and QUTAYBA A. HAMID[§]
*Imperial College School of Medicine at the National Heart and Lung Institute, London UK, [†]The Randall Institute, King's College London, London UK, and [§]Meakins-Christie Laboratories, McGill University, Montreal, Canada

2.1 INTRODUCTION

IgE-dependent mechanisms involving mast cells and eosinophils (1, 2) are hallmarks of allergic inflammation (1). Both mast cells and eosinophils express high affinity receptors for IgE (FcεR1) and have the potential for direct IgE-dependent activation following triggering by allergen presenting at mucosal surfaces. Human IgE-dependent activation following allergen provocation may result in an immediate reaction which peaks at 15–30 min. Depending on the level of allergen exposure and the IgE sensitivity of the subject, a large proportion of individuals go on to develop a late-phase response at 6–24 hr after challenge. Whereas the early response may depend largely on mast cell activation, there is now strong evidence that the late phase of allergic inflammation is T cell dependent (3). Furthermore, both mast cell activation and the recruitment, activation and persistence of eosinophils at allergic tissue sites are dependent upon generation of cytokines produced by a variety of cells, particularly T lymphocytes. Both IgE synthesis and tissue eosinophilia are dependent upon cytokines produced by a distinct subset of T lymphocytes, so called 'Th2-type' helper T cells (4).

In this chapter, evidence relating to activation of a distinct subset of T-cells producing particularly IL-4 and IL-5 *in vivo* in man will be summarised. There follows evidence relating to the upregulation and clinical expression of high affinity IgE receptors at allergic tissue sites, consistent with local IgE-dependent events. These data lead logically to an appraisal of previous studies examining the possibility of local IgE synthesis in tissues and recent work from our own group confirming local IgE synthesis in the nasal mucosa at least at RNA level. Finally the influence of treatment including topical corticosteroids and immunotherapy on these events will be considered, particularly in relation to novel therapeutic strategies.

2.2 HUMAN T LYMPHOCYTE TH2 RESPONSES

Studies of murine models originally demonstrated the existence of distinct helper T lymphocyte subsets, based on the profile of cytokines produced (4, 5). These

IgE Regulation: Molecular Mechanisms. Edited by D. Vercelli. © 1997 John Wiley & Sons Ltd.

observations were subsequently confirmed using human peripheral blood mono-nuclear cells and T-cell clones (6). Th1-type cells which characterise delayed-type hypersensitivity reactions produce predominantly interleukin (IL)-2 and interferon (IFN)-γ (7). In contrast, human atopic allergy is characterised by Th2-type cells with production of preferentially IL-4 and IL-5. Thus, human allergen-specific T-cell clones derived from atopic donors have been shown to exhibit a Th2-type cytokine profile following stimulation by extracts of the relevant aeroallergen (6) (see also Chapters 1 and 5).

Th2-type cytokines were originally described as products of T lymphocytes. However more recent studies have identified human mast cells, basophils and eosinophils as alternative sources (8, 9, 10). Recent studies *in vivo* have confirmed preferential generation of Th2-type cytokines at both RNA and protein levels, during natural disease and following allergen provocation in the bronchi, skin and nose (11).

2.3 BRONCHIAL MUCOSA

T lymphocytes are prominent in the epithelial layer and submucosa of the human respiratory tract (12, 13). We tested the hypothesis that T lymphocyte recruitment, activation and cytokine production within the bronchial mucosa may contribute to eosinophil recruitment and IgE-dependent events which may result in airway nar-rowing and bronchial hyper-responsiveness which characterise bronchial asthma. We performed a series of controlled clinical studies in patients with atopic and non-atopic asthma and controls. Their atopic status was confirmed by skin testing and radioallergosorbent test (RAST). Their asthma severity was measured by ques-tionnaire (Aas score) and airway histamine responsiveness. By use of immunohis-tochemistry of bronchial biopsies obtained at fibreoptic bronchoscopy, T-cell subsets were characterised and their activation status assessed using expression of IL-2 receptor (CD25). Cytokine synthesis was assessed at mRNA level using the tech-nique of *in situ* hybridisation. The cell source of Th2-type cytokines was determined by double immunohistochemistry/*in situ* hybridisation studies. We observed the following:

(1) T lymphocyte and eosinophil numbers and activation status in the bronchial mucosa were increased in asthmatic compared with normal non-atopic normal control subjects (13).

(2) T-cell activation and the level of cytokine mRNA expression correlated with asthma severity as determined by a symptom score (Aas score) and airway methacholine responsiveness (14, 15, 16).

(3) Allergen provocation by bronchial inhalation resulted in increased T-cell acti-vation and preferential increased expression of both IL-4 and IL-5 in cells in bronchoalveolar lavage fluid (3) and bronchial biopsies (17) obtained 24 hours after challenge.

(4) In a double-blind placebo-controlled study of oral prednisolone therapy in a group of moderately severe asthmatics, in whom an elective trial of cortico-steroids was indicated, there was a selective decrease in CD25 expression and a reduction in tissue eosinophilia and IL-4 and IL-5 mRNA-positive cells, both in bronchoalveolar lavage fluid (18) and in bronchial mucosal biopsies (19) (Figure 2.1).

(5) Asthma of different aetiology including atopic, occupational (20) and intrinsic (non-atopic) (21) asthma exhibited the same immunopathological features and, surprisingly, intrinsic asthma (as well as extrinsic asthma) was characterised by increased expression of IL-4 and IL-5 at both mRNA (using *in situ* hybridisation and a semi-quantitative polymerase chain reaction (PCR)-based method) and protein levels (by immunohistochemistry) (22, 23).

(6) The specificity of these changes for asthma is supported by the lack of Th2-type cytokines and a predominance of IFN-γ producing cells in bronchoalveolar lavage obtained from patients with pulmonary tuberculosis (24).

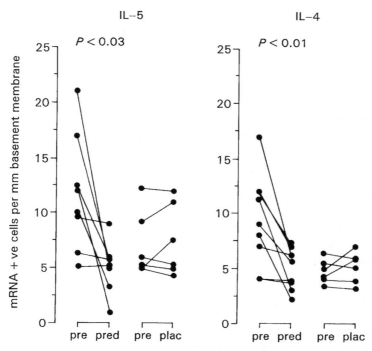

Figure 2.1. A double-blind placebo-controlled trial of 2 weeks prednisolone (0.6 mg/kg) in patients with moderately severe asthma in whom an elective trial of corticosteroid was indi-cated. Fibreoptic broncoscopic bronchial biopsies were taken before and after prednisolone or placebo treatment. *in situ* hybridisation detected cytokine mRNA$^+$ cells for IL-5 and IL-4. (Reproduced by kind permission of the editor, *Am J Resp Crit Care Med* 1996; **153**:551–556)

(7) Double immunohistochemistry/hybridisation confirmed that, at least at mRNA level, the principal cell source of Th2 cytokines in human asthma is the T lymphocyte (approximately 70%), with lesser contributions from mast cells (particularly IL-4, approximately 20–25%) and eosinophils (10%) (10).

We have recently investigated the tissue distribution and cell phenotype of cells expressing the high affinity IgE receptor FcεR1. We employed both polyclonal and monoclonal antibodies directed against the α chain of FcεR1 (kindly supplied by Dr J.P. Kinet). These studies demonstrated increased expression of FcεR1 in the bronchial mucosa in asthma. FcεR1 was expressed predominantly on mast cells but also on tissue macrophages and eosinophils. FcεR1 expression was also increased in patients with so-called intrinsic (non-atopic) asthma (25). These features were in keeping with local IgE-dependent events and raised the possibility that local IgE expression may occur in 'non-atopic' asthma even in the absence of a raised serum total IgE or allergen-specific IgE.

2.4 SKIN

Cutaneous allergen-induced responses, unlike in the bronchi, are not biphasic. The immediate weal and flare blends imperceptibly into the more persistent reddened, oedematous and indurated late-phase response at 6–24 hours. The advantage of studying allergen-induced cutaneous responses is the ability to study the time course of evolution of cell recruitment and cytokine gene expression during the allergic response (26). Thus, tissue eosinophilia peaks at 6 hours whereas T lymphocyte recruitment after allergen is also increased at 6 hours but maximal at 24 hours. The peak of Th2-type cytokine expression occurs at 6–24 hours and parallels the clinical response. In contrast, delayed-type tuberculin-induced responses and expression of Th1-type cytokines (IL-2 and IFN-γ) peaked at 48 hours after challenge (26). Thus, both allergic and delayed-typed hypersensitivity reactions are characterised by T-cell recruitment and activation. However, the profile of cytokines is distinct and the time course of their production also differs and parallels closely the evolution of the clinical late (or delayed) response. Both IL-4 (via upregulation of vascular cell adhesion molecule 1 (VCAM-1)) and IL-5 (via prolonged survival) produced after allergen in the skin may promote tissue eosinophilia.

2.5 NASAL MUCOSA

Allergic rhinitis is common and frequently troublesome. The nasal mucosa is an attractive model since it represents the target organ, is more accessible than bronchial tissue and is largely a mirror of events in the lower respiratory tract. We have studied patients with severe summer hay fever after allergen provocation and during natural seasonal exposure to grass pollen. We have confirmed T-lymphocyte activation and eosinophil recruitment at 24 hours after allergen provocation (27). These results

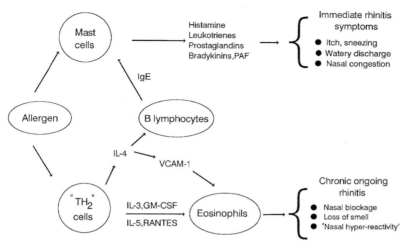

Figure 2.2. Hypothesis on mechanism of allergen-induced early and late nasal responses (Reproduced with kind permission of the editor, *Allergy* 1994; **49**:Suppl 19:1–34. Copyright © 1994 Munksgaard International Publishers Ltd, Copenhagen, Denmark.

were confirmed during natural seasonal exposure and, additionally, the transepithelial migration of tryptase only (mucosal type) mast cells was observed (28). Increased numbers of cytokine mRNA positive cells for IL-3, granulocyte–macrophage colony-stimulating factor (GM-CSF) as well as IL-4 and IL-5 were observed (29). These results suggest the scheme outlined in Figure 2.2 as a possible mechanism of allergen-induced early and late nasal responses. We demonstrated that topical steroid therapy may inhibit early and late nasal responses (Figure 2.3) and the associated increase in IL-4 mRNA expression (Figure 2.4) (30). More recently we

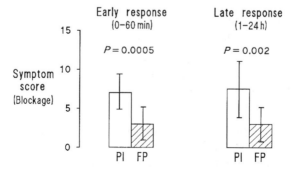

Figure 2.3. Influence of topical corticosteroid (fluticasone propionate 200 µg twice daily for 6 weeks) (FP) or matched placebo nasal spray (PL) on allergen-induced subjective nasal blockage during early and late nasal responses. Results represent median plus interquartile ranges. Levels of significance (Mann–Whitney *U* test) are shown

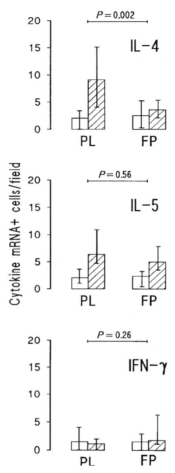

Figure 2.4. Influence of topical nasal corticosteroid (fluticasone propionate 200 μg twice daily for 6 weeks) (FP) or matched placebo nasal spray (PL) on the number of cytokine mRNA$^+$ cells in the nasal mucosa 24 hours after allergen provocation [hatched bars compared to baseline (open bars)]. Significant increases in IL-4 and IL-5 mRNA$^+$ cells were observed, but only IL-4$^+$ cells were inhibited following fluticasone treatment. IFN-γ^+ cells did not change after allergen and were uninfluenced by topical steroid treatment

demonstrated increases in the C–C chemokine RANTES at both mRNA and protein level in the nasal mucosa after allergen challenge (31). These events raised the possibility of local IgE synthesis. IL-4 induces increased expression of Cε germline transcripts, a necessary first step in B-cell IgE switch recombination (see also Chapters 7–10). Moreover RANTES (as well as MIP1-α) has been shown to selectively enhance IgE (and IgG4) production by human B cells (32).

2.6 LOCAL IgE

2.6.1 Background

Following the recognition of IgE as 'reaginic antibody', this immunoglobulin iso-type has been detected in nasal secretions by a number of investigators, which raises the possibility that IgE may be synthesised locally in the 'target' organ (33, 34, 35). IgE antibody has also been demonstrated in nasal tissue homogenates. Platts-Mills demonstrated the presence of grass-pollen specific IgE in nasal but not salivary secretions of hay fever patients (36). However, although he was able to determine a disproportionate increase in grass pollen-specific immunoglobulin compared to total immunoglobulin for IgA and IgM in nasal secretions compared with plasma, IgE levels in nasal secretions were either undetectable or present in too low concentration to allow comparison.

Brostoff suspected local IgE synthesis on clinical grounds in patients who described seasonal hay fever symptoms but who were negative on skin prick testing with grass pollen and grass-pollen specific IgE was undetectable in their serum (33). Within this group, grass-pollen sensitivity was confirmed by nasal provocation with a grass-pollen extract and specific IgE was detected in nasal fluid in amounts comparable to hay fever sufferers who also showed positive skin tests and raised allergen-specific IgE.

These observations, whilst demonstrating IgE locally, could not determine whe-ther IgE resulted from plasma exudation of IgE, recruitment of mast cells with IgE on their surface, migratory IgE-producing plasma cells from the bone marrow or regional lymph glands or *in situ* production of IgE by B lymphocytes within the nasal mucosa (37). The possibility of local IgE synthesis was questioned by Ganzer by use of immunohistology (38). He detected low numbers of IgE-positive B cells in cervical lymph glands and tonsillar tissue but not within the nasal mucosa of hay fever patients. However anti-IgE also stains mast cells and basophils and the marker he employed for B cells (CD19) may possibly interfere with anti-IgE binding.

The provenance of IgE which is detectable within the target organ assumes great importance for a number of reasons. First, atopy refers only to a predisposition to develop exaggerated IgE responses to common aeroallergens. Atopy is defined clinically by a positive skin prick test to one or more common aeroallergens. Allergy, however, refers to the clinical manifestations (asthma, eczema, rhinitis etc) which may or may not be present in atopic subjects. For example, some patients develop summer hay fever but never wheeze. Similarly bronchial asthma and atopic eczema may occur separately or in combination within the same individual. The local occurrence of IgE synthesis following allergen provocation may explain why some atopic individuals develop rhinitis whereas others have either no clinical manifes-tations or develop atopic disease elsewhere.

Second, asthma is traditionally referred to as 'atopic', extrinsic or allergic asthma or 'late-onset' non-atopic 'intrinsic' asthma. Non-atopic asthma may occur for the first time in older individuals with no personal or family history of allergies and tends to be more severe and less responsive to corticosteroids (39). However an epidemiological study identified a close association between total serum IgE levels (adjusted for age and gender) and the presence of asthma, independent of the atopic state as defined by skin tests and allergen-specific IgE concentrations in serum (40). More recent studies have confirmed a close relationship between total IgE levels and asthma severity defined by FEV_1. Total IgE levels in serum increase during asthma exacerbations. Taken together with our observation that cells expressing IL-4 are detectable in the bronchial mucosa in both atopic and non-atopic asthma, these observations lend further support to the hypothesis that local IgE synthesis may occur in both atopic and so-called 'intrinsic' asthma in the absence of positive skin tests (22). Presumably in non-atopic asthma IgE synthesis locally might result from either unidentified allergens or other non-allergenic triggers, viruses etc.

Third, topical anti-inflammatory therapy with agents such as corticosteroids and disodium cromoglycate are effective in treating mucosal allergy. These agents are known to exert potent effects on IgE synthesis. Disodium cromoglycate inhibits IL-4-induced IgE synthesis *in vitro* (41). Whereas corticosteroids increase IL-4-induced IgE synthesis *in vitro*, this effect of corticosteroids may be pre-empted *in vivo* by their known potent inhibitory effects on cytokine synthesis (42), including IL-4 (see below). These observations raise the possibility that strategies developed locally against IgE synthesis may be effective, thereby avoiding potential systemic side effects.

2.6.2 IgE Synthesis

IgE is produced by a small proportion of B cells that have undergone heavy chain switching to IgE. The heavy chain switch is the mechanism by which the effector function of an antibody is modified without change in the antigen specificity (1). It is effected by genetic recombination between the V region of an expressed heavy chain gene coding for the μ or γ chain of an IgM or IgG antibody initially produced by the B cell, and the ε germline gene. Heavy chain switching is known to occur in germinal centres along with somatic mutation of immunoglobulin genes and affinity maturation of B cells (43) (see also Chapter 10 in this book).

Two signals are required for heavy chain gene switching to IgE (44). IL-4 targets the ε gene for recombination (step 1) whereas cross-linking of CD40 on the B cell membrane allows recombination to proceed (step 2). Step 1 involves generation of a sterile RNA transcript which includes the $I\varepsilon$ exon. Exposure to IL-4 induces transcription of the ε germline gene from the promoter site. Transcription proceeds through the constant region coding exons $C\varepsilon 1$–$C\varepsilon 4$ but RNA splicing joins the $I\varepsilon$ and $C\varepsilon 1$ exons. During step 2, the DNA between the recombined sequences in the homologous switch regions including the $I\varepsilon$ exon is deleted and replaced by a transcription unit containing the variable region coding exons. The $I\varepsilon$ probe thus detects the transient appearance of ε germline gene transcripts, which precedes the synthesis of mature messenger RNA, while the $C\varepsilon$ probe detects both the germline transcript and ε chain mRNA (45) (see also Chapters 7–11 in this book).

2.6.3 Local IgE Synthesis

IL-4 is present within the atopic nasal mucosa and is increased after allergen challenge (29) and in patients with perennial rhinitis (46). IL-4 is released from cytoplasmic stores following mast-cell activation and is secreted by helper Th1 type cells. We have shown that the latter represent the principal source of IL-4 message within the nasal mucosa (9). CD40 ligand (CD40L) is constitutively expressed by mast cells (47) and induced on T cells following antigen activation. We have also shown (unpublished observations) that CD40L is also expressed within the nasal mucosa. Based on our observation that topical corticosteroids inhibit allergen-induced early and late nasal responses and associated IL-4 synthesis (30), we have pursued the possibility of local IgE synthesis using gene probes which detect cells that express ε chain RNA (the Cε probe) and those that have been targeted for heavy chain switching to IgE by IL-4 but have not yet undergone genetic recombination (the Iε probe) (45).

In a double-blind trial 21 patients with summer hay fever received 6 weeks treatment with either topical corticosteroid (fluticasone propionate 200 μg b.d.) or matched placebo nasal sprays. Nasal biopsies were taken from the inferior turbinate at baseline out of season and 24 hours after allergen following 6 weeks treatment. Nasal provocation resulted in early and late increases in sneezing, nasal secretions

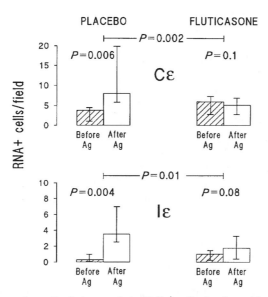

Figure 2.5. Changes in antibody heavy chain RNA$^+$ cells for Cε and Iε before and 24 hours after local nasal allergen challenge in patients with hay fever. Highly significant increases were observed in both Cε RNA$^+$ cells and Iε RNA$^+$ cells. In contrast, 6 weeks treatment with a topical corticosteroid (fluticasone propionate 200 μg twice daily) inhibited increases in both Cε and Iε$^+$ cells

and nasal blockage (Figure 2.3). In the actively-treated group these effects were markedly inhibited following topical steroid treatment (48).

B cells ($CD20^+$) were present within the nasal epithelium and submucosa. $C\varepsilon^+$ cells increased markedly 24 hours after allergen challenge (Figure 2.5). Similarly Iε cells were clearly detectable after allergen. Double immunohistochemistry/*in situ* hybridisation showed that the vast majority of these $C\varepsilon^+$ cells were $CD20^+$ B cells. Increases in both Cε and Iε^+ cells ($P < 0.01$) were accompanied by parallel increases in $IL-4^+$ cells (data not shown). These changes were isotype specific; an oligonucleotide probe directed against the heavy chain of IgG (Cγ) confirmed isotype specificity. In contrast to Cε a small decrease in immunoglobulin G (Cγ) RNA^+ cells was observed (data not shown).

Since Cε also detects the Iε-containing sterile germline transcript these data did not confirm production of mature Cε RNA. However, we also detected an increase in $C\varepsilon^+$ but not Iε^+ cells in atopic rhinitic grass-pollen sensitive patients out of the pollen season when compared with normal non-atopic control subjects, which confirms that the Cε signal must represent productive ε chain RNA.

The influence of topical corticosteroids on these changes is shown in Figure 2.5. Allergen-induced increases in $C\varepsilon^+$ and Iε^+ cells were completely inhibited by 6 weeks treatment with topical fluticasone propionate. This was accompanied by a marked reduction in IL-4 RNA^+ cells. Given the requirement for IL-4 for heavy chain switching to IgE this is probably the mechanism, *in vivo*, by which IgE expression is controlled locally and is susceptible to topical steroids.

2.7 INFLUENCE OF TREATMENT ON IgE SYNTHESIS

We have shown that topical corticosteroids *in vivo* inhibit allergen-induced increases in IL-4, IgE germline transcripts and synthesis of mature Cε RNA within the nasal mucosa. We are currently investigating the possible influence of allergen injection immunotherapy on local cytokine expression and antibody production. Immunotherapy involves the stepwise incremental subcutaneous injection of allergen extract to which the patient is sensitive over a period of days or weeks. In selected patients this may result in a state of clinical tolerance following subsequent natural allergen exposure. This form of treatment is confined to carefully selected patients with clearly defined IgE-mediated disease (49, 50). Immunotherapy is associated with marked increases in allergen-specific serum IgG concentrations. In contrast, allergen-specific IgE concentrations (51) may initially increase and subsequently fall to baseline levels whereas seasonal increases in IgE may be reduced (52). The mechanism of immunotherapy is largely unknown. The 'blocking antibody' theory suggests that IgG may prevent the binding of allergen to IgE on mast cells. Several investigators have shown a reduction in allergen-induced tissue recruitment of effector cells including eosinophils following a course of successful immunotherapy (53). Moreover immunotherapy may inhibit the epithelial migration of mucosal-type mast cells following antigenic exposure 54).

In grass-pollen sensitive patients we showed that allergen-injection immunotherapy was successful and inhibited allergen-induced late responses occurring in the skin (55) and nose (56). Inhibition of the late response was accompanied by a reduction in tissue eosinophilia and, in the skin, a reduction in tissue mast cells, whereas CD8$^+$ T lymphocyte numbers were increased. Cytokine expression in the skin was studied locally by use of *in situ* hybridisation and probes directed against IL-4, IL-5, IL-2 and IFN-γ (55). In contrast to our expectations, neither IL-4 nor IL-5 mRNA$^+$ cells were inhibited following immunotherapy (in contrast to topical corticosteroids). However, we identified a marked increase in markers of macrophage activation including increased expression of MHC class II molecules (HLA-DR) and IL-2 receptor expression (CD25 also expressed on macrophages as well as activated T cells). This raised the possibility that immunotherapy, rather than suppressing Th2 responses, may upregulate Th1 responses, in a fashion comparable to natural immunization with tuberculin. Thus we identified highly significant increases in IFN-γ expression in the nasal mucosa which corresponded to inhibition of the late response. This inhibition of IFN-γ which accompanied inhibition of the late response in the nose correlated closely with clinical improvement. Thus in patients who had received grass pollen immunotherapy IFN-γ mRNA$^+$ cells in the nasal mucosa 24 hours after allergen correlated inversely with their seasonal symptoms and 'rescue' medication requirements.

IL-12 is a novel cytokine produced by activated macrophages and B lymphocytes. IL-12 is a primary growth factor which may initiate and sustain Th1-lymphocyte responses following *in vitro* antigenic stimulation. In the same subjects we recently showed that IL-12 expression after intradermal allergen was upregulated following grass pollen immunotherapy (Figure 2.6). IL-12 expression correlated closely with IFN-γ expression in these biopsies and, interestingly, inversely with IL-4 expression (57).

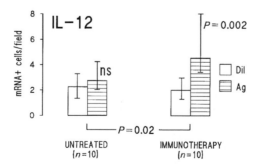

Figure 2.6. The influence of immunotherapy on cytokine mRNA$^+$ cells for IL-12 in cutaneous biopsies taken before and 24 hours after intradermal grass-pollen allergen challenge in patients who had received 9 months treatment with grass-pollen immunotherapy compared with untreated control subjects. Results are expressed as median values ($\pm$ interquartile ranges). Dil, diluent; Ag, antigen; ns, not significant

Th1 and Th2-type clones are known to show reciprocal inhibition. These observations support the view that one way in which immunotherapy may act is to promote additional Th1 responses. These responses may be sustained by altered antigen presentation from macrophages, the principal source of IL-12 in the skin. IFN-γ might act by inhibiting local IL-4-induced IgE expression. Furthermore, IFN-γ has been shown to preferentially promote IgG production by human B lymphocytes cloned from bee-venom sensitive patients, cultured in the presence of the major allergen, phospholipase A2 (58).

These observations suggest that topical corticosteroids and immunotherapy, both extremely effective agents in treating seasonal hay fever and in inhibiting late responses, may be acting by distinct mechanisms (Figure 2.7). Topical steroids, on the one hand, may act at least in part by suppressing IL-4 production and local IgE expression. In contrast allergen injection immunotherapy may act by promoting additional Th1 responses with local generation of IFN-γ. IFN-γ in turn may possibly inhibit local IgE and promote IgG synthesis, raising the possibility of 'local blocking IgG antibody' (Figure 2.7). These possibilities are currently under investigation.

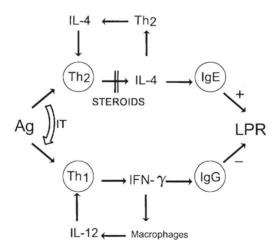

Figure 2.7. Hypothesis on mechanism of action of allergen injection immunotherapy (IT) compared with topical corticosteroids on allergen-induced late nasal responses. In atopic subjects allergen induces 'Th2' responses which are amplified by IL-4 production stimulating preferentially 'Th2'-type clones. IL-4 may generate local IgE synthesis. Late responses are known to be IgE-dependent. 'Th1' responses promote IFN-γ production, macrophage activation and production of IL-12 which promotes and sustains 'Th1'-type responses. IFN-γ may inhibit IL-4 induced IgE synthesis and also promote IgG production by B cells. IgG may possibly 'block' IgE-dependent activation with inhibition of the late response. Topical steroids may act by inhibiting 'Th2'-type cytokine production whereas immunotherapy induces preferential allergen-induced increases in 'Th1' responses

2.8 CONCLUSIONS

IgE mediates allergic reactions by binding to the high affinity IgE receptor on mast cells and basophils at mucosal surfaces. The provenance of IgE has not been established. However, our observations challenge the conventional wisdom that antibodies are synthesised by plasma cells in the bone marrow or regional glands and reach various tissues by diffusion through the blood or by way of migrating cells. We and others have highlighted the prominence of Th2-type responses in human allergic inflammation. Our results imply that IL-4 may be necessary but not sufficient for human allergic manifestations, whereas IL-5, additionally, may promote local tissue eosinophilia which may correlate possibly more closely with tissue damage and expression of clinical symptoms. We and others (59) have also provided evidence for allergen-induced IgE synthesis by resident B cells. Our data also suggest that rather than a scenario of migration of IgE-producing B cells, B cells may undergo switch recombination at mucosal surfaces locally in response to allergen provocation. Topical corticosteroids may act, at least in part, by preventing this process.

In contrast, immunotherapy upregulates Th1 responses with increases in local IFN-γ production. We hypothesise that this may either inhibit IL-4-induced IgE locally or alternatively upregulate IgG antibody synthesis (60).

Finally, local IgE synthesis may explain why some atopic individuals develop rhinitis whereas others have either no clinical manifestations or develop atopic disease elsewhere. There are clear implications for therapy in that topical treatments of whatever kind which downregulate heavy chain switching to IgE locally may control allergic diseases including hay fever.

ACKNOWLEDGEMENTS

This work was supported by The National Asthma Campaign and Medical Research Council, UK. We are grateful to Glaxo International Research for financial assistance and for supplying fluticasone and matched-placebo nasal sprays.

REFERENCES

1. Sutton BJ and Gould HJ (1993) The human IgE network. *Nature* **366**:421–428.
2. Gounni AS, Lamkhioued B, Ochiai K *et al* (1994) High affinity IgE receptor on eosinophils is involved in defence against parasites. *Nature* **367**:183–186.
3. Robinson DS, Hamid Q, Bentley A, Sun Y, Kay AB and Durham SR (1993) Activation of CD4$^+$ T cells, increased Th2-type cytokine mRNA expression, and eosinophil recruitment in bronchoalveolar lavage after allergen inhalation challenge in atopic asthmatics. *J Allergy Clin Immunol* **92**:313–324.
4. Mosmann TR, Cherwinski H, Bond MW, Giedlin M and Coffman RL (1986) Two types of murine helper T cell clone. I. Definition according to profiles of lymphokine activities and secreted proteins. *J Immunol* **136**:2348–2357.
5. Mossman TR and Coffman RL (1989) Th1 and Th2 cells: different patterns of lymphokine secretion lead to different functional properties. *Annu Rev Immunol* **7**:145–173.

6. Wierenga EA, Snoek M, de Groot C *et al* (1990) Evidence for compartmentalization of functional subsets of CD4[+] T lymphocytes in atopic patients. *J Immunol* **144**:4651–4656.
7. Cher DJ and Mossman TR (1987) Two types of murine helper T-cell clone. II. Delayed-type hypersensitivity is mediated by Th1 clones. *J Immunol* **138**:3688–3694.
8. Ying S, Durham SR, Barkans J *et al* (1993) T cells are the principal source of interleukin-5 mRNA in allergen-induced rhinitis. *Am J Resp Cell Mol Biol* **9**:356–360.
9. Ying S, Durham SR, Jacobson MR *et al* (1994) T lymphocytes and mast cells express messenger RNA for interleukin-4 in the nasal mucosa in allergen-induced rhinitis. *Immunology* **82**:200–206.
10. Ying S, Durham SR, Corrigan CJ, Hamid Q and Kay AB (1995) Phenotype of cells expressing mRNA for TH2-type (interleukin 4 and interleukin 5) and TH1-type (interleukin 2 and interferon γ) cytokines in bronchoalveolar lavage and bronchial biopsies from atopic asthmatic and normal control subjects. *Am J Resp Cell Mol Biol* **12**:477–487.
11. Robinson DS, Hamid Q, Jacobson M, Ying S, Kay AB and Durham SR (1993) Evidence for Th2-type T helper cell control of allergic disease *in vivo*. *Springer Semin Immunopathol* **15**:17–27.
12. Azzawi M, Bradley B, Jeffery PK *et al* (1990) Identification of activated T lymphocytes and eosinophils in bronchial biopsies in stable atopic asthma. *Am Rev Resp Dis* **142**:1407–1413.
13. Bradley BL, Azzawi M, Jacobson M *et al* (1991) Eosinophils, T-lymphocytes, mast cells, neutrophils, and macrophages in bronchial biopsy specimens from atopic subjects with asthma: comparison with biopsy specimens from atopic subjects without asthma and normal control subjects and relationship to bronchial hyperresponsiveness. *J Allergy Clin Immunol* **88**:661–674.
14. Robinson DS, Hamid Q, Ying S *et al* (1992) Predominant TH2-like bronchoalveolar T-lymphocyte population in atopic asthma. *N Engl J Med* **326**:298–304.
15. Robinson DS, Bentley AM, Hartnell A, Kay AB and Durham SR (1993) Activated memory T helper cells in bronchoalveolar lavage fluid from patients with atopic asthma: relation to asthma symptoms, lung function, and bronchial responsiveness. *Thorax* **48**:26–32.
16. Robinson DS, Ying S, Bentley AM *et al* (1993) Relationships among numbers of bronchoalveolar lavage cells expressing messenger ribonucleic acid for cytokines, asthma symptoms, and airway methacholine responsiveness in atopic asthma. *J Allergy Clin Immunol* **92**:397–403.
17. Bentley AM, Meng Q, Robinson DS, Hamid Q, Kay AB and Durham SR (1993) Increases in activated T lymphocytes, eosinophils, and cytokine mRNA expression for interleukin-5 and granulocyte/macrophage colony-stimulating factor in bronchial biopsies after allergen inhalation challenge in atopic asthmatics. *Am J Resp Cell Mol Biol* **8**:35–42.
18. Robinson D, Hamid Q, Ying S *et al* (1993) Prednisolone treatment in asthma is associated with modulation of bronchoalveolar lavage cell IL-4, IL-5 and IFN-γ cytokine gene expression. *Am Rev Respir Dis* **148**:401–406.
19. Bentley AM, Hamid Q, Robinson DS *et al* (1996) Prednisolone treatment in asthma. Reduction in the numbers of eosinophils, T cells, tryptase-only positive mast cells, and modulation of IL-4, IL-5, and interferon-γ cytokine gene expression within the bronchial mucosa. *Am J Resp Crit Care Med* **153**:551–556.
20. Bentley AM, Maestrelli P, Saetta M *et al* (1992) Activated T-lymphocytes and eosinophils in the bronchial mucosa in isocyanate-induced asthma. *J Allergy Clin Immunol* **89**:821–829.
21. Bentley AM, Menz G, Storz C *et al* (1992) Identification of T lymphocytes, macrophages, and activated eosinophils in the bronchial mucosa in intrinsic asthma. Relationship to symptoms and bronchial responsiveness. *Am Rev Resp Dis* **146**:500–506.

22. Humbert M, Durham SR, Corrigan CJ *et al* (1996) IL-4 and IL-5 mRNA and protein in bronchial biopsies from atopic and non-atopic asthmatics: evidence against 'intrinsic' asthma being a distinct immunopathological entity. *Am J Resp Crit Care Med* **145**:1497–1504.

23. Humbert M, Durham SR, Kimmit P *et al* (1997) Elevated expression of mRNA encoding interleukin-13 in the bronchial mucosa of atopic and non-atopic asthmatics. *J Allergy Clin Immunol* (in press).

24. Robinson DS, Ying S, Taylor IK *et al* (1994) Evidence for a TH1-like bronchoalveolar T-cell subset and predominance of interferon-γ gene activation in pulmonary tuberculosis. *Am J Resp Crit Care Med* **149**:989–993.

25. Humbert M, Grant JA, Taborda-Barata L *et al* (1996) High-affinity IgE receptor-bearing cells in bronchial biopsies from atopic and nonatopic asthma. *Am J Resp Crit Care Med* **153**:1931–1937.

26. Tsicopoulos A, Hamid Q, Haczku A *et al* (1994) Kinetics of cell infiltration and cytokine messenger RNA expression after intradermal challenge with allergen and tuberculin in the same atopic individuals. *J Allergy Clin Immunol* **94**:764–772.

27. Varney VA, Jacobson MR, Sudderick RM *et al* (1992) Immunohistology of the nasal mucosa following allergen-induced rhinitis. Identification of activated T lymphocytes, eosinophils, and neutrophils. *Am Rev Resp Dis* **146**:170–176.

28. Bentley AM, Jacobson MR, Cumberworth V *et al* (1992) Immunohistology of the nasal mucosa in seasonal allergic rhinitis: increases in activated eosinophils and epithelial mast cells. *J Allergy Clin Immunol* **89**:877–883.

29. Durham SR, Ying S, Varney VA *et al* (1992) Cytokine messenger RNA expression for IL-3, IL-4, IL-5, and granulocyte/macrophage colony-stimulating factor in the nasal mucosa after local allergen provocation: relationship to tissue eosinophilia. *J Immunol* **148**:2390–2394.

30. Masuyama K, Jacobson MR, Rak S *et al* (1994) Topical glucocorticosteroid (fluticasone propionate) inhibits cells expressing cytokine mRNA for interleukin-4 in the nasal mucosa in allergen-induced rhinitis. *Immunology* **82**:192–199.

31. Rajakulasingam K, Hamid Q, O'Brien F *et al* (1997) RANTES in human disease: cellular source and relationship to tissue eosinophilia. *Am J Resp Crit Care Med* **155**: 254–260.

32. Kimata H, Yoshida A, Ishioka C, Fujimoto M, Lindley I and Furusho K (1996) RANTES and macrophage inflammatory protein 1α selectively enhance IgE and IgG4 production in human B cells. *J Exp Med* **183**:2397–2402.

33. Huggins KG and Brostoff J (1975) Local production of specific IgE antibodies in allergic-rhinitis patients with negative skin tests. *Lancet* **2**:148–150.

34. Merrett TG, Houri M, Mayer ALR and Merrett J (1976) Measurement of specific IgE antibodies in nasal secretion—evidence for local production. *Clin Allergy* **6**:69–73.

35. Illum P and Balle V (1978) Immunoglobulins in nasal secretions and nasal mucosa in perennial rhinitis. *Acta Otolaryngol* **86**:135–141.

36. Platts-Mills TAE (1979) Local production of IgG, IgA and IgE antibodies in grass pollen hayfever. *J Immunol* **122**:2218–2225.

37. Gillon J (1981) Where do mucosal mast cells acquire IgE? *Immunol Today* **2**:80–81.

38. Ganzer U and Bachert U (1988) Localisation of IgE synthesis in immediate-type allergy to the upper respiratory tract. *Otorhinolaryngology* **50**:257–264.

39. Rackemann FM (1947) A working classification of asthma. *Am J Med* **3**:601–606.

40. Burrows B, Martinez FD, Halonen M, Barbee RA and Cline MG (1989) Association of asthma with serum IgE levels and skin test reactivity to allergens. *N Engl J Med* **320**:271–277.

41. Geha RS, Jabara HH and Loh RK (1994) Disodium cromoglycate inhibits Sμ–Sε deletional switch recombination and IgE synthesis in human B cells. *J Exp Med* **180**:663–671.

42. Daynes RA and Araneo BA (1989) Contrasting effects of glucocorticoids on the capacity of T cells to produce the growth factors interleukin 2 and interleukin 4. *Eur J Immunol* **19**:2319–2325.
43. Feuillard JD, Taylor D, Casamayor-Palleja M, Johnson GD and MacLennan ICM (1995) Isolation and characteristics of tonsil centroblasts with reference to Ig class switching. *Int Immunol* **7**:121–130.
44. Vercelli D and Geha RS (1989) Regulation of IgE synthesis in man. *J Clin Immunol* **9**:75–83.
45. Durham SR, Gould HJ, Thienes CP *et al* (1996) Local control of ε gene expression in B cells of the nasal mucosa in hayfever patients following allergen challenge. *J Allergy Clin Immunol* **97**:297 (abstr.).
46. Bradding P, Feather IH, Howarth PH *et al* (1992) Interleukin-4 is localised to and released by human mast cells. *J Exp Med* **176**:1381–1386.
47. Gauchat J-F, Henchoz S, Mazzei G *et al* (1993) Induction of human IgE synthesis in B cells by mast cells and basophils. *Nature* **365**:340–343.
48. Rak S, Jacobson MR, Sudderick RM *et al* (1994) Influence of prolonged treatment with topical corticosteroid (fluticasone propionate) on early and late phase nasal responses and cellular infiltration in the nasal mucosa after allergen challenge. *Clin Exp Allergy* **24**:930–939.
49. Varney VA, Gaga M, Frew AJ, Aber VR, Kay AB and Durham SR (1991) Usefulness of immunotherapy in patients with severe summer hay fever uncontrolled by antiallergic drugs. *Br Med J* **302**:265–269.
50. Walker SM, Varney VA, Gaga M, Jacobson MR and Durham SR (1995) Grass pollen immunotherapy: efficacy and safety during a 4-year follow-up study. *Allergy* **50**:405–413.
51. Lichtenstein LM, Ishizaka K, Norman PS, Sobotka AK and Hill BM (1973) IgE antibody measurements in ragweed hayfever. Relationship to clinical severity and the results of immunotherapy. *J Clin Invest* **52**:472–482.
52. Djurup R (1985) The subclass nature and clinical significance of the IgE antibody response in patients undergoing allergen-specific immunotherapy. *Allergy* **40**:469–486.
53. Furin MJ, Norman PS, Creticos P *et al* (1991) Immunotherapy decreases antigen-induced eosinophil migration into the nasal cavity. *J Allergy Clin Immunol* **88**:27–32.
54. Otsuka H, Mezawa A, Ohnishi M, Okubo K, Seki H and Okuda M (1991) Changes in nasal metachromatic cells during allergen immunotherapy. *Clin Exp Allergy* **21**:115–119.
55. Varney VA, Hamid QA, Gaga M *et al* (1993) Influence of grass pollen immunotherapy on cellular infiltration and cytokine mRNA expression during allergen-induced late-phase cutaneous responses. *J Clin Invest* **92**:644–651.
56. Durham SR, Ying S, Varney VA *et al* (1996) Grass pollen immunotherapy inhibits allergen-induced infiltration of CD4$^+$ T lymphocytes and eosinophils in the nasal mucosa and increases the number of cells expressing messenger RNA for interferon-γ. *J Allergy Clin Immunol* **97**:1356–1365.
57. Hamid Q, Schotman E, Jacobson MR, Walker SM and Durham SR (1997) Increases in IL-12 cells accompany inhibition of allergen-induced late skin responses following successful grass pollen immunotherapy. *J Allergy Clin Immunol* **99**: 254–260.
58. Carballido JM, Carballido-Perrig N, Oberli-Schrammli A, Heusser CH and Blaser K (1994) Regulation of IgE and IgG4 responses by allergen-specific T cell clones to bee venom phospholipase A2 *in vitro*. *J Allergy Clin Immunol* **93**:758–767.
59. Diaz-Sanchez D, Dotson AR, Takenaka H and Saxon A (1994) Diesel exhaust particles induce local IgE production *in vivo* and alter the pattern of IgE messenger RNA isoforms. *J Clin Invest* **94**:1417–1425.
60. Durham SR (1995) New concepts of the mechanism of allergen-specific immunotherapy. In: Proceedings of the XVI European Congress of Allergology and Clinical Immunology, Basomba A and Sastre J (eds), pp. 701–707. Monduzzi Editore, Bologna.

3 IgE Homeostasis: is CD23 the Safety Switch?

HANNAH J. GOULD, REBECCA L. BEAVIL, RAJKO RELJIĆ,
JIANGUO SHI, CHECK W. MA, BRIAN J. SUTTON
and RODOLFO GHIRLANDO*

*The Randall Institute, King's College London, London UK and *Centre de
Biochimie Structurale, Faculté de Pharmacie, Montpellier, France*

3.1 THE STARTING POINT

Allergy afflicts one in five of the population and is associated with the over-production of IgE. It is therefore essential to understand the physiological mechanisms of IgE regulation. A major advance in the study of IgE regulation came with the discovery that IL-4 is required for IgE expression (1–3). The multiple activities of IL-4 that influence IgE expression are summarized in Figure 3.1. We shall be concerned here with the consequences of the upregulation of CD23, the low-affinity receptor for IgE, in B cells, T cells and immune effector cells in Th2 cell-mediated inflammatory reactions. In this chapter we review the evidence that CD23 participates in the regulation of IgE synthesis. Paradoxically, CD23 has been implicated in both the upregulation (in humans, but not mice) and downregulation of IgE synthesis (4). This can be rationalized by reference to the structure of CD23 and its dichotomous functions as a receptor on B cells for IgE and an exogenous ligand for CD21 on B cells. We conjecture that the opposing activities are part of a unique mechanism for the feedback control of IgE synthesis which underlies homeostasis.

3.2 DISCOVERY OF FCεRII/CD23 AND ITS B CELL FUNCTIONS

3.2.1 Molecule With a Split Personality

CD23 was first identified as a ligand for IgE on B cells and monocytes (5), whence the original name FcεRII (FcεRI having been discovered earlier). The two IgE receptors are also known as the high-affinity receptor (FcεRI) and the low-affinity receptor (CD23), reflecting the difference in their affinities for IgE ($K_A = 10^{10}$ and $\sim 10^7$ M^{-1}, respectively; see Ref. 4 for a review). CD23 has been found on a wide

IgE Regulation: Molecular Mechanisms. Edited by D. Vercelli. © 1997 John Wiley & Sons Ltd.

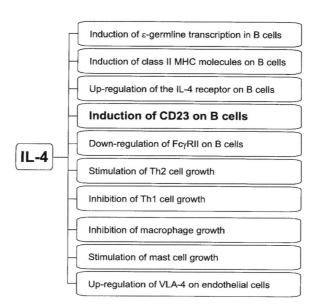

Figure 3.1. Influence of IL-4 on IgE expression. IL-4 is a multi-functional lymphokine. This is an abbreviated list of the various activities that may influence the level of IgE expression *in vivo*. For further information see Refs. 1 and 57. We highlight the influence of IL-4 on the expression of CD23 and expand on the consequences of this in Figure 3.2, and in the text

range of cells (see Ref. 6 for a review), but its expression on monocytes/macrophages, eosinophils and platelets in particular, suggested that it may participate in IgE antibody effector functions, and it was indeed shown to mediate IgE antibody-dependent killing of parasites by several types of effector cells (7). Certain types of cells that express CD23 are not normally available in the circulation, however, nor do they participate directly in cell killing.

CD23 was independently discovered on B cells activated by Epstein–Barr virus (EBV) infection (8, 9) and as an antigen on follicular dendritic cells (10, 11). It has come to be recognized as a marker for antigen-activated B cells, expressed at high levels prior to heavy chain switching (12), and for the follicular dendritic cells that occupy the apical layer of the light zone within germinal centers of a lymphoid follicle (see also Chapter 10). CD23 is also detected on bone marrow stromal epithelium. The topographically restricted specific expression on cells of these latter lineages points to a role in lymphoid development. Not surprisingly, therefore, the efforts of B-cell immunologists have focused on the function of CD23 in B-cell development and activation. The proteins designated CD23 and FcεRII were found to be identical in experiments carried out to test the inhibition of IgE binding to B cells by various monoclonal antibodies (mAbs) against all CD antigens (13, 14).

CD23 fragments are found in the supernatants of cells cultured *in vitro* and in body fluids, and there are indeed many reports that soluble CD23 (sCD23) may serve as a marker for a wide variety of pathological conditions, including chronic lymphocytic leukemia, bone marrow graft rejection, rheumatoid arthritis and atopy (15). These reports do not reveal whether sCD23 is an active agent in the disease or only a by-product of inflammation.

Figure 3.2 summarizes the various activities that have been ascribed to CD23. We distinguish between the activities that are triggered by IgE with membrane CD23 as the receptor, and those that are elicited by exogenous CD23 acting on CD21 (also known as complement receptor 2, CR2) or other complement receptors CD11b–CD18 (CR3) and CD11c–CD18 (CR4). Since we are concerned here with B-cell functions in the synthesis of antibodies, we shall refer only in passing to the interesting recent work, which showed that CD23 binds to CD11 b or c/CD18 on monocytes and is thereby linked to the pathogenesis of rheumatoid arthritis (16, 17).

3.2.2 Growth and Differentiation of B cells, and Upregulation of IgE Synthesis

The significance of CD23 expression on activated B cells became apparent when it was shown that isolated CD23 serves as a growth factor for 'primed' (antigen-

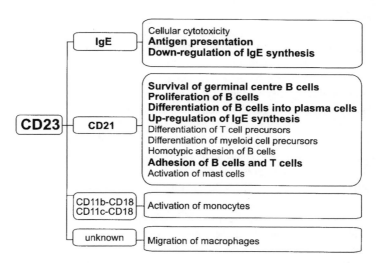

Figure 3.2. Activities of CD23 with its alternative ligands. The known activities of CD23 are enumerated and classified according to whether they require IgE, CD21 or CD11b–CD18/CD11c–CD18 as the ligand. We highlight the activities that are considered to be important in IgE regulation

activated or phorbol ester-treated) B cells in culture (18). Soluble CD23 also has a profound effect on germinal center B cells (centrocytes). These cells undergo apoptosis *in vivo* without antigen stimulation and *in vitro* upon isolation and culture. Soluble CD23, in association with IL-1, arrests the process of apoptosis and allows the centrocytes to differentiate into plasma cells *in vitro* (19, 20). The same mixture also promotes differentiation of pro-thymocytes into T cells and myeloid precursors into basophils *in vitro* (21, 22). The survival of centrocytes in the presence of sCD23 and IL-1 has been correlated with the upregulation of bcl-2, a member of the well-characterized family of B-cell survival proteins (23). While it is reasonable to infer that bcl-2 may be the protective agent in centrocytes rescued from apoptosis by CD23, the evidence in this case remains circumstantial.

To test the effect of sCD23 on IgE synthesis, Delespesse and co-workers (24) first used B cells from atopic individuals, that produce IgE *in vitro*. Following the demonstration that IL-4 induces heavy chain switching to IgE in resting B cells in culture, several groups also tested the effects of sCD23 on the production of IgE in these systems. It was found that sCD23 augments ongoing spontaneous IgE production by cells from atopic patients (24) and acts synergistically with sub-optimal concentrations of IL-4 to induce IgE production by normal resting B cells (25, 26). sCD23 induced increased levels of the ε germline gene transcript, as well as increased levels of IgE (26), indicating that it acted upon cells before (as well as possibly after) genetic recombination.

Antibodies directed to CD23 have the opposite effect to that of sCD23: they inhibit the synthesis of IgE by peripheral blood mononuclear cells (PBMC) from atopic patients (27) and IL-4 induction of IgE synthesis in normal PBMC (25). It has also been shown that antibodies against CD23 inhibit IgE synthesis *in vivo* in rats (28). Although the effects of these antibodies were at first thought to derive from their ability to neutralize sCD23 activity, there is at least one alternative interpretation in view of the involvement of membrane CD23 in the downregulation of IgE synthesis (see below), namely that the antibodies might rather, or in addition, activate this inhibitory mechanism. There is nevertheless ample support for positive regulation by sCD23 without the evidence from antibodies.

The frequency of IgE-expressing B cells in the circulation of normal individuals is exceedingly low at around one in ten thousand (29), although higher frequencies may occur in specialized tissues, such as the nasal mucosa (30). Cells that have switched to IgE will first express mainly membrane-bound IgE, but may differentiate into plasma cells, which will then express much larger amounts of the secreted form of IgE. Membrane IgE could, in principle, serve as a receptor for exogenous CD23. There are probably too few IgE-expressing cells in PBMC or germinal center centrocytes, however, to account for the general effects of CD23 on B-cell growth and differentiation.

To search for a different ligand, Bonnefoy and co-workers (31) examined the adherence of fluorescent liposomes containing CD23 to B cells from several lines, using flow cytometry. Having identified a suitable line, they then tested mAbs against a comprehensive panel of 129 CD antigens for their ability to inhibit the interaction between the B cells and the CD23-liposomes. Only anti-CD21 antibodies proved to be effective inhibitors. Next, they isolated proteins from the B cells and analyzed them by Western blotting with labelled CD23-liposomes and anti-CD21. The antibody labelled a small number of proteins of similar size (> 100 kDa), assumed to be differently glycosylated forms of CD21. The CD23 liposomes labelled a protein with the same size as one of the CD21 species, thus confirming the identity of CD21 as the principal receptor for CD23 on resting B cells. Further studies revealed that anti-CD21, as well as sCD23, could stimulate the synthesis of IgE by PBMC incubated with IL-4 *in vitro*. These studies further revealed that the stimulation of IgE synthesis by CD23 in a minority of the B cell population is mediated by CD21, rather than, for example, membrane IgE or any other hetero-geneously expressed membrane protein in the absence of CD21.

3.2.3 Suppression of B-cell Activation and Downregulation of IgE Synthesis

A different view comes from the work of Saxon and Delespesse and their co-workers showing that membrane CD23 on B cells can transmit signals which inhibit B-cell growth and differentiation, as well as basal IgE synthesis in committed B cells, in response to inducing agents. Luo *et al* (32) found that cross-linking membrane CD23, whether by anti-CD23 mAbs, polymeric IgE or IgE immune complexes, suppressed the growth and differentiation of peripheral blood B cells in culture induced by anti-IgM or *Staphylococcus aureus* Cowan A strain together with IL-4 (but not with IL-2). The cross-linking agents were effective only if (i) they were present in the early stage of the incubations, and (ii) if CD23 were expressed at a high density on the B cells. The requirement for IL-4, and the inefficacy of IL-2, were probably related to the threshold level of membrane CD23 expression for the negative response, as IL-4 but not IL-2 induces the expression of CD23 (1). Earlier workers had reported that a subset of anti-CD23 mAbs stimulated, rather than suppressed, B cell proliferation, but this was equally true of their univalent Fab fragments (33), whereas divalent F(ab)$_2$ fragments of the inhibitory mAbs were inactive (32). Luo *et al* (32) argued that the anti-CD23 mAbs were not acting to neutralize sCD23, partly on the grounds that intact antibody or F(ab)$_2$ fragments were required for suppression, and also because they could not confirm the activities of sCD23 on B-cell proliferation.

This group also reported that anti-CD23 suppressed the basal synthesis of IgE by B cells from atopic donors and the induction of IgE synthesis by normal B cells cultured in the presence of IL-4 (34). Sherr *et al* (35) confirmed the downregulation of basal IgE synthesis in B cells from atopic donors and in IgE myeloma cells, and showed further that in myeloma cells the cross-linking of membrane CD23 alone (with no cross-linking of IgE to itself or to CD23), was sufficient. Interestingly, the expression of membrane IgE was unaffected by anti-CD23 (36). In a related study, Campbell *et al* (37) found that co-cross-linking CD23 and membrane Ig blocks the stimulation of proliferation and Ig secretion by IL-4 in mouse primary B cell cultures. It is difficult to envisage how IgE could be excluded from the company of CD23 molecules, cross-linked by an antigen-IgE complex; both cross-linking of CD23 and co-cross-linking of CD23 and IgE may therefore contribute to the inhibition of IgE secretion from primary B cells (Figure 3.3).

Experiments with CD23 knockout and transgenic mice conclusively support these models for negative regulation by membrane CD23. The most striking phenotype of the CD23 knockout mice is their IgE antibody response to T-dependent antigens. CD23-deficient mice produce 10- to 100-fold higher levels of IgE than wild-type mice, while expression of other antibody classes, except IgG1—classically co-regulated with IgE—are unchanged (38). Conversely, transgenic mice over-expressing membrane CD23, but not sCD23 exhibit a weaker IgE response than wild type mice (39). There was no evidence in favor of positive regulation by CD23, either of B- or T-cell growth and differentiation or of immune competence. The lack of general effects on the immune system of mice was confirmed in two other CD23 knockout studies (40, 41). These observations may betray a true difference between the murine and human immune systems. It has not been possible to demonstrate that murine CD23 binds to CD21 (42) or that soluble fragments have any cytokine activity in mice (43).

In sum, the experiments on both the human and mouse systems indicate that IgE can transmit, through membrane CD23, signals which interfere with the induction of B cell growth and differentiation by IL-4 and the secretion of IgE. There is a striking similarity between this function of CD23 and that of one form of the low-affinity

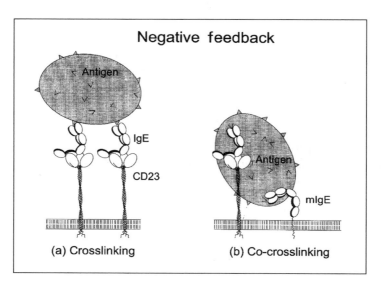

Figure 3.3. Mechanisms proposed to account for the down-regulation of IgE synthesis: (a) proposed by Sherr *et al* (35); (b) Proposed by Campbell *et al* (37). Membrane IgE is abbreviated mIgE

IgG receptor, CD32 or FcγRII. Antigen–IgG complexes inhibit blastogenesis of B cells expressing this receptor and also inhibit the synthesis of IgG (44, 45). Ravetch and co-workers have identified the receptor as FcγRIIb (46). Signal transduction through FcγRIIb leads to the apoptosis of B cells (47). If the mechanism of signal transduction through membrane CD23 is analogous to that of the low-affinity IgG receptor, there may be a nexus between separate signaling pathways, induced by CD23 and sCD23, that governs apoptosis.

3.2.4 IgE-dependent Antigen Presentation

The work of Kehry and Yamashita (48) on the mouse system and Pirron et al (49) on the human system first demonstrated that CD23 efficiently focuses protein antigens bound to IgE for presentation to antigen-specific T cells in vitro. Similar results were obtained in the mouse system with anti-CD23, cross-linked to an antigen (50), and with allergen–IgE complexes from atopic individuals (51). Antigen presentation was shown to be up to 10 000 times more efficient with CD23 than with an IgG antigen receptor in vitro.

By immunizing mice with haptenated carrier protein and simultaneously injecting them with IgE mAb against the hapten, Heyman and co-workers (52, 53) found a 100-fold higher immune response to the carrier than in control mice that had not been given IgE. Unlike the in vitro systems, in which the activation of antigen-specific T cells was assayed, the criterion in vivo was the production of antigen-specific antibodies. The results implied that only antigen-specific B cells could be stimulated to antibody production by the cognate T cells. The authors were unable to distinguish between two possible mechanisms: (i) that the antigen–IgE complex must be recognized and captured both by membrane Ig and by CD23 (cf. Figure 3.3b), whereupon only specific B cells, susceptible to subsequent help from antigen-specific T cells, would be allowed to present the antigen; or (ii) that all B cells expressing CD23 could present the antigen to specific T cells, but only B cells able to recognize the antigen would be susceptible to help from these T cells.

Luo et al (32) have suggested a possible basis for the second mechanism, namely that cross-linking of membrane CD23 by antigen–IgE complexes on B cells, which are not specific for the antigen, will downregulate Ig production, thus restricting the production of antibodies of unrelated specificities. The corollary is that antigen-specific T cells, expanded by stimulation through the CD23/IgE-dependent B-cell pathway, will preferentially promote antibody production by 'CD23-low' memory B cells, which have undergone heavy chain switching. Memory B cells in the nasal mucosa are predominantly IgE producers (30). Thus, with help from the activated T cells and allergen stimulation, they may be induced to differentiate into plasma cells and secrete IgE (see also Chapter 2).

Recent work of Grosjean and co-workers (54) suggests that CD23 may have two separate functions in antigen presentation, one to capture the antigen–IgE complex, and the other to induce the expression of CD21 resulting in stimulation of antigen-specific T cells. Expression of CD21 may enable T cells to present antigen in turn to specific B cells via CD21 and C3 (cf. Figure 3.4c). It is also conceivable that CD23, expressed on T cells at a significantly higher level in allergic as compared with normal individuals (55, 56), may present antigen–IgE complexes in turn to specific B cells. Secrist *et al* (57) have reported that antigen presentation by B cells favors T helper 2 (Th2) cell activation. Thus, one might envisage a concerted reaction, wherein B cells presenting antigen by the CD23/IgE-dependent pathway induce Ag-specific T cells to differentiate into Th2 cells; if the B cell involved in this interaction also expresses an antigen receptor, the T cell may then induce heavy chain switching to IgE and differentiation of the B cells into an IgE antibody-secreting cell. Whether or not separate B cells are required for antigen capture and antibody production, it appears likely that antigen presentation by allergen–IgE complexes through CD23 may bias the secondary (memory) immune response towards production of antibodies of the IgE class. Were a concerted mechanism to prevail, it could account for the fact that allergen-specific IgE constitutes a high proportion (30–50%) of total IgE in an allergic response, which differs fundamentally from an IgG response (58).

3.3 THE FUNCTION OF CD21 IN B-CELL ACTIVATION

Exogenous CD23 induces growth and differentiation of B cells and stimulates IgE synthesis in B cells by binding to CD21. CD21 is expressed on mature B cells up to the stage of their differentiation into plasma cells; it is not expressed on immature (bone marrow) B cells (see Refs 59 and 60 for reviews). Before its identification as the CD23 receptor on B cells, CD21 was already familiar as receptor for the activated products of the third component of complement, C3, for EBV and interferon-α. C3 is a critical component of the immune response in mammals. C3 deficiency in experimental animals, as well as in humans, leads to extreme vulnerability to microbial infections (61–64), and CD21-deficient mice are similarly compromised (65, 66).

The mechanism of C3 enhancement of the immune response is understood (67–69). The classical and alternative pathways of complement activation both result in covalent attachment of the C3 fragments, C3b or C3d, to antigen through a thioester bond. C3b-antigen adducts bind to CD35 (or complement receptor 1, CR1), while C3d-antigen adducts bind to CD21 (or CR2). In the form of adduct with an antigen, C3d acts as an adjuvant, that is to say it lowers the threshold concentration of antigen which will cause mature resting, membrane-antibody expressing B cells, capable of recognizing that antigen, to enter the cell cycle. This effect is contingent on the co-ligation of the antigen receptor complex (membrane-bound antibody and its four associated signaling subunits, comprising two α–β chain heterodimers) and the CD21/CD19/TAPA-1 complex in the plane of the B cell membrane (Figure 3.4a). Such an association between the two kinds of complexes in the cell membrane is required for synergistic signaling.

The experimental approach first used to test the proposed mechanism is illustrated in Figure 3.4b (67): we have used a similar scheme to examine the activity of CD23.

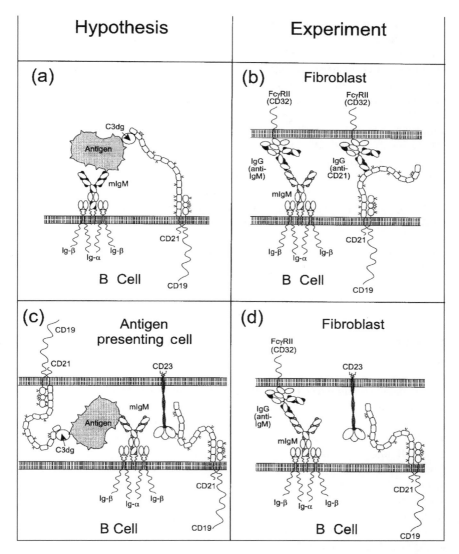

Figure 3.4. Hypotheses and model systems: (a) hypothesis and (b) model system for the activation of B cells by C3dg; (c) hypothesis and (d) model system for activation of B cells by CD23 (see Section 3.3 for further description)

A fibroblast cell line that expressed a recombinant receptor for IgG (FcγRII/CD32) was used to mimic the C3-antigen adducts, by presenting a surrogate antigen (anti-IgM) and a surrogate C3d molecule (anti-CD19 or anti-CD21) to tonsil B cells. The fibroblasts were treated with mitomycin to block DNA synthesis, mixed with the B cells and incubated with anti-IgM at varying concentrations in the presence or absence of a saturating amount of anti-CD19 or anti-CD21. It emerged that the anti-CD19 reduces the threshold concentration of anti-IgM required to stimulate tonsil B cell proliferation by three orders of magnitude, from 10^{-8} to 10^{-11} M; this supports the proposed co-ligation mechanism. Recently, Dempsey *et al* (68) confirmed this result by a more direct experimental approach, taking advantage of a recombinant model antigen containing hen egg lysozyme fused to one, two or three molecules of C3d. The fusion products were much more immunogenic than the unmodified antigen; the immunogenicity increased by a factor of 10^3 when two molecules of C3d were fused with the antigen and by a further factor of 10 when the third molecule was included.

Figure 3.4c depicts a hypothetical scheme for the activation of B cells by exogenous CD23, which we have tested by a strategy (Figure 3.4d) similar to that used for C3 by Carter and Fearon (67) (Figure 3.4b). The fibroblast cell line expressing CD32 was stably transformed with an expression vector for CD23 and then used in the same manner as the untransfected line reacted with anti-CD19. As expected the outcome was quite similar, although the magnitude of the effect was somewhat smaller (70). These results support the representation of CD21 as a conduit for multiple ligands, including C3d, EBV, interferon-α and CD23, to signal for B-cell survival, growth and differentiation (71).

3.4 STRUCTURE OF CD23 AND ITS COMPLEXES WITH IgE AND CD21

The modeled structure of CD23 is illustrated in Figure 3.5. Unlike other antibody Fc receptors which are all members of the Ig superfamily, CD23 belongs to a group of proteins known as calcium-dependent or C-type lectins, exemplified by the more widely known asialoglycoprotein receptor (ASGPR) (72, 73). Like ASGPR, CD23 is a type II integral membrane protein, with an extracellular C-terminus and cytoplasmic N-terminus. The lectin domain is near the C-terminal end of the extracellular sequence. Its three-dimensional structure has not been determined, but has been modeled by several groups (4, 74, 75) on the basis of the structure of the C-type lectin domain of mannose binding protein (MBP) (76, 77) and E-selectin (78). The presence of at least one 'calcium pocket' is a feature of this protein family and is found in CD23, as shown (Figure 3.5). Binding to both IgE and CD21 is dependent on calcium (79, 80), but this does not imply that the binding sites encompass the calcium pockets, since the calcium ion probably stabilizes the native fold of the domain.

The lectin domain is flanked on the C-terminal side by a sequence containing, in human, though not murine CD23, an inverse RGD sequence (DGR). This may function as an integrin receptor, as indicated by the fact that an anti-fibronectin antibody binds to eosinophils bearing CD23 and this interaction is inhibited by the tetrapeptides RGDS and SDGR (81). On the N-terminal side of the lectin domain is a sequence of 112 amino acids which has the capacity to self-associate by forming a

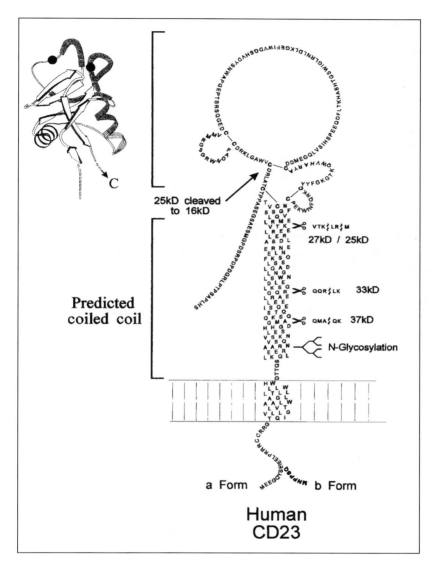

Figure 3.5. Predicted structure of CD23. The predicted coiled-coil region is represented by the 3–4 heptad repeats. Sites of cleavage by endogenous proteases and of glycosylation and the alternative isoforms a and b are indicated. Ca^{2+} binding sites are indicated by filled circles.

three-stranded α-helical coiled-coil (82–85). The lectin domains of such a trimer project outwards from the cell membrane at the end of a 10 nm stalk in the form of a bouquet, reminiscent of the arrangement of the globular domain of certain other C-type lectins and the complement protein C1q (86). It had appeared that the 12 amino acids connecting the lectin domains to the stalk were unstructured, so as to allow the lectin domains flexional freedom. A sequence of similar length, corresponding to the 'neck' that links the lectin domain of MBP to its collagenous stalk, had also been represented in this way. However, the neck of MBP is now known to form a triple-stranded α-helical coiled-coil (87, 88). The coiled-coil structure extends right up to the boundary with the lectin domain and the terminal lectin domains all make non-covalent contacts with the neck of the adjacent subunit. The structure of the trimer is evidently much more compact and rigid than had been supposed. On re-examination of the corresponding linker sequence in CD23, we have found that it conforms to the criteria for a three-stranded α-helical coiled-coil, which could be continuous with the lower stalk (with a skip residue, accommodated in the structure) and contiguous with the lectin domain. We now envisage that in the CD23 trimer the three lectin domains are packed tightly together, as in MBP (Figure 3.6a).

Each subunit of human CD23 contains a single site for *N*-glycosylation, located near the membrane-proximal end of the sequence which forms the coiled-coil stalk. In the trimer the three carbohydrate attachment sites lie on the surface of the stalk

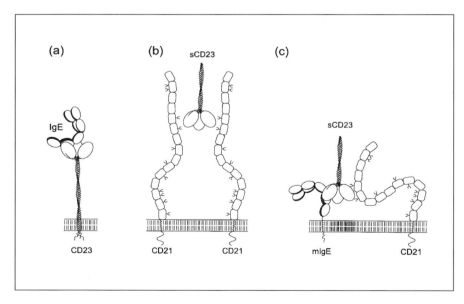

Figure 3.6. Models for the complexes of trimeric CD23 with IgE and CD21: (a) 1:1 complex with IgE, occupying two lectin domains in CD23; (b) 1:2 (or up to 3) complex with CD21; (c) cross-linking of membrane IgE (mIgE) and CD21 by a fragment of CD23, occupying all three lectin domains

(Figure 3.5). *N*-glycosylation sites are conserved in the stalks of human, mouse and rat CD23, although their number and locations along the surface of the stalks differ. The carbohydrate chains may stabilize the trimers in the membrane against dissociation. The fragments of human CD23 (see below) do not contain the N-linked carbohydrate and may therefore dissociate more readily.

Another feature of the stalk sequence are the three histidines on the inside of the coiled-coil (Figure 3.5). At physiological pH these may be uncharged, but in a low pH compartment, such as the endosome, they may become protonated, thereby perhaps disrupting the structure. ASGPR also contains histidines in its predicted coiled-coil 'stalk' and it is known that they are involved in the process by which ASGPR discharges its glycoprotein ligands in endosomes before returning to the surface of the liver cell (89).

Closer to the N-terminus of CD23 is the single transmembrane sequence and the short (20/21 amino acid) cytoplasmic sequence. The latter occurs in two forms, CD23a, which is constitutively expressed in activated B cells, and CD23b, which is induced by IL-4 in a wide range of cells, including B cells (90). The two forms differ in the N-terminal 6/7 amino acids; they originate from mRNAs initiated from different promotors, but are spliced in the same reading frame to the common sequence. CD23a, but not CD23b, contains the YSEI motif, which is a targeting signal for coated pits. Both CD23a and CD23b have been expressed in monocytes and it has been shown that only the former is active in the internalization of antigen-IgE complexes for presentation to T cells, while only the latter mediates phagocytosis of red cells coated with IgE (91). CD23b then must be the form that generally mediates the effector functions of IgE (7).

The 45 kDa CD23 is cleaved at the cell membrane by endogenous protease into specific fragments of 37, 33, 29, 25 and 16 kDa apparent molecular weight (6, 92). The initial cleavage releases the larger fragment and then progressively more of the stalk is removed from the free end. The 25 kDa fragment (comprising the C-terminal tail, lectin domain and the neck of CD23) is relatively stable and found in serum at concentrations of ≈ 2 ng/ml (15). The 16 kDa fragment is the C-type lectin domain, devoid of 'tail' and stalk sequences. All the fragments bind to both IgE and CD21, although the full length CD23 and larger fragments bind more tightly than the smaller fragments (see Ref. 6 and Reljić *et al*, unpublished results). The binding sites for both IgE and CD21 are therefore thought to reside entirely within the lectin domain. The proteases responsible for the cleavage of CD23 *in vivo* have not been identified. Interestingly, IgE inhibits the proteolysis of CD23 (93, 94), even though its binding site is far from the initial site of cleavage (Figure 3.5). We have shown that the formation of trimeric fragments is concentration dependent in solution, and we therefore believe an equilibrium may prevail in the cell membrane. Proteases may attack the dissociated subunits and IgE may protect CD23 by stabilizing the trimers. Antibodies may either stabilize or destabilize the trimers, depending on the location of their epitopes in CD23. Unglycosylated CD23 appears to be more susceptible to proteolysis than native CD23 (92, 95, 96), suggesting that the carbohydrate chain may be a barrier to dissociation of the trimer.

The structure of IgE is likely to be similar to that of IgG, since the expected features of the sequence are conserved between the two Igs (see Ref. 4 for a review). IgE has an additional domain (Cε2) in place of the hinge region in IgG. Unlike IgG, which is planar, IgE appears to have an inflexible bend between Cε2 and Cε3, so that Cε2 and Fab regions come into close apposition at one side of the molecule (97), as illustrated in Figure 3.6a. We have recently shown that the complex of the mono- meric recombinant 16 kDa fragment of CD23 with IgE contains two molecules of CD23 and one of IgE (98). This leads to the model shown in Figure 3.6a in which two of the lectin domains in CD23 bind on the opposite sides of two Cε3 domains in IgE. This geometry implies that one of the three lectin domains in CD23 is not engaged in the complex. It may thus be free to bind to another IgE molecule or to CD21 (Figure 3.6c).

CD21 is a type I integral membrane protein with an extracellular sequence comprising 15/16 repeats of a sequence motif of 60–75 amino acids, known as the short consensus repeat (SCR; see Refs. 59 and 60 for reviews). The SCRs are numbered 1–16 from the extracellular N-terminus. The missing domain in the shorter form is eliminated by RNA splicing and is not known to alter the function of CD21. In the mouse CD21 forms part of a larger protein (CD35), as well as being expressed on its own by elimination of the N-terminal repeats of the precursor mRNA. The parent protein (also known as CR1) additionally functions as a com- plement receptor, though for C3b.

The location of the CD23 binding site in CD21 has been mapped to two regions of the molecule, SCR 1–2 and SCR 5–8 (99, 100). Glycosylation of SCR 5 and 6 appears to contribute to the binding affinity. All other biological ligands for CD21, C3d, EBV and interferon-α, and all the antibodies that signal through CD21 bind to SCR 1 and 2 (60, 100). How the binding to SCRs 1 and 2, but not other SCR in this flexible structure, results in signal transduction remains unknown. The observation that the carbohydrate moiety of CD21 is recognized by CD23 resolved the question of why CD23 alone, among the antibody receptors, is a C-type lectin. When IgE was the only known ligand it was assumed that CD23 recognized the IgE-bound carbohydrate chains. IgE is unusually heavily glycosylated, with three N-linked chains at two external sites that are specific to Fcε and a buried site that is conserved in all antibody Fcs. We found however that these carbohydrate chains are not essential for binding to CD23 and appear even to weaken the interaction (101, 102).

It is well established that the aggregation state of C3 is important for signaling (see Ref. 60 for a review). The EBV ligand, the major membrane envelope glyco- protein gp350/220, is also expressed in multiple copies on the virus (103). The trimeric state of CD23 on the cell membrane and, at least for a time, after it is cleaved from the cell membrane, may afford an important clue to its function. The 16 kDa lectin domain, which we have shown to be a monomer (98), suppresses the synthesis of IgE by PBMC in vitro, unlike the larger fragments with parts of the coiled-coil stalk, which are stimulatory (104). The oligomeric form of CD23 thus appears to be essential for its cytokine functions.

3.5 MODEL OF CD23 FUNCTION IN IgE HOMEOSTASIS

Figure 3.7 illustrates, in a highly schematic form, one of the processes that we believe to be responsible for an upward spiral of IgE synthesis in an allergic reaction, taking the nasal mucosa in hay fever patients as the paradigm (4, 105, 30). Research on this tissue has led us to suggest that the resident B cells in the nasal mucosa provide a local source of IgE antibodies that keep the mast cells continuously sensitized (30). Thus, as the IgE antibodies, attached to FcεRI on the mast cells, slowly dissociate or turn over in the tissue, they may be immediately replaced by IgE secreted by these B cells. Upon allergen challenge, the mast cells release IL-4 and tumor necrosis factor (TNF)-α and there are at least five consequences, all of which may drive up the levels of IgE. Thus: (i) IL-4 and TNF-α upregulate vascular cell adhesion molecule 1 (VCAM-1) and perhaps other vascular addressins on the local

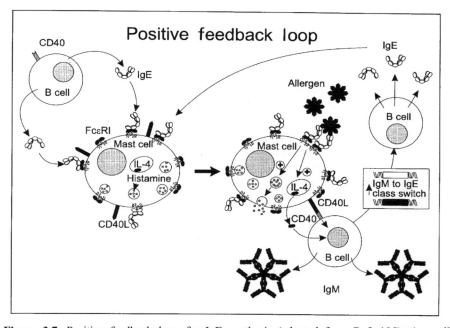

Figure 3.7. Positive feedback loop for IgE synthesis (adapted from Ref. 105). A small number of B cells have been induced by Th2 cells to produce allergen-specific IgE, which binds to FcεRI on the surface of mast cells. The mast cells can now bind allergen, which stimulates them to release histamine and to secrete IL-4. IL-4 and the CD40–CD40 ligand interactions together induce more B cells to switch to IgE production, thus creating a local feedback loop. This scheme is greatly over-simplified, since it fails to indicate the contribution of B cells and T cells in antigen focusing (Section 3.2.4). A more complete scheme is shown in Sutton and Gould (Ref. 4, Fig. 8). Moreover, Schmitz *et al* (109) have demonstrated that *in vivo* only T cells are the initial source of IL-4 and induce an IgE class switch in (murine) B cells. The activation of mast cells however results in the recruitment of T cells to the tissue (30)

endothelium to induce the extravasation of leukocytes into the tissue (106, 107); (ii) IL-4 induces the differentiation of Th0 cells to Th2 cells, which also produce IL-4 (1); (iii) IL-4, mainly from the T cells, but perhaps also from mast cells, may upregulate its own receptor and MHC class II molecules on B cells, allowing IL-4 to transmit signals to the B cell and to present antigens to T cells (1); (iv) IL-4 would also upregulate CD23 on eosinophils and monocytes, as well as on B cells and T cells (1, 6), to provide a local source of sCD23; (v) sCD23 may be expected, in synergy with IL-4, to increase expression of the ε germline gene in B cells that have not yet switched to IgE (26). Another requirement for switching will be met by the expression of CD40 ligand on activated T cells and mast cells. How may the T cells be activated? As has been mentioned (Section 3.2.4), the identities of the cells that give help to and receive help from the T cells remain to be clarified.

Returning to Figure 3.7, and assuming that our hypothesis of local switching and IgE synthesis is correct, we see that the nascent IgE secreted by the B cells may then sensitize the mast cells. The latter, freshly sensitized by IgE and exposed to allergen, would be activated, and would release IL-4 and TNF-α to stimulate the synthesis of more IgE, leading to an amplified response. This constitutes a positive feedback loop, dependent on IL-4 and CD23, as well as any subsidiary factors in the various 'black boxes' in the cell that are required for the expression of these molecules. Amplification of the response by antigen focusing is not included in Figure 3.7, but is likely to be an essential component (Section 3.2.4.).

How might one then terminate this upward spiral? Membrane-bound, as opposed to soluble fragmented CD23 appears to be crucial (38, 108). From our knowledge of the affinity of IgE for its high- and low-affinity receptors, FcεRI and CD23, it is apparent that there would be a range of concentrations, lying between the half-saturation levels for the two, within which positive regulation of IgE synthesis may occur following activation of the mast cell. At a concentration near the K_D of the low-affinity receptor the various mechanisms that depend on its occupancy (see below) could come into play. These are enumerated in Table 3.1.

After antigen challenge the concentration of IgE antibodies in the blood and presumably in the tissue falls to a low level. Subsequent antigen challenge will now lead to a situation, as described above, in which IL-4 is produced and CD23 is

Table 3.1. Basis of the paradoxical positive and negative activities of CD23

Trimeric CD23 fragments bind to membrane-bound IgE and CD21 to up-regulate IgE synthesis in committed (membrane-bound IgE$^+$) B cells	+
Secreted IgE binds to soluble fragments of CD23 to block their binding to membrane-bound IgE	−
IgE binds to membrane-bound CD23 to block proteolysis and release of soluble fragments	−

Antigen-IgE antibody complexes bind to membrane-bound CD23
  (a) Initiates a negative signaling pathway
  (b) Steals membrane-bound IgE away from CR2 to terminate positive signaling
	−

upregulated on the bystander cells. In the absence of IgE to protect membrane CD23, sCD23 will be released by proteases and captured by CD21 on the B cells. As indicated, these fragments can participate in the positive feedback mechanism, in which we envisage CD23 co-ligating IgE and CD21 in the B-cell membrane. As its concentration in the tissue rises above 10^{-7} M the IgE and its complexes with antigen will bind to both soluble fragments of CD23 and to membrane CD23. This will result in downregulation of IgE synthesis by multiple mechanisms (Table 3.1). (1) By binding to soluble fragments of CD23 the IgE can prevent their binding to membrane IgE, which we speculate may be required for the specific effect on IgE synthesis. (2) By binding to membrane CD23, IgE and its complexes would protect the CD23 from proteolytic cleavage and so prevent any further release of the stimulatory fragments. (3) The co-ligation of membrane CD23 molecules and/or CD23 and membrane IgE by antigen–IgE complexes triggers a negative signaling pathway that results in the downregulation of IgE synthesis. (4) The co-ligation of membrane CD23 and membrane IgE would also sequester the latter, and make it unavailable to CD21 in the B cell membrane. This would in turn abrogate the synergy between membrane IgE and CD21 in positive signaling. This scenario can be viewed as a competition between CD23 and CD21 for IgE in the B cell membrane (Figure 3.8).

Some, if not all, of these conjectural mechanisms may be involved in IgE homeostasis. The action of CD23 in negative feedback control of IgE synthesis may be essential to counterbalance the various factors that contribute to the positive feedback loop, including (in humans at least) the contribution of CD23 fragments. We suggest that CD23 may constitute an on–off switch to upregulate IgE synthesis at

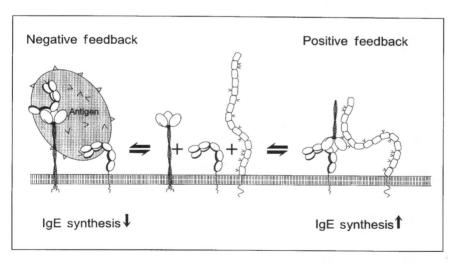

Figure 3.8. Competition between membrane CD23 and CD21 for IgE in the B-cell membrane. IgE shunts between CD21 (positive regulation) and CD23 (negative regulation) as the local concentration of IgE/antigen–IgE complex varies between the K_D values of FcεRI and CD23

low IgE concentrations and to shut down the mechanism when the concentration of IgE rises above the safe limit.

REFERENCES

1. Paul WE (1991) Interleukin-4: A prototypic immunoregulatory lymphokine. *Blood* **77:**1859–1870.
2. Tepper RI, Levinson DA, Stranger BZ, Campos-Torres J, Abbas AK and Leder P (1990) IL-4 induces allergic-like inflammatory disease and alters T cell development in transgenic mice. *Cell* **62:**457–467.
3. Kühn R, Rajewsky K and Müller W (1991) Generation and analysis of interleukin-4 deficient mice. *Science* **254:**707–710.
4. Sutton BJ and Gould HJ (1993) The human IgE network. *Nature* **366:**421–428.
5. Lawrence DA, Weigle WO and Spiegelberg HL (1975) Immunoglobulins cytophilic for human lymphocytes, monocytes and neutrophils. *J Clin Invest* **55:**368–376.
6. Delespesse G, Suter U, Mossalayi D *et al* (1991) Expression, structure and function of the CD23 antigen. *Adv Immunol* **49:**149–191.
7. Capron A, Dessaint JP, Capron M, Joseph M, Ameisen JC and Tonnel AB (1986) From parasites to allergy: a second receptor for IgE. *Immunol Today* **7:**15–18.
8. Kintner C and Sugden B (1981) Identification of antigenic determinants unique to the surface of cells transformed by Epstein–Barr virus. *Nature* **294:**458–460.
9. Thorley-Lawson DA, Nadler LM, Bhan AK and Schooley RT (1985) Blast-2 (EBVCS), an early cell surface marker of human B cell activation, is superinduced by Epstein–Barr virus. *J Immunol* **134:**3007–3012.
10. Nadler L (1986) In: Reinherz ER *et al* (Eds) *Leukocyte Typing II*, volume 2, pp. 3–42. Springer, Berlin.
11. Gordon J, Cairns JA, Liu YJ *et al* (1991) Role of membrane and soluble CD23 in lymphocyte physiology. In: Gordon J (Ed.) *CD23. A novel multifunctional regulator of the immune system that binds IgE. Monographs in Allergy*, volume 29, pp. 156–168. Karger, Basel.
12. Kikutani H, Suemura M, Owaki H *et al* (1986) Fcε receptor, a specific differentiation marker transiently expressed on mature B cells before isotype switching. *J Exp Med* **164:**1455–1469.
13. Yukawa K, Kikutani H, Owaki H *et al* (1987) A B cell-specific differentiation antigen, CD23, is a receptor for IgE (FcεR) on lymphocytes. *J Immunol* **138:**2576–2580.
14. Bonnefoy J-Y, Aubry J-P, Peronne C, Wijdenes J and Banchereau J (1987) Production and characterization of a monoclonal antibody specific for the human lymphocyte low affinity receptor for IgE: CD23 is a low affinity receptor for IgE. *J Immunol* **138:**2970–2978.
15. Gordon J (1991) CD23: Novel disease marker with a split personality. *Clin Exp Immunol* **86:**356–359.
16. Lecoanet-Henchoz S, Gauchat J-F, Aubry J-P *et al* (1995) CD23 regulates monocyte activation through a novel interaction with the adhesion molecules CD11b–CD18 and CD11c–CD18. *Immunity* **3:**119–125.
17. Plater-Zyberk C and Bonnefoy J-Y (1995) Marked amelioration of established collagen-induced arthritis by treatment with antibodies to CD23 *in vivo*. *Nature Med* **1:**781–785.
18. Cairns JA and Gordon J (1990) Intact 45 kDa (membrane) form of CD23 is consistently mitogenic for normal and transformed B lymphoblasts. *Eur J Immunol* **20:**539–543.
19. Liu Y-J, Cairns JA, Holder MJ *et al* (1991) Recombinant 25 kDa CD23 and interleukin-1α promote the survival of germinal center B cells: evidence for bifurcation in the development of centrocytes rescued from apoptosis. *Eur J Immunol* **21:**1107–1114.

20. Arpin C, Déchanet J, van Kooten C *et al* (1995) Generation of memory B cells and plasma cells *in vitro*. *Science* **268**:720–722.

21. Mossalayi MD, Lecron J-C, Dalloul AH *et al* (1990) Soluble CD23 (FcεRII) and interleukin-1 synergistically induce early human thymocyte maturation. *J Exp Med* **171**:959–964.

22. Mossalayi MD, Arock M, Bertho JM *et al* (1990) Proliferation of early human myeloid precursors induced by interleukin-1 and recombinant soluble CD23. *Blood* **75**:1924–1927.

23. Cory S (1995) Regulation of lymphocyte survival by the Bcl-2 gene family. *Annu Rev Immunol* **13**:513–543.

24. Sarfati M, Rector E, Wong K, Rubio-Trujillo M, Sehon AH and Delespesse G (1984) *In vitro* synthesis of IgE by human lymphocytes. II: Enhancement of the spontaneous IgE synthesis by IgE-binding factors secreted by RPMI 8866 lymphoblastoid B cells. *Immunology* **53**:197–205.

25. Péne J, Rousset F, Brière F *et al* (1988) IgE production by normal human lymphocytes is induced by interleukin-4 and suppressed by interferon γ and α and prostaglandin E2. *Proc Natl Acad Sci USA* **85**:6880–6884.

26. Henchoz, S. Gauchat J-F, Aubry J-P, Graber P, Pochon S and Bonnefoy J-Y (1994) Stimulation of human IgE production by a subset of anti-CD21 monoclonal antibodies: requirement of a co-signal to modulate ε transcripts. *Immunology* **81**:285–290.

27. Sarfati M, Bron D, Lagneaux L, Fonteyn C, Frost H and Delespesse G (1988) Elevation of IgE binding factors in serum of patients with B cell-derived chronic lymphocytic leukemia. *Blood* **71**:94–98.

28. Flores-Romo L, Shields J, Humbert Y *et al* (1993) Inhibition of an *in vivo* antigen-specific IgE response by antibodies to CD23. *Science* **261**:1038–1041.

29. King CL, Poindexter RW, Ragunathan J, Fleisher TA, Ottesen EA and Nutman TB (1991) Frequency analysis of IgE-secreting B lymphocytes in persons with normal or elevated serum IgE levels. *J Immunol* **146**:1478–1483.

30. Durham SR, Gould H and Hamid Q. IgE regulation in tissues. This volume, Chapter 2.

31. Aubry JP, Pochon S, Graber P, Jansen KU and Bonnefoy JY (1992) CD21 is a ligand for CD23 and regulates IgE production. *Nature* **358**:505–507.

32. Luo H, Hofstetter H, Banchereau J and Delespesse G (1991) Cross-linking of CD23 antigen by its natural ligand (IgE) or by anti-CD23 antibody prevents B lymphocyte proliferation and differentiation. *J Immunol* **146**:2122–2129.

33. Gordon J, Webb AJ, Guy GR and Walker L (1987) Triggering of B lymphocytes through CD23: epitope mapping and studies using antibody derivatives indicate an allosteric mechanism of signalling. *Immunology* **60**:517–521.

34. Sarfati M and Delespesse G (1988) Possible role of human lymphocyte receptor for IgE (CD23) or its soluble fragments in the *in vitro* synthesis of human IgE. *J Immunol* **141**:2195–2199.

35. Sherr E, Macy E, Kimata H, Gilly M and Saxon A (1989) Binding the low affinity FcεR on B cells suppresses ongoing human IgE synthesis. *J Immunol* **142**:481–489.

36. Saxon A, Kurbe-Leamer M, Behle K, Max EE and Zhang K (1991) Inhibition of human IgE production via FcεRII stimulation results from a decrease in the mRNA for secreted but not membrane εH-chains. *J Immunol* **147**:4000–4006.

37. Campbell KA, Lees A, Finkelman FD and Conrad DH (1992) Co-crosslinking FcεRII/CD23 and B cell surface immunoglobulin modulates B cell activation. *Eur J Immunol* **22**:2107–2112.

38. Yu P, Kosco-Vilbois M, Richards M, Köhler G and Lamers MC (1994) Negative feedback regulation of IgE synthesis by murine CD23. *Nature* **369**:753–756.

39. Texido G, Eibel H, Le Gros G and van der Putten H (1994) Transgene CD23 expression on lymphoid cells modulates IgE and IgG1 responses. *J Immunol* **153**:3028–3042.

40. Fujiwara H, Kikutani H, Suematsu S *et al* (1994) The absence of IgE-mediated augmentation of immune responses in CD23-deficient mice. *Proc Natl Acad Sci USA* **91**:6835–6839.

41. Stief A, Texido G, Sansig G, Eibel H, Le Gros G and van der Putten H (1994) Mice deficient in CD23 reveal its modulatory role in IgE production, but no role in T-cell and B-cell development. *J Immunol* **152**:3378–3390.

42. Bartlett WC, Graber P, Bonnefoy J-Y, Ahearn JM and Conrad DH (1993) Evidence for lack of species specificity for the CD23/CD21 interaction. *J Immunol* **150**:1274 (abstr.).

43. Bartlett WC and Conrad DH (1992) Murine soluble FcεRII—a molecule in search of a function. *Res Immunol* **143**:431–436.

44. Phillips NE and Parker DC (1984) Cross-linking of B lymphocyte Fcγ receptors and membrane immunoglobulin inhibits anti-immunoglobulin-induced blastogenesis. *J Immunol* **132**:627–632.

45. Phillips NE, Gravel KA, Tumas GK and Parker DC (1988) IL-4 (B-cell stimulatory factor-1) overcomes Fcγ receptor-mediated inhibition of mouse B lymphocyte proliferation without affecting inhibition of c-myc mRNA induction. *J Immunol* **141**:4243–4249.

46. Muta T, Kurosaki T, Misulovin Z, Sanchez M, Nussenzweig MC and Ravetch JV (1994) A 13-amino-acid motif in the cytoplasmic domain of FcγRIIB modulates B-cell receptor signalling. *Nature* **368**:70–73.

47. Ashman RF, Peckham D and Stunz LL (1996) Fc receptor off-signal in the B cell involves apoptosis. *J Immunol* **157**:5–11.

48. Kehry M and Yamashita LC (1989) Low-affinity IgE receptor (CD23) function on mouse B cells: role in IgE-dependent antigen focusing. *Proc Natl Acad Sci USA* **86**:7556–7560.

49. Pirron U, Schlunck T, Prinz JC and Rieber EP (1990) IgE-dependent antigen focusing by human B lymphocytes is mediated by the low-affinity receptor for IgE. *Eur J Immunol* **20**:1547–1551.

50. Squire CM, Studer EJ, Lees A, Finkelman FD and Conrad DH (1994) Antigen presentation is enhanced by targeting antigen to the FcεRII by antigen–anti-FcεRII conjugates. *J Immunol* **152**:4388–4396.

51. van der Heijden FL, Joost van Neerven RJ, van Katwijk M, Bos JD and Kapsenberg ML (1993) Serum-IgE-facilitated allergen presentation in atopic disease. *J Immunol* **150**:3643–3650.

52. Heyman B, Liu TM and Gustavsson S (1993) *In vivo* enhancement of the specific antibody response via the low-affinity receptor for IgE. *Eur J Immunol* **23**:1739–1742.

53. Gustavsson S, Hjulström S, Tianmin L and Heyman B (1994) CD23/IgE-mediated regulation of the specific antibody response *in vivo*. *J Immunol* **152**:4793–4800.

54. Grosjean I, Lachaux A, Bella C, Aubry J-P, Bonnefoy J-Y and Kaiserlian D (1994) CD23/CD21 interaction is required for presentation of soluble protein antigen by lymphoblastoid B cell lines to specific CD4$^+$ T cell clones. *Eur J Immunol* **24**:2982–2986.

55. Gagro A and Rabatić S (1994) Allergen-induced CD23 on CD4$^+$ T lymphocytes and CD21 on B lymphocytes in patients with allergic asthma: evidence and regulation. *Eur J Immunol* **24**:1109–1114.

56. Prinz JC, Baur X, Mazur G and Rieber EP (1990) Allergen-directed expression of Fc receptors for IgE (CD23) on human T lymphocytes is modulated by interleukin 4 and interferon γ. *Eur J Immunol* **20**:1259–1264.

57. Secrist H, DeKruyff RH and Umetsu DT (1995) Interleukin 4 production by CD4$^+$ T cells from allergic individuals is modulated by antigen concentration and antigen-presenting cell type. *J Exp Med* **181**:1081–1089.

58. Gleich GS and Jacob GL (1975) Immunoglobulin E antibodies to pollen allergens account for high percentages of total immunoglobulin E protein. *Science* **190**:1106–1108.

59. Ahearn JM and Fearon DT (1989) Structure and function of the complement receptors CR1 (CD35) and CR2 (CD21). *Adv Immunol* **46**:183–219.

60. Fearon DT and Carter RH (1995) The CD19/CR2/TAPA-1 complex of B lymphocytes: linking natural to acquired immunity. *Ann Rev Immunol* **13**:127–149.

61. Pepys MB (1976) Role of complement in the induction of immunological responses. *Transplant Rev* **32**:93–120.

62. Alper CA, Colten HR, Rosen FS, Rabson AR, Macnab GM and Gear JSS (1972) Homozygous deficiency of C3 in a patient with repeated infections. *Lancet* **2**:1179–1181.

63. Wessels MR, Butko P, Ma MM, Warren HB, Lage AL, Carroll MC (1995) Studies of group B streptococcal infection in mice deficient in complement component C3 or C4 demonstrate an essential role for complement in both innate and acquired immunity. *Proc Natl Acad Sci USA* **92**:11490–11494.

64. Villiers C (1995) C3, protéine du complément: une molécule aux multiples capacités. *Medicine/Sciences* **11**:1419–1429.

65. Ahearn JM, Fisher MB, Croix D *et al* (1996) Disruption of the Cr2 locus results in a reduction in B-1a cells and in an impaired B cell response to T-dependent antigen. *Immunity* **4**:251–262.

66. Molina H, Holers VM, Li B *et al* (1996) Markedly impaired humoral immune response in mice deficient in complement receptors 1 and 2. *Proc Natl Acad Sci USA* **93**:3357–3361.

67. Carter RH and Fearon DT (1992) CD19: lowering the threshold for antigen receptor stimulation of B lymphocytes. *Science* **256**:105–107.

68. Dempsey PW, Allison MED, Akkaraju S, Goodnow CC and Fearon DT (1996) C3d of complement as a molecular adjuvant: bridging innate and acquired immunity. *Science* **271**:348–350.

69. de Franco AL (1995) Transmembrane signaling by antigen receptors of B and T lymphocytes. *Curr Opin Cell Biol* **7**:163–175.

70. Reljić R, Cosentino G and Gould HJ (1997) Function of CD23 in the response of human B cells to antigen. *Eur J Immunol* **27**:572–575.

71. Gordon J (1993) Factors and receptors regulating the survival and selection of B lymphocytes: implications for the evolution and management of follicular lymphoma. *FORUM Trends Exp Med* **3**:334–340.

72. Drickamer K (1993) Evolution of Ca^{2+}-dependent animal lectins. *Prog Nucl Acid Res Mol Biol* **45**:207–232.

73. Drickamer K (1993) Ca^{2+}-dependent carbohydrate-recognition domains in animal proteins. *Curr Opin Struct Biol* **3**:393–400.

74. Padlan EA and Helm BA (1993) Modelling of the lectin-homology domains of the human and murine low-affinity Fcε receptor (FcεRII/CD23). *Receptor* **3**:325–341.

75. Bajorath J and Aruffo A (1996) Structure-based modeling of the ligand binding domain of the human cell surface receptor CD23 and comparison of two independently derived molecular models. *Protein Sci* **5**:240–247.

76. Weis WI, Kahn R, Fourme R, Drickamer K and Hendrickson WA (1991) Structure of the calcium-dependent lectin domain from a rat mannose-binding protein determined by MAD Phasing. *Science* **254**:1608–1615.

77. Weis WI, Drickamer K and Hendrickson WA (1992) Structure of a C-type mannose-binding protein complexed with an oligosaccharide. *Nature* **360**:127–134.

78. Graves BJ, Crowther R, Chandran C *et al* (1994) Insight into E selectin/ligand inter-action from the crystal structure and mutagenesis of the lec EGF domains. *Nature* **367**:532–538.

79. Richards ML and Katz DH (1990) The binding of IgE to murine FcεRII is calcium-dependent but not inhibited by carbohydrate. *J Immunol* **144**:2638–2646.

80. Pochon S, Graber P, Yeager M *et al* (1992) Demonstration of a second ligand for the low affinity receptor for immunoglobulin E (CD23) using recombinant CD23 reconstituted into fluorescent liposomes. *J Exp Med* **176**:389–397.

81. Grangette C, Gruart V, Ouaissi MA *et al* (1989) IgE receptor on human eosinophils (FcεRII): comparison with B cell CD23 and association with an adhesion molecule. *J Immunol* **143**:3580–3588.

82. Gould H, Sutton B, Edmeades R and Beavil A (1991) CD23/FcεRII: C-type lectin membrane protein with a split personality? In: Gordon J (Ed.) *CD23. A novel multi-functional regulator of the immune system that binds IgE. Monographs in Allergy*, volume 29, pp. 28–49. Karger, Basel.

83. Beavil AJ, Edmeades RL, Gould HJ and Sutton BJ (1992) α-helical coiled-coil stalks in the low-affinity receptor for IgE (FcεRII/CD23) and related C-type lectins. *Proc Natl Acad Sci USA* **89**:753–757.

84. Dierks SE, Bartlett WC, Edmeades RL, Gould HJ, Rao M and Conrad DH (1993) The oligomeric nature of the murine FcεRII/CD23 – implications for function. *J Immunol* **150**:2372–2382.

85. Beavil RL, Graber P, Aubonney N, Bonnefoy JY and Gould HJ (1995) CD23/FcεRII and its soluble fragments can form oligomers on the cell surface and in solution. *Immunology* **84**:202–206.

86. Hoppe HJ and Reid KBM (1994) Trimeric C-type lectin domains in host defence. *Structure* **2**:1129–1133.

87. Weis WI and Drickamer K (1994) Trimeric structure of a C-type mannose-binding protein. *Structure* **2**:1227–1240.

88. Sheriff S, Chang CYY and Ezekowitz RAB (1994) Human mannose-binding protein carbohydrate recognition domain trimerizes through a triple α-helical coiled-coil. *Struct Biol* **1**:789–794.

89. DiPaola M and Maxfield FR (1984) Conformational changes in the receptors for epi-dermal growth factor and asialoglycoproteins induced by the mildly acidic pH found in endocytic vesicles. *J Biol Chem* **259**:9163–9171.

90. Yokota A, Kikutani H, Tanaka T *et al* (1988) Two species of human Fcε receptor II (FcεRII/CD23): tissue-specific and IL-4-specific regulation of gene expression. *Cell* **55**:611–618.

91. Yokota A, Yukawa K, Yamamoto A *et al* (1992) Two forms of the low-affinity Fc receptor for IgE differentially mediate endocytosis and phagocytosis: Identification of the critical cytoplasmic domains. *Proc Natl Acad Sci USA* **89**:5030–5034.

92. Letellier M, Sarfati M and Delespesse G (1989) Mechanisms of formation of IgE-binding factors (soluble CD23). I. FcεRII bearing B cells generate IgE-binding factors of different molecular weights. *Mol Immunol* **26**:1105–1112.

93. Delespesse G, Sarfati M, Rubio-Trujillo M and Wolowiec T (1986) IgE receptors on human lymphocytes. III. Expression of IgE receptors on mitogen-stimulated human mononuclear cells. *Eur J Immunol* **16**:1043–1047.

94. Lee WT, Rao M and Conrad DH (1987) The murine lymphocyte receptor for IgE. IV. The mechanism of ligand-specific receptor upregulation on B cells. *J Immunol* **139**:1191–1198.

95. Letellier M, Nakajima T and Delespesse G (1988) IgE receptor on human lymphocytes. IV. Further analysis of its structure and of the role of N-linked carbohydrates. *J Immunol* **141**:2374–2381.

96. Conrad DH, Keegan AD, Rao M and Lee WT (1987) Synthesis and regulation of the IgE receptor on B lymphocyte cell lines. *Int Arch Allergy Appl Immunol* **82**:402–404.

97. Beavil AJ, Young RJ, Sutton BJ and Perkins SJ (1995) Bent domain structure of recombinant human IgE-Fc in solution by X-ray and neutron scattering in conjuction with an automated curve fitting procedure. *Biochemistry* **34**:14449–14461.

98. Shi J, Ghirlando R, Beavil RL *et al.* (1997) Interaction of the low-affinity receptor CD23/FcεRII lectin domain with the Fcε3-4 fragment of human immunoglobulin E. *Biochemistry* **36**:2112–2122.

99. Aubry J-P, Pochon S, Gauchat JF *et al* (1994) CD23 interacts with a new functional extracytoplasmic domain involving N-linked oligosaccharides on CD21. *J Immunol* **152**:5806–5813.

100. Henchoz-Lecoanet S, Jeannin, P, Aubry J-P *et al* (1996) The Epstein–Barr virus-binding site on CD21 is involved in CD23 binding and interleukin-4-induced IgE and IgG4 production by human B cells. *Immunology* **88**:35–39.

101. Vercelli D, Helm B, Marsh P, Padlan E, Geha RS and Gould HJ (1989) The B-cell binding site on human immunoglobulin E. *Nature* **338**:649–651.

102. Young RJ, Owens RJ, Mackay GA *et al* (1995) Secretion of recombinant human IgE-Fc by mammalian cells and biological activity of glycosylation site mutants. *Prot Engin* **8**:193–199.

103. Tanner J, Weis J, Fearon D, Whang Y and Kieff E (1987) Epstein–Barr virus gp350/220 binding to the B lymphocyte C3d receptor mediates adsorption, capping, and endocytosis. *Cell* **50**:203–213.

104. Sarfati M, Bettler B, Letellier M *et al* (1992) Native and recombinant soluble CD23 fragments with IgE suppressive activity. *Immunology* **76**:662–667.

105. Scharenberg AM and Kinet J-P (1994) Is localized immunoglobulin E synthesis the problem? *Curr Biol* **4**:140–142.

106. Moser R, Fehr J and Bruijnzeel PLB (1992) IL-4 controls the selective endothelium-driven transmigration of eosinophils from allergic individuals. *J Immunol* **149**:1432–1438.

107. Klein LM, Lavker RM, Matis WL and Murphy GF (1989) Degranulation of human mast cells induces an endothelial antigen central to leukocyte adhesion. *Proc Natl Acad Sci USA* **86**:8972–8976.

108. Lamers MC and Yu P (1995) Regulation of IgE synthesis. Lessons from the study of IgE transgenic and CD23-deficient mice. *Immunol Rev* **148**:71–95.

109. Schmitz J, Thiel A, Kühn R *et al* (1994) Induction of interleukin-4 (IL-4) expression in T-helper (Th) cells is not dependent on IL-4 from non-Th cells. *J Exp Med* **179**:1349–1353.

4 Genetic Regulation of Total Serum IgE Levels and Linkage to Chromosome 5q

DEBORAH A. MEYERS and EUGENE R. BLEECKER

University of Maryland School of Medicine, Baltimore MD, USA

4.1 INTRODUCTION

High total serum IgE levels correlate with the clinical expression of both allergy and asthma (1–4). Most patients with asthma, a respiratory disease that is characterized by variable airways obstruction, airways inflammation and bronchial hyper-responsiveness have clinical and serologic evidence of atopy (5). Even in children who are asymptomatic, there is an association between total serum IgE levels and bronchial hyperresponsiveness (3, 6, 7). Approximately 30% of the variance in bronchial responsiveness is explained by an individual's total serum IgE levels (2, 3). There has been a recent increase in morbidity associated with asthma (8), and epidemiological studies have provided strong evidence that asthma and allergic disorders are increasing both in prevalence and severity (9, 10). While the precise reasons for these changes are unknown, there is some evidence to indicate that these rising trends are associated with increased levels of sensitization to common environmental allergens and early life exposure to factors including air pollutants and viruses in susceptible individuals (11). An approach to understanding the underlying mechanisms responsible for the development of asthma and allergic disorders is to investigate the causes that produce susceptibility to these conditions.

Therefore, the results from genetic studies on total serum IgE levels will be important for mapping genes for the allergic and asthmatic phenotypes. Delineating the basic genetic mechanisms responsible for individual susceptibility to allergy and asthma has widespread public health consequences, since it may lead to improved preventive measures and new therapeutic approaches.

4.2 GENETIC EPIDEMIOLOGY AND FAMILIAL AGGREGATION

There are age-related changes with total serum IgE levels. Levels tend to rise rapidly in infancy and gradually increase until puberty and then slowly decrease with age

IgE Regulation: Molecular Mechanisms. Edited by D. Vercelli. © 1997 John Wiley & Sons Ltd.

(12–16). Total serum IgE levels are certainly affected by environmental factors such as parasitic infections, recent allergen exposure and smoking as well as by gender and ethnicity (17–20).

The presence of familial aggregation for total serum IgE levels provides preliminary evidence for an important genetic component, especially after adjusting for all known environmental factors. Meyers *et al* (21) investigated the association of total serum IgE levels in 278 individuals from 42 random families, and showed a significant correlation between parents and offspring ($P < 0.05$), and an even stronger correlation among siblings ($P < 0.001$). Of course, environmental factors may be responsible for some of the observed correlation and an interactive effect between genes and the environment may also be involved.

Twin studies provide additional evidence that total serum IgE levels are under strong genetic control. The observed difference between the disease frequency in monozygotic (MZ) and dizygotic (DZ) twins provides an indication for heritability, while the difference within MZ twins is a measure of the environmental influence. Heritability, the ratio of genetic variance to the total variance, is used to measure the degree of familial aggregation due to a genetic component. In a twin study by Hopp *et al* the intrapair correlation coefficient for IgE levels was 82% in the 61 MZ twins and 52% in the 46 DZ twins, showing an overall heritability of 61% (22). While studies of relatives are helpful in determining whether a genetic component is important, usually they do not provide insight into the mode of inheritance or the specific location of the disease genes in the genome.

4.3 SEGREGATION ANALYSIS

Segregation analysis is used to determine the mode of inheritance of a specific trait such as total serum IgE levels or a disease such as asthma. The observed number of family members with the trait is compared to the expected number using various Mendelian modes of inheritance (e.g. recessive, dominant, etc.). For example, if high IgE levels are inherited in a recessive manner, then children of two parents with high levels would also be expected to have high levels. The method of ascertainment of families is very important in segregation analysis since it directly influences the results. If families were selected through an affected parent and an affected child, the results would be biased in favor of a dominant model of inheritance. Thus, one needs to adjust for ascertainment in the analysis. The best fitting model is determined by comparing the likelihoods from the different models tested (i.e. dominant, recessive, polygenic, environmental) with the likelihood of a general model. Models that significantly differ from this general model can be rejected. Estimates of gene frequency, frequency of each genotype and mean IgE levels are obtained. The best fitting model and its resulting parameter estimates can then be used in subsequent linkage analysis.

For total serum IgE levels, segregation analysis has been performed to test whether the segregation of IgE levels is consistent with a major gene model with two alleles, 'L' for 'low' levels (gene frequency = q_L) and 'H' for 'high' levels. For each model, the means (μ_{LL}, μ_{LH}, μ_{HH}) and variances for the three distributions representing the three types of individuals (LL, LH, HH) are estimated. Individuals of types LL, LH, HH transmit the L allele with probabilities τ_{LL}, τ_{LH} and τ_{HH}, respectively. Under a Mendelian model, these parameters are restricted to $\tau_{LL} = 1.0$, $\tau_{LH} = 0.5$, $\tau_{HH} = 0.0$. The parent–offspring (ρ_{po}) and sib–sib (ρ_{ss}) correlations may be constrained to be equal because this represents the conventional 'mixed model' (23). The likelihood ratio test is used to compare hierarchical models and approximates a χ^2 distribution. To compare non-hierarchical models, the Akaike's Information Criterion (AIC) (24) is used ($-2 \ln L + 2k$ where k is the number of parameters estimated in the model).

First, a general model is tested where all parameters are estimated without restrictions. This model by definition gives the best fit to the data, and the best likelihood. There are three Mendelian models, recessive, dominant and codominant, that are usually tested. To fit a model of dominant inheritance of high IgE levels, means for two distributions are estimated from the family data, one distribution representing HH and LH individuals and one representing family members with a low IgE value (genotype: LL). To test for recessive inheritance of high levels, the mean value for LH individuals is set equal to that for LL family members. Means for each of the three genotypes (HH, LH, LL) are estimated in the codominant model. In a polygenic model, many genes are involved so it is not possible to estimate the separate distributions. In the environmental, or sporadic model, the transmission probability (τ) is the same as the gene frequency, while the means (μ) are not restricted. The best fitting model can be determined by comparing the likelihoods from the several models tested with the likelihood of the general model. Models that significantly differ from this general model can be rejected. Estimates of gene frequency, and mean values for 'high' and 'low' IgE phenotypes are obtained.

Our analyses on data from 92 Dutch families will be described as an example of this type of analysis. Ninety-two families (ascertained through a parent, the proband) with asthma diagnosed approximately 25 years ago in Holland were studied (25). The probands were restudied and all available family members were characterized in regards to the asthma and atopy phenotypes. Total serum IgE (IU) was measured by solid phase immunoassay (Pharmacy IgE EIA, Pharmacy Diagnostics AB, Sweden). The mean of duplicate tests was used for the IgE level. The test was repeated if the difference between duplicates was > 5%.

The log[IgE] data were analyzed by fitting the class D regressive models of Bonney (26) as implemented in SAGE (27). Age was included as a covariate since there was a significant correlation between age and total serum IgE levels in the overall sample. There was no significant correlation between gender and log[IgE] levels in this sample, and similar results were obtained when the segregation analysis was repeated including gender as a covariate. An ascertainment correction was not used because the families were ascertained through one parent with asthma, and not through affected offspring. Since individuals with asthma may have an increased IgE level, this may bias the estimate of the gene frequency but should not affect the segregation pattern (genetic model) observed in the offspring. The results of the analysis are shown graphically in Figure 4.1. The general model is the most likely and both the recessive model of high levels and the codominant model have very similar likelihoods although there is one more degree of freedom in the χ^2 test for the codominant model (Figure 4.1). Clearly, both the models of dominant inheritance of high levels and sporadic inheritance are unlikely. The estimates for the various parameters for these six models are shown in Table 4.1. The AIC (a measure of likelihood) for the recessive model is the lowest, and this is the most parsimonious model for inheritance of serum IgE levels. The estimates of the mean levels for the low and high phenotypes appear reasonable and clinically relevant (38 IU and 437 IU, respectively). In this study, only recessive inheritance of high levels gave a good fit to the data; the other genetic and nongenetic models could be rejected. The codominant model had a similar likelihood but since an additional parameter was estimated, similar results to the recessive model were obtained but not significantly better (AIC).

In several previous studies, evidence for recessive inheritance of high total serum IgE levels has been observed with different estimates for gene frequency and for mean levels in the low and high phenotypes (28–30). From a study of several large pedigrees, evidence was obtained suggesting genetic heterogeneity in the mode of inheritance; the most parsimonious genetic model was different in the different pedigrees (31). In a sample of families from the Amish community, which is genetically isolated and inbred, evidence for codominant inheritance has been reported (32). However, evidence for polygenic inheritance was obtained from a study of large Mormon families which are more representative of the general population than the Amish (33).

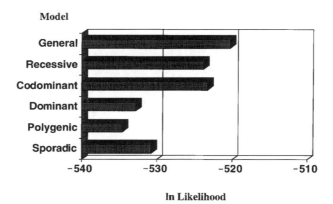

Figure 4.1. The likelihood of each segregation model is shown in this bar graph. The general model is the most likely since additional parameters are estimated in this model. Both the models of recessive inheritance of high IgE levels and of codominant inheritance gave similar likelihoods. The model of recessive inheritance was the most parsimonious

Table 4.1. Segregation analysis of total serum log [IgE] levels in 92 Dutch families

Model	q_L	μ_{LL}	μ_{LH}	μ_{HH}	σ_{LL}^2	σ_{LH}^2	σ_{HH}^2	τ_{LL}	τ_{LH}	τ_{HH}	ρ_{sp}	ρ_{ss}	$-2\ln(L)$	AIC	χ^2
General	0.60 ±0.04	1.26 ±0.11	1.60 ±0.09	2.65 ±0.09	0.41 ±0.07	0.16 ±0.03	0.14 ±0.03	1.00*	0.30 ±0.06	0.00*	−0.19 ±0.13	0.07 ±0.06	1040.7	1062.7	
Recessive	0.46 ±0.09	1.58 ±0.09	$=\mu_{LL}$	2.64 ±0.15	0.19 ±0.11	0.32 ±0.06	0.21 ±0.07	[1.0]	[0.5]	[0.0]	0.03 ±0.15	0.27 ±0.07	1047.6	1061.6	6.9 3 d.f.
Codominant	0.39 ±0.08	1.66 ±0.11	1.49 ±0.10	2.53 ±0.14	0.13 ±0.07	0.29 ±0.05	0.26 ±0.07	[1.0]	[0.5]	[0.0]	−0.02 ±0.16	0.29 ±0.07	1046.6	1062.6	5.9 4 d.f.
Dominant	0.84 ±0.11	1.62 ±0.16	2.55 ±0.27	$=\mu_{LH}$	0.33 ±0.07	0.30 ±0.12	0.23 ±0.18	[1.0]	[0.5]	[0.0]	−0.07 ±0.14	0.18 ±0.07	1065.7	1079.7	25.0 3 d.f.
Polygenic	[1]	1.89 ±0.07			0.49 ±0.03	$=\sigma_{LL}^2$				±0.09	−0.01 ±0.04	0.30	1069.2	1079.2 6 d.f.	28.5
Sporadic	0.31 ±0.07	1.43 ±0.08	1.65 ±0.22	2.11 ±0.24	0.04 ±0.02	0.51 ±0.11	0.44 ±0.12	$=q_L$	$=q_L$	$=q_L$	−0.02 ±0.11	0.36 ±0.09	1061.6	1077.6	20.9 3 d.f.

* Estimate converged to a boundary. Abstracted from Meyers et al. (25).
See text for explanation of column headings.

In a recent, large study of 50 Hispanic families and 241 non-Hispanic white families, Martinez and co-workers showed significant familial correlation coefficients between mother and offspring, father and offspring and between sibs; the resulting P values were all less than 0.0001 (34). Segregation analysis using a similar method to that used in the Dutch family study showed evidence for a codominant mode of inheritance. For their analyses, they used the logarithm of the total serum IgE levels adjusted for age and gender. Evidence favoring the codominant model was found in both ethnic groups and no significant evidence for genetic heterogeneity across the ethnic groups was obtained.

It is important to note that the difference in the best fitting models of inheritance in the mentioned studies do not necessarily represent conflicting results. It rather reflects the inability to distinguish between two or three underlying distributions of the mode of inheritance of total serum IgE levels, which display substantial overlap. In the smaller study of Meyers *et al*, the recessive model was the most parsimonious although the codominant model had a very similar likelihood but an additional degree of freedom (25). However, in the larger study of Martinez and co-workers, means and variances for three distributions were estimated fitting a codominant model of inheritance (34). Basically, it reflects whether or not it is possible to distinguish gene carriers from unaffected family members or for total IgE levels, whether it is possible to distinguish heterozygous individuals (LH) from homozygous family members (LL or HH).

Although evidence for a major gene was obtained from single-locus segregation analysis, this does not mean that only one locus is involved in regulation of total serum IgE levels. In the Dutch asthma family data, the estimate of the residual variance was significant from the segregation analysis, suggesting an additional genetic influence. Therefore, two-locus segregation analysis was performed to determine whether a portion of this residual variance was due to a second major locus (35). The log[IgE] data were analyzed by fitting two-locus models using the computer package PAP (36). Analysis was performed to determine whether the segregation of IgE levels was consistent with two loci (D1, D2) each with two alleles (A,a and B,b). The difficulty with two-locus analysis is that it is very computer intensive because there are many possible two-locus models. Alleles at each locus may act in a dominant or recessive manner with regards to determining the resulting phenotype (IgE levels) and the effects from the two loci may be additive or independent of each other. For each model, the following parameters were estimated: gene frequency for the alleles at each locus (qA, qa $= 1 - $ qA; qB, qb $= 1 - $ qB), the recombination fraction between the two loci (v), the means (μ) for the nine possible distributions representing the nine types of individuals (AABB, AABb, AAbb, AaBB, AaBb, Aabb, aaBB, aaBb, aabb) with a common standard deviation (σ), and heritability (h^2) which is a measure of the residual variance. Different two locus models were tested by constraining means for different phenotypes to be equal. Multiple two-locus models including dominant models were tested; however, the two-locus recessive models with epistasis were the most parsimonious (Table 4.2). As reported in Table 4.2, there were five different recessive models (II–VI) with

Table 4.2. Two-locus analysis for log [total serum IgE] levels 92 Dutch families

Model	q_A	q_B	AABB AABb AAbb	AaBB AaBb Aabb	aaBB aaBb aabb	σ	h^2	$-2 \ln L$ (AIC)
			means (μ)					
2-locus								
I. Codominant	0.54	0.36	1.31 1.04 1.71	0.45 1.39 2.05	1.89 2.63 2.82	0.30	0.09	1031.3 (1057.3)
Recessive inheritance of 'high' levels with epistasis								
II.	0.54	0.36	1.34 1.05 1.71	0.46 1.40 2.05	1.97 (2.73) (2.73)	0.31	0.15	1032.1 (1056.6)
III.	0.56	0.31	1.37 0.96 1.57	0.42 1.40 2.02	(2.71) (2.71) (2.71)	0.32	0.13	1033.6 (1055.6)
IV.	0.44	0.72	1.45 0.56 [2.09]	1.29 1.59 (2.68)	[2.09] (2.68) (2.68)	0.36	0.40	1034.3 (1054.3)
V.	0.74	0.43	1.47 1.27 2.08	0.54 1.60 (2.68)	(2.68) (2.68) (2.68)	0.37	0.42	1034.4 (1054.4)
Heterogeneity								
VI.	0.50	0.76	1.48 1.46 (2.52)	0.66 1.60 (2.52)	(2.52) (2.52) (2.52)	0.41	0.46	1037.6 (1055.6)

( ), [ ] represents means that were constrained to be equal under the given model. Abstracted from Xu *et al*. (35).

similar likelihoods (AICs all between 1054.3 and 1056.1) although Models IV and V were the most parsimonious. Both of these models and a heterogeneity model (Model VI) had relatively high residual variances ($h^2 = 0.40, 0.42, 0.46$, respectively) compared to Models II and III ($h^2 = 0.15, 0.13$, respectively). These five models were more likely, based on their AICs, than the two-locus codominant (general) model. The two locus model was significantly more likely than the one-locus recessive model. No evidence for linkage between the two loci was observed for any of the models; therefore these two loci are probably on different chromosomes, or at least on different arms of the same chromosome.

The first locus explains 50.6% of the variance in total IgE levels, and the second locus explains 19% of the variance. Considered jointly, the two loci account for 78.4% of the variance in total serum IgE levels. However, this may represent an overestimate since the families were ascertained through an asthmatic parent. This study provides evidence that there are at least two loci involved in regulation of total serum IgE levels. Individuals who are homozygous for the recessive alleles at the first loci have the highest mean IgE levels (513 IU) while mean levels ranged from 3 to 105 IU, depending on their genotype at each locus.

4.4 LINKAGE ANALYSIS

Linkage analysis is performed to determine the chromosomal location of suscept-ibility gene(s) by demonstrating cosegregation of the trait or disease with known inherited factors such as blood groups or polymorphic DNA markers. A poly-morphic marker is usually not a specific disease-related gene but is a segment of DNA with multiple alleles that can be characterized in all family members and followed through different generations. For example, one can test whether children with high total serum IgE level inherited the same marker allele from their parent with high levels, and that the unaffected offspring inherited the other allele for a specific marker with a known chromosomal location. There are two general approaches for linkage analysis: performing a genome-wide search and studying candidate regions, areas of the genome where candidate genes for the disorder have already been mapped. In a genome-wide search, polymorphic markers that are distributed at relatively equal distances throughout the genome are examined. If desired, one can initiate a genome search by first investigating regions with known candidate genes.

To utilize the very powerful method of maximum likelihood for linkage analysis (LOD score), a model of inheritance for the trait or disease is required and may be obtained from previous segregation analysis. For analysis of total serum IgE levels in the Dutch families, two-point LOD scores were calculated using the best fitting genetic model using the findings from the segregation analysis. Results of these analyses are expressed as a LOD score (logarithm of the odds for the two hypotheses of linkage versus no linkage or independent assortment). For Mendelian disorders, a LOD > 3.0 (odds 1000:1) at a specific recombination fraction is considered to be significant evidence for linkage (37, 38) while a LOD of 3.3 is considered evidence for linkage when performing a genome screen for a complex disorder (39).

For complex genetic disorders where multiple genes are probably involved in disease susceptibility, there are alternative methods for testing for genetic linkage. For example sib-pair analysis, which tests for deviation from the expected Mendelian distribution of haplotypes shared by descent among affected sibs, is a commonly used method. Siblings on average share 50% of their genes 'identical by descent' meaning that the same gene was transmitted from a parent to both children. Increased sharing provides evidence that a susceptibility locus maps to the region of the genome where the DNA marker tested is mapped. For a quantitative measure such as total serum IgE levels, a regression analysis is performed for the squared difference in log[IgE] levels between sibs and the estimated proportion of marker alleles identical by descent. In the presence of linkage, sibs who are identical by descent for the marker alleles would be expected to have similar IgE levels and those not sharing marker alleles would be expected to have a larger difference in their IgE levels.

4.4.1 Mapping to Chromosome 5q

To illustrate these approaches, the findings from linkage studies on chromosome 5q for total IgE levels will be described. There are several genes on chromosome 5q that may be important in the regulation of IgE and the development or progression of inflammation associated with allergy and asthma. They include interleukin (IL)-3, IL-4, IL-5, IL-9, IL-13, granulocyte–macrophage colony-stimulating factor (GM-CSF), a receptor for macrophage colony stimulating factor (CSF-1R) and fibroblast growth factor acidic (FGFA) (40). The genes for the IL-4-related cytokines stimulate B-cell growth and regulate specific immunoglobulin synthesis (41, 42).

In the Dutch study, sib-pair analysis for total serum IgE levels was performed for multiple markers in this large candidate region. Significant evidence for linkage was obtained with the highly polymorphic marker D5S436 and with the flanking loci, D5S393 and CSF-1R (25). The FGFA polymorphism that was typed was not very informative in these families (both parents were homozygous in approximately one third of the families) resulting in little evidence for or against linkage (Figure 4.2). The LOD score analysis using the recessive model from the segregation analysis showed similar results. The highest LOD (3.56) was obtained for D5S436 with 9% recombination. Lower LOD scores were observed for the flanking markers: D5S393 and CSF-1R. The IL-9 polymorphism maps below but relatively close to the other interleukin gene candidates, and resulted in a LOD of 0.98 (Figure 4.2).

Marsh and co-workers described evidence for linkage of a locus for total serum IgE levels to chromosome 5q in an isolated population consisting of 11 Amish pedigrees (43). Segregation analysis similar to that described for the Dutch families was performed and the Mendelian models fitted the data better than a non-Mendelian model, although there was not significant evidence favoring a specific Mendelian model for the inheritance of total serum IgE levels. In testing for linkage to 5q, sib-pair analysis was performed showing a P-value of 0.002 with D5S399, a marker tightly linked to D5S393, one of the markers typed in the Dutch study (Figure 4.2). LOD score analysis was performed assuming dominant inheritance of 'high' serum IgE levels. For D5S399 a LOD score of 1.3 at 0.0 recombination was obtained. The highest LOD score reported was 1.84 for the marker D5S210 with a recombination fraction of 0.0 (Figure 4.3). Five other markers spanning over 20 cM also showed 0.0 recombination with total serum IgE levels probably because of the marked overlap between the distributions of low and high IgE levels in this inbred population. Thus, although both studies reported evidence for linkage to 5q, the results do not appear to specify one gene candidate within this large region containing multiple candidate genes.

Additional markers were genotyped in this region of 5q in the Dutch study. For total serum IgE levels, 60% of families are linked to this region with a multipoint LOD of 7.6 at 6 cM from D5S1480. The cytokine cluster of genes fall within the confidence interval for this linkage. Other investigators have shown an association with IL-9 and IgE levels in a set of randomly ascertained families (44). Therefore, further studies of IL-9 as a candidate gene were performed (45). A novel polymorphism in exon 5, C to T nucleotide substitution at position 4130, that results in an amino acid change (Thr to Met) was found by direct DNA sequencing of probands. Probands and spouses (non-asthmatic) were evaluated in the 26 families that

70

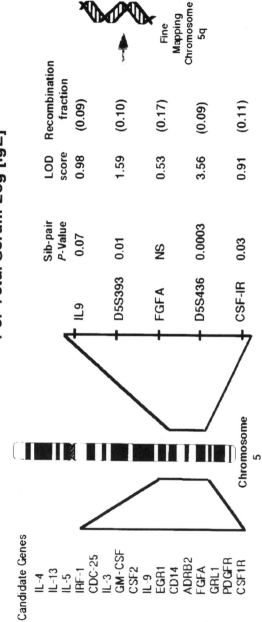

Figure 4.2. Results of sib-pair and LOD score linkage analysis for a major locus regulating total serum IgE levels mapping to 5q in the Dutch families. The markers tested are shown in map order on 5q

Summary of sib-pair analysis and two-point LOD scores for log total serum IgE levels

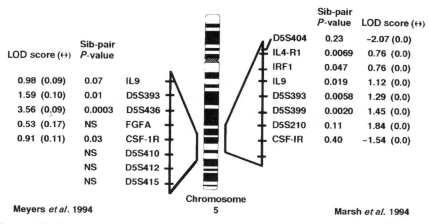

Figure 4.3. Comparison of results from two studies (25, 43) both showing evidence for a major locus for regulation of total serum IgE levels mapping to 5q. The markers used in each study are shown in map order

show the strongest evidence for linkage to 5q. The frequency of this polymorphism is similar in probands (21.7% are CT, freq(T) = 10.9%) and in spouses (19.5% are CT, freq(T) = 9.8%). Geometric mean IgE levels were low in both groups (< 100 IU) and not significantly different (47 IU in CC individuals versus 38 IU in CT individuals). Thus, this IL-9 polymorphism is not related to the regulation of elevated IgE levels in these asthmatic Dutch families.

After performing two-locus segregation analyses on the Dutch asthma families, two-locus linkage analysis was used to test the hypothesis that there are two unlinked loci, and only one of these map to chromosome 5q (35). As previously described, there was significant evidence favoring the two-locus models, but it was not possible from the segregation analysis alone to determine the best two-locus model. Therefore, LOD scores were calculated for D5S436 (the marker with the highest LOD from the previous one-locus analysis (25)) for the most likely two-locus models. This procedure is described as the MOD score method, maximizing the LOD score over several genetic models (46). Except for the general model where more parameters were estimated, the recessive model III from Table 4.2 had the highest LOD score (4.67 at 9% recombination compared to 3.00 at 10% recombination), increasing the evidence for linkage to this region. An increase in the LOD was also observed for D5S393 and FGFA. No positive LODs were obtained when the second locus was tested for linkage to 5q. Therefore, it appears that only the first locus which accounts for the highest percentage of the variability in the total serum IgE levels maps to this candidate region, and that there is at least one additional locus mapping elsewhere in the genome.

Linkage of a susceptibility locus for bronchial hyper-responsiveness mapping to this same region of 5q in the Dutch families has been reported (47). When total serum IgE levels were included as a covariate, significant evidence for linkage for bronchial hyper-responsiveness was obtained suggesting that there may be separate loci on 5q for these two important components of the asthma phenotype. Evidence for linkage of the asthma phenotype to this region has also been obtained in the same set of families (48). These findings support the importance of this region in regulating aspects of the allergic and asthmatic phenotype.

Once linkage is confirmed in complex genetic disorders such as asthma or clinical allergic disease, finding the actual gene is a complex process that calls for close integration between clinical approaches and disease identification, genetic analysis using techniques that include linkage disequilibrium, and molecular and physical mapping with detection of mutations.

4.5 CONCLUSIONS

Since total serum IgE levels are correlated with the clinical expression of allergy, bronchial hyper-responsiveness and asthma, it represents an important quantitative parameter that can be used to map genes for these complex disorders. From segregation analyses it appears that there are at least two major loci involved in determining an individual's total serum IgE level in addition to environmental factors.

The locus with the strongest influence on total serum IgE levels has been mapped to chromosome 5q, a region with multiple candidate genes. Fine mapping studies are underway, multiple genes on 5q may be involved. In addition, genome searches are being performed to map additional genes. Once these studies are completed the relationships between these loci and other measures of the asthma phenotype can be investigated. All these studies are important in investigating the complex nature of the genetics of asthma and atopic disease.

These findings will be useful in dissecting the complex genetic relationship between susceptibility to bronchial hyper-responsiveness, allergic disorders and asthma. Additional studies replicating previous studies and positional cloning studies will further define the genes important in the regulation of inflammatory processes in asthma and allergy. These combined genetic and clinical studies will lead to improved therapies and better techniques for early diagnosis of these disorders.

REFERENCES

1. Johansson SG, Bennich HH and Berg T (1972) The clinical significance of IgE. *Prog Clin Immunol* **1**:157–181.
2. Burrows B, Martinez FD, Halonen M, Barbee RA and Cline MG (1989) Association of asthma with serum IgE levels and skin-test reactivity to allergens. *N Engl J Med* **320**:271–277.

3. Sears MR, Burrows B, Flannery EM, Herbison GP, Hewitt CJ and Holdaway MD (1991) Relation between airway responsiveness and serum IgE in children with asthma and in apparently normal children. *N Engl J Med* **325**:1067–1071.

4. Halonen M, Stern D, Taussig LM, Wright A, Ray CG and Martinez FD (1992) The predictive relationship between serum IgE levels at birth and subsequent incidences of lower respiratory illnesses and eczema in infants. *Am Rev Respir Dis* **146**:866–870.

5. Holgate ST, Beasley R and Twentyman OP (1987) The pathogenesis and significance of bronchial hyperresponsiveness in airway disease. *Clin Sci* **73**:561–572.

6. Hopp RJ, Townley RG, Biven RE, Bewtra AK and Nair NM (1990) The presence of airway reactivity before the development of asthma. *Am Rev Respir Dis* **141**:2–8.

7. Burrows B, Sears MR, Flannery EM, Herbison GP and Holdaway MD (1992) Relationships of bronchial responsiveness assessed by methacholine to serum IgE, lung function, symptoms, and diagnoses in 11-year-old New Zealand children. *J Allergy Clin Immunol* **90**:376–385.

8. Gergen PJ and Weiss KB (1992) The increasing problem of asthma in the United States. *Am Rev Respir Dis* **146**:823–824.

9. Peat JK, Van den Berg RH, Green WF, Mellis CM, Leeder SR and Woolcock AJ (1994) Changing prevalence of asthma in Australian children. *Br Med J* **308**:1591–1596.

10. Ninan TK and Russel G (1992) Respiratory symptoms and atopy in Aberdeen school children: evidence from two surveys 25 years apart. *Br Med J* **304**:873–875.

11. Burr ML (1993) Epidemiology of clinical allergy. *Monogr Allergy* **31**:1–8.

12. Barbee RA, Lebowitz MD, Thompson HC and Burrows B (1976) Immediate skin-test reactivity in a general population sample. *Ann Intern Med* **84**:129–133.

13. Gerrard JW and Brook D (1977) Serum IgE levels in forty families studied for two or three years. *Ann Allergy* **38**:396–399.

14. Halonen M, Stern D, Lyle S, Wright A, Taussig L and Martinez FD (1991) Relationship of total serum IgE levels in cord and 9-month sera of infants. *Clin Exp Allergy* **21**:235–241.

15. Stoy PJ, Roitman-Johnson B, Walsh G *et al* (1981) Aging and serum immunoglobulin E levels, immediate skin tests, RAST. *J Allergy Clin Immunol* **68**:421–426.

16. Kjellman NI (1988) Epidemiology and prevention of allergy. *Allergy* **43, Suppl 8**:39–40.

17. Halonen M, Barbee RA, Lebowitz MD and Burrows B (1982) An epidemiologic study of interrelationships of total serum immunoglobulin E, allergy skin-test reactivity, and eosinophilia. *J Allergy Clin Immunol* **69**:221–228.

18. Croner S and Kjellman NI (1986) Predictors of atopic disease: cord blood IgE and month of birth. *Allergy* **41**:68–70.

19. Marsh DG, Meyers DA and Bias WB (1981) The epidemiology and genetics of atopic allergy. *N Engl J Med* **305**:1551–1559.

20. Burrows B, Halonen M, Barbee RA and Lebowitz MD (1981) The relationship of serum immunoglobulin E to cigarette smoking. *Am Rev Respir Dis* **124**:523–525.

21. Meyers DA, Beaty TH, Freidhoff LR and Marsh DG (1987) Inheritance of total serum IgE (basal levels) in man. *Am J Hum Genet* **41**:51–62.

22. Hopp RJ, Bewtra AK, Watt GD, Nair NM and Townley RG (1984) Genetic analysis of allergic disease in twins. *J Allergy Clin Immunol* **73**:265–270.

23. Demenais FM and Bonney GE (1989) Equivalence of the mixed and regressive models for genetic analysis. I. Continuous traits [published erratum appears in *Genet Epidemiol* (1990) **7**:103]. *Genet Epidemiol* **6**:597–617.

24. Akaike H (1974) A new look at the statistical model identification. *IEEE Trans Automatic Control* **19**:716–723.

25. Meyers DA, Postma DS, Panhuysen CI *et al* (1994) Evidence for a locus regulating total serum IgE levels mapping to chromosome 5. *Genomics* **23**:464–470.

26. Bonney GE (1986) Regressive logistic models for familial disease and other binary traits. *Biometrics* **42**:611–625.
27. SAGE, Statistical Analysis for Genetic Epidemiology. (1992) (2.1) Department of Biometry and Genetics, LSU Medical Center, New Orleans, LA.
28. Marsh DG, Bias WB and Ishizaka K (1974) Genetic control of basal serum immunoglobulin E level and its effect on specific reaginic sensitivity. *Proc Natl Acad Sci USA* **71**:3588–3592.
29. Gerrard JW, Rao DC and Morton NE (1978) A genetic study of immunoglobulin E. *Am J Hum Genet* **30**:46–58.
30. Meyers DA, Hasstedt SJ, Marsh DG *et al* (1983) The inheritance of immunoglobulin E: genetic linkage analysis. *Am J Med Genet* **16**:575–581.
31. Blumenthal MN, Namboodiri K, Mendell N, Gleich G, Elston RC and Yunis E (1981) Genetic transmission of serum IgE levels. *Am J Med Genet* **10**:219–228.
32. Meyers DA, Bias WB and Marsh DG (1982) A genetic study of total IgE levels in the Amish. *Hum Hered* **32**:15–23.
33. Hasstedt SJ, Meyers DA and Marsh DG (1983) Inheritance of immunoglobulin E: genetic model fitting. *Am J Med Genet* **14**:61–66.
34. Martinez FD, Holberg CJ, Halonen M, Morgan WJ, Wright AL and Taussig LM (1994) Evidence for Mendelian inheritance of serum IgE levels in Hispanic and non-Hispanic white families. *Am J Hum Genet* **55**:555–565.
35. Xu J, Levitt RC, Panhuysen CI *et al* (1995) Evidence for two unlinked loci regulating total serum IgE levels. *Am J Hum Genet* **57**:425–430.
36. PAP: Pedigree Analysis Package (1994) Rev. 4, Hasstedt SJ, Department of Human Genetics, University of Utah, Salt Lake City, UT.
37. Ott J (1991) *Analysis of Human Genetics*. The Johns Hopkins University Press, Baltimore, MD.
38. Morton NE (1955) Sequential tests for the detection of linkage. *Am J Human Genet* **7**:277–318.
39. Lander ES and Kruglyak L (1996) Genetic dissection of complex traits: guidelines for interpreting and reporting linkage results. *Nature Genet* **11**:241–247.
40. Chandrasekharappa SC, Rebelsky MS, Firak TA, Le Beau MM and Westbrook CA (1990) A long-range restriction map of the interleukin-4 and interleukin-5 linkage group on chromosome 5. *Genomics* **6**:94–99.
41. Kelley J (1990) Cytokines of the lung. *Am Rev Respir Dis* **141**:765–788.
42. Boulay JL and Paul WE (1992) The interleukin-4-related lymphokines and their binding to hematopoietin receptors. *J Biol Chem* **267**:20525–20528.
43. Marsh DG, Neely JD, Breazeale DR *et al* (1994) Linkage analysis of IL-4 and other chromosome 5q31.1 markers and total serum immunoglobulin E concentrations. *Science* **264**:1152–1156.
44. Doull IJM, Lawrence S, Watson M *et al* (1996) Allelic association of gene markers on chromosomes 5q and 11q with atopy and bronchial hyperresponsiveness. *Am J Respir Crit Care Med* **153**:1280–1284.
45. Bleecker ER, Scott AF, Xu J, Panhuysen CIM, Postma DS and Meyers DA (1996) Fine mapping of asthma susceptibility locus to 5q31–33. *Am Soc Genet* **A213**.
46. Hodge SE and Elston RC (1994) Lods, wrods, and mods: the interpretation of lod scores calculated under different models. *Genet Epidemiol* **11**:329–42.
47. Postma DS, Bleecker ER, Amelung PJ *et al* (1995) Genetic susceptibility to asthma—bronchial hyperresponsiveness coinherited with a major gene for atopy. *N Engl J Med* **333**:894–900.
48. Panhuysen CIM, Levitt RC, Postma DS *et al* (1995) Evidence for a susceptibility locus for asthma mapping to chromosome 5q. *J Invest Med* **43**:281A.

5 IL-4 and IL-13 in Atopy: Regulation of Production and Effects

VOLKER BRINKMANN and **BERND KINZEL**
Novastis Pharma Inc., Research Department, Therapeutic Area Respiratory Diseases, CH 4002 Basel, Switzerland

5.1 INTRODUCTION

The cytokines interleukin (IL)-4 and IL-13 are produced by activated T cells (1–7) and mast cells/basophils (8–12), and display multiple common effects on the immune system. Both cytokines induce proliferation, differentiation, and IgE isotype switching of human B cells (13–21), and therefore may be central to the pathophysiology of allergy and asthma (22–24). Indeed, a significant inheritable component of allergy and asthma is linked to genetic markers within the 5q31 chromosomal region, where the genes for IL-4 and IL-13 are encoded (25, 26), and to increased total serum IgE levels (27). Besides the striking effects of IL-4 and IL-13 on B cells, both cytokines inhibit the production of pro-inflammatory cytokines and chemokines by monocytes/macrophages (6, 28–30). Furthermore, IL-4 and IL-13 modulate expression of adhesion molecules on endothelial cells (31, 32), which may have consequences on the transmigration of lymphoid cells from the periphery to inflamed tissues. The overlapping biological properties of IL-4 and IL-13 relate to the fact that their receptors share the IL-4 receptor α chain (33–35). In contrast to IL-4, IL-13 may not act directly on T cells, since functional IL-13 receptors (IL-13R) could not be detected on these cells (6, 35). Although both IL-4 and IL-13 were initially classified as T helper type 2 (Th2) cytokines (2, 36, 37), it became clear that their phylogenetically similar genes can be independently expressed and that IL-13 is also produced by Th1 cells (5). Compared to IL-4, IL-13 is produced by activated T cells in larger quantities and for longer periods of time (5, 38), and T cells secreting IL-13, but not IL-4, can induce IgE isotype switching of human B cells (39). However, the differential regulatory mechanisms leading to IL-4 and/or IL-13 expression by T cells and to IL-4 and/or IL-13-dependent IgE production by B cells are only now beginning to be elucidated.

It is well established that stimulation of uncommitted naive T cells by antigens presented on specialized antigen-presenting cells (APC) induces the T cells to express IL-2R, to secrete IL-2, and to proliferate in response to IL-2 (1). The cytokines present during this activation process critically affect differentiation of the

IgE Regulation: Molecular Mechanisms. Edited by D. Vercelli. © 1997 John Wiley & Sons Ltd.

naive T cells into Th1 or Th2 effector cells (1–3). Within a complex cytokine network, IL-4 is the major cytokine that amplifies Th2 immunity by accelerating production of IL-13 (38, 40) and IL-4 (41, 42). Moreover, IL-4 counteracts Th1 immunity by suppressing production of interferon (IFN)-γ (43). Both IL-4 and IL-13 may also indirectly support Th2 cell development by inhibiting macrophage production of IL-12 and IFN-α, cytokines which reportedly induce Th1 cell differentiation (44, 45). In allergy and asthma, allergen-specific Th2 cells (secreting IL-3, IL-4, IL-5, IL-10, IL-13, and granulocyte–macrophage colony-stimulating factor (GM-CSF)) are responsible for the excessive IgE production by B cells, as well as for the hyperactivation of mast cells and eosinophils (3, 4). In contrast, Th1 cells (secreting IL-2 and IFN-γ) are involved mainly in delayed-type hypersensitivity reactions, as well as in the activation of macrophages in response to intracellular pathogens (1–4, 22).

From the current literature it appears that the mechanisms initiating Th2 differentiation in uncommitted naive T cells (in the absence of preformed IL-4) may differ from those which amplify established Th2 immunity in an IL-4-dependent manner. Furthermore it has been shown that the genes for Th2 cytokines, including those for IL-4 and IL-13, can be independently regulated. We shall discuss and compare the expression of IL-4 and IL-13 in T cells, the structure of IL-4R and IL-13R, and the possible role of different IL-4- or IL-13-secreting cell populations in the regulation of IgE production in atopy.

5.2 REGULATION OF IL-4 AND IL-13 EXPRESSION

5.2.1 Localization and Structure of the Genes for IL-4 and IL-13

The human IL-4 and IL-13 genes are located in the chromosomal region 5q31. This region contains a gene cluster of haematopoietic and immunoregulatory growth factors that include the genes for IL-3, IL-4, IL-5, IL-9, IL-13, and GM-CSF (25, 26, 46). Additional genes clustered in the 5q31–q33 region include those for interferon regulatory factor-1, the receptors for glucocorticoids, macrophage-colony stimulating factor, platelet-derived growth factor, and the β2-adrenergic receptor (26, 46). Interestingly, recent studies have demonstrated a significant inheritable component to allergy and asthma, and a linkage of these diseases to increased total serum IgE levels (27) and to genetic markers on chromosome 5q31–q33 in humans (26, 46). Like IL-4, IL-13 occurs as a single copy gene and is composed of four exons and three introns (47, 48). The common exon/intron structure, also shared by IL-5 and GM-CSF, is highly conserved in the murine genome, where these genes map to a region on chromosome 11. Recently it was shown that IL-13 is separated from IL-4 by as little as 12 kb of chromosomal region (48), suggesting that the two genes may share regulatory DNA elements. Although there is little homology between the IL-4 and IL-13 genes or the proteins they encode, the close proximity of the genes, the similar protein structure, and the biological function suggest that they have evolved by gene duplication from a common ancestor. However, because of their divergence, the duplication events must have occurred early in evolution. Several ancient regulatory mechanisms might still allow for co-regulation during distinct T-cell activation stages, but others were adapted to allow for specific expression of IL-4 or IL-13.

5.2.2 Transcriptional Control of IL-4 and IL-13 in Uncommitted T Cells

The transcription of cytokine genes in T cells is induced by binding of ligand molecules to their specific membrane receptors. These receptors induce a complex cascade of intracellular events, leading to the activation of specific nuclear factors which selectively induce or suppress gene transcription (49). A growing body of evidence suggests that the mechanisms which initiate Th2 differentiation in uncommitted naive T cells may differ from those which amplify established Th2 immunity in an IL-4-dependent manner. In the absence of preformed IL-4, the initial activation of the IL-4 gene may depend on the type of the stimulating antigen/allergen, the co-stimulatory signals given by the APC to the T cell via cytokines or surface molecules, and the type of the APC (1–4, 44, 45).

Molecular studies of the IL-4 promoter in T cells have identified a set of regulatory elements located 5' of the IL-4 transcription initiation site. Close to the TATA-box (where transcription of IL-4 is initiated by RNA polymerase II) a *cis*-regulatory DNA element (named P element) was found to induce IL-4 transcription by binding the nuclear factor NF(P), which by itself is activated by T-cell receptor (TCR) signals (50). In the human IL-4 promoter three P elements have been identified, whereas five P elements are located within the murine IL-4 promoter, of which at least four contribute to inducible IL-4 expression. The locations and sequences of each P element are highly conserved between the mouse and human genome (51). Interestingly there is a significant homology between the NF(P) binding region in the IL-4 promoter and two sites for nuclear factor of activated T cells (NF-AT) in the promoters of the human or murine IL-2 gene (52). NF-AT is a cytoplasmatic protein whose dephosphorylation and nuclear translocation is catalysed by the Ca^{2+}/calmodulin-dependent phosphatase calcineurin. Based on a similar function and close structural homologies it was postulated that NF-AT is identical to NF(P). However, NF(P) differs from NF-AT in that it lacks a protein kinase C (PKC) activation-dependent activator-protein-1 (AP-1) component, i.e. a heterodimer of Fos and Jun oncoproteins thought to be required for IL-2 expression. This may explain why NF(P) complex formation and IL-4 transcription is dependent solely on an increase in intracellular free Ca^{2+} levels ($[Ca^{2+}]_i$) (53, 54). A sustained increase in $[Ca^{2+}]_i$ may on the other hand activate Ca^{2+}-dependent protein kinase II (CaM-K II), which reportedly inhibits IL-2 promoter activity by interfering with the PKC-dependent AP-1 and NF-AT transactivating pathways (55).

Several other studies suggested that stimulation of PKC may lead to an active repression of the IL-4 gene and an induction of IL-2 transcription (a model is depicted in Figure 5.1a). Receptor-mediated activation of phospholipase C (PLC)

78

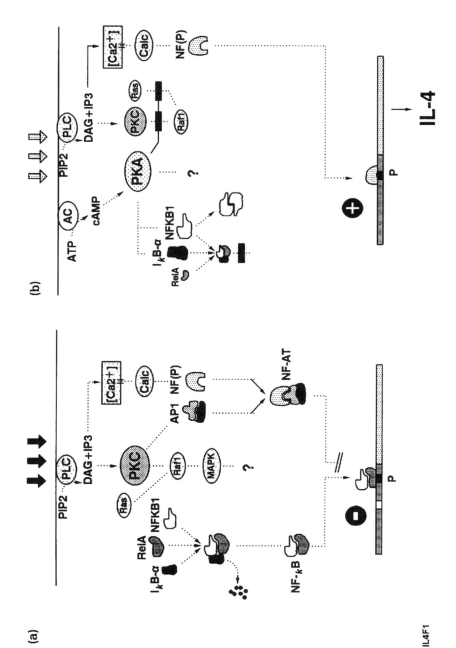

IL4F1

Figure 5.1. (a) Repression of the IL-4 gene. Receptor-mediated activation of phospholipase C (PLC) causes the release of inositol triphosphate (IP$_3$) and diacylglycerol (DAG) from membrane phosphatidyl inositol biphosphate (PIP$_2$). DAG increases the activity of protein kinase C (PKC). PKC activates Raf1 kinase, and this is followed by activation of a cascade of other protein kinases (MAP kinases). Moreover, activation of the PKC pathway induces formation of AP-1 from Fos and Jun oncoproteins, and of NF-κB from RelA and NFKB1. In parallel, IP$_3$ induces release of Ca^{2+} from intracellular stores, and thereby activates the Ca^{2+}/calmodulin-dependent phosphatase calcineurin (Calc) and in turn the nuclear factor NF(P). NF(P) and AP1 form the NF-AT complex, which initiates IL-2 transcription (not shown). Furthermore, PKC ζ catalyses degradation of the NF-κB inhibitor IκB-α, the factor that retains NF-κB in the cytoplasm. As a consequence, NF-κB translocates to the nucleus and represses the IL-4 promoter by displacing NF-AT from its positive regulatory P element. In contrast, NF-κB plays a permissive role in NF-AT-dependent IL-2 transcription (not shown). In naive T cells, this process may help initiate Th1 cell differentiation. (b) Activation of the IL-4 gene. Receptor-mediated stimulation of adenylate cyclase (AC) catalyses the formation of cAMP from ATP, and cAMP supports activation of protein kinase A (PKA). PKA suppresses activation of Raf1 by PKC (or by Ras), thereby abrogating the activation of downstream kinases. Moreover, PKA enhances *de novo* synthesis of the NF-κB subunit NFKB1, but not of RelA. This reduces formation of the IL-4-repressive NF-κB heterodimer (RelA/NFKB1), and favors formation of the IL-2-repressive NFKB1 homodimer. Furthermore, PKA enhances expression of IκB-α, which retains the NF-κB hetero- dimer in the cytoplasm, and this process further counteracts repression of IL-4. In parallel, activation of PLC induces a rise in [Ca^{2+}]$_i$, and this stimulates the Ca^{2+}/calmodulin-dependent phosphatase calcineurin (Calc) and leads to the activation of NF(P). Finally, NF(P) binds to the P sequence in the IL-4 promoter and induces IL-4 gene transcription. In T cells, this pathway may help initiate differentiation of Th2 cells

causes the release of inositol triphosphate (IP_3) and diacyl glycerol (DAG) from membrane phosphatidyl inositol biphosphate (PIP_2). IP_3 mobilizes Ca^{2+}, which is followed by an activation of the Ca^{2+}/calmodulin-dependent phosphatase calcineurin and an activation of NF(P), which by itself could function as an IL-4 promoter activator (57). However, NF(P) action is counteracted by a PKC-dependent mechanism. DAG increases the activity of PKC, and this leads to a sequential activation of further downstream protein kinases, collectively termed the mitogen-activated protein (MAP) kinase cascade (49, 56). This process further activates the nuclear factor AP-1 and supports formation of NF-AT from NF(P) and AP-1. Furthermore, PKC activation supports formation of the transcription factor NF-κB, a heterodimer consisting of the subunits RelA (p65) and NFKB1 (p50) (57). The PKC ζ isoform catalyses degradation of IκB-α, a factor which retains NF-κB in the cytoplasm, thereby supporting nuclear translocation of NF-κB (58, 59). Once in the nucleus, NF-κB represses human IL-4 promoter activity by displacing NF(P) (or NF-AT) from its positive regulatory P element (57), whereas it plays a permissive role in NF-AT-induced IL-2 transcription (57, 60). In line with these results, production of IL-4 in murine Th2 clones has been related to the failure of these cells to generate active NF-κB heterodimers (61). These data suggest that strong TCR stimulation (in the absence of accessory signalling) may preferentially activate the PKC pathway and induce nuclear translocation of the RelA/NFKB1 heterodimer NF-κB, which represses the IL-4 gene and induces transcription of IL-2, and thereby promotes Th1 immunity (see also Chapter 6).

Interestingly, the IL-4-suppressive activity of NF-κB may be counteracted by another major signalling pathway involving cyclic adenosine monophosphate (cAMP)-dependent protein kinase A (PKA) (Figure 5.1b). It is known that receptor-mediated stimulation of adenylate cyclase (AC) catalyses formation of cAMP from adenosine triphosphate (ATP), and that cAMP supports activation of PKA (56). There is now increasing evidence that PKA counter-acts activation of Raf1 by Ras or PKC (49, 56, 62), which as a consequence abrogates activation of further downstream kinases and exerts an inhibitory effect on the proliferation of numerous cells, including T cells (63). Moreover, PKA enhances *de novo* synthesis of the NF-κB subunit NFKB1 (but not of RelA), which reduces formation of the NF-κB heterodimer RelA/NFKB1 and favours formation of NFKB1 homodimers (57, 64). Furthermore, PKA enhances expression of the NF-κB inhibitor IκB-α, which retains the IL-4-repressive NF-κB heterodimer in the cytoplasm (63). In parallel, activation of PLC induces a rise in $[Ca^{2+}]_i$, which is followed by an activation of the Ca^{2+}/calmodulin-dependent phosphatase calcineurin and an activation of NF(P), which (in the absence of NF-κB) acts as an IL-4 promoter activator. These molecular data are confirmed by functional studies showing that activation of PKA by forskolin inhibits TCR/PKC-mediated IL-2 production and proliferation of Th1 cells, while the same reagent fails to block IL-4 production and proliferation of Th2 cells (65, 66). Furthermore, prostaglandin E_2 (PGE_2), a stimulator of cAMP, abolishes binding of NF-κB to its target sequence and increases production of IL-4, whereas it suppresses production of IL-2 (66, 67). At the same time the IL-4 inducer PGE_2 counteracts excessive IgE production by inhibiting the Ig switch at the B cell level (68). Collectively the data strongly suggest a predominant role for the NF-κB component RelA as a repressor of the IL-4 gene, and a role of the cAMP-dependent PKA pathway in the elimination of this repression. Accordingly, the induction of Th2 cell differentiation may coincide with preferential activation of the PKA pathway rather than PKC, and a reduced RelA/NF-κB activity (see also Chapter 6).

Besides the mechanisms described above, IL-4 gene expression may be regulated by other *cis* regulatory DNA elements and additional nuclear factors. Candidates are the positive regulatory element PRE (69), and the negative regulatory element NRE (70), as well as an additional binding site which partially overlaps with the NF(P) site and interacts with the novel proximal constitutive complex PCC (71). Furthermore, a palindromic promoter element containing two symmetrical inverted repeats was recently identified in the upstream region of the GM-CSF gene. This palindrome contains a core sequence shared by the promoters of IL-2, IL-4, IL-5, IL-13, and GM-CSF (72), and this sequence may be involved in the simultaneous expression of these cytokines in Th0 cells.

The involvement of the nuclear factors described above in the regulation of the IL-13 gene is only partially elucidated. Sequence analysis of the 5' untranslated IL-13 region has revealed a set of recognition sites for transcription factors, several of which are shared by IL-4 and IL-13 and are localized in promoter regions and in the biggest introns of these genes (48). IL-4 and IL-13 show about 50% overall homology in their 5' flanking region but there is also a region of higher homology, suggesting that there may be conserved regulatory elements. In line with these findings, functional studies provided evidence that IL-4 and IL-13 can be coregulated or separately expressed in T cells (5, 38–40).

IL-4 and IL-13 are produced, not only by T cells, but also by basophils and mast cells. Because of their distinct tissue distribution mast cells may play a different role in local inflammatory immune responses, and IL-4 production might be differently regulated in these cells. In fact a mast cell-specific enhancer region located within the first intron of the IL-4 gene may contribute to high basal IL-4 expression in these cells (73). It is possible that mast cell-derived IL-4 may play a role in local Th2 immunity. As mentioned above, IL-4 secreted by committed Th2 cells (or by mast cells/basophils) amplifies its own release, and thereby maintains established Th2 immunity (see also Chapter 6).

5.2.3 Production of IL-13 by CD8$^+$ and CD4$^+$ Th0, Th1 and Th2 T Cells

Recent functional studies demonstrated that both CD4$^+$ and CD8$^+$ T cells can produce IL-4 and IL-13 (5, 38), but that the genes for IL-4 and IL-13 are not necessarily coregulated. If naive uncommitted human CD4$^+$ 45RO$^-$ T cells are primed and restimulated by anti-CD3 monoclonal antibody (mAb) and IL-2, they secrete large amounts of IL-13 and IFN-γ, but no IL-4 (39). The development of these IL-13-producers is IL-4 independent, since it can occur in the presence of neutralizing anti-IL-4 mAbs. Interestingly, stimulation of human CD4 or CD8 T cells by the PKC activator phorbol myristate acetate (PMA) induces co-expression of IL-13 and IFN-γ without IL-4, whereas activation by calcium ionophores induces co-expression of IL-4 and IL-13 without IFN-γ. Furthermore, costimulation of ionomycin-treated human CD4 T cells with PMA downregulates IL-4, whereas it increases IL-13 and induces IFN-γ (Brinkmann, unpublished). Similar cytokine secretion patterns are observed in a large panel of long-term Th1 and Th2 clones restimulated by their specific antigens (5). Th1 clones specific for purified protein derivative (PPD) express IL-13 and IFN-γ without IL-4, whereas Th2 clones specific for the allergen *Dermatophagoides pteronyssinus* 1 (Der p1) express IL-4 and IL-13 without IFN-γ. In contrast, tetanus-toxoid (TT)-specific Th0 clones co-express all three cytokines. It should also be noted that the levels of secreted IL-13 are comparably high in T-cell clones of all three phenotypes (5). These data show that IL-13 can be expressed by CD4$^+$ T cells of Th0, Th1, and Th2 phenotype, and also by CD8$^+$ T cells. It appears that IL-13 transcription may be less sensitive to signals that repress the IL-4 gene, and that IL-13 can be induced via the Ca^{2+}/calmodulin-dependent as well as the PKC-dependent signalling pathways.

Earlier studies already indicated that Th2 cytokines can be further separated into groups which are independently expressed. It was found that expression of IL-3, IL-4 and GM-CSF by the murine Th2 clone D10.G4.1 involves the Ca^{2+}/calmodulin-dependent phosphatase calcineurin, the activity of which is inhibited by a complex formed between cyclosporin A (CSA) and its intracellular target, cyclophilin (54). In contrast, expression of IL-5, IL-6 and IL-10 is relatively resistant to suppression by CSA, and can be induced optimally by PMA, suggesting that the PKC signalling pathway can independently regulate this group of cytokine genes. We further found that in human CD4 T cells, ionomycin induces co-expression of IL-4 and IL-13 without IL-5, whereas PMA induces IL-5 and IL-13 without IL-4. Moreover, in contrast to IL-5, optimal production of IL-13 requires both high [Ca^{2+}]$_i$ and activation of PKC. These data further underline a differential regulation of the genes for IL-4, IL-5, and IL-13.

In this context it may also be of interest that *in vitro* low concentrations of glucocorticosteroids (CS) induce uncommitted TCR-stimulated CD4$^+$ CD45RO$^-$ T cells to secrete IL-4 and IL-10, but not IL-5 and IFN-γ (74). On the other hand, CS block production of IL-4, IL-5, and IL-10, but not IFN-γ, in CD4$^+$ CD45RO$^+$ T cells, which contain *in vivo* preactivated memory T cells. Moreover, CS strongly inhibit clonal expansion of primary but not memory T cells (74). These data support the concept that the regulation of individual cytokine genes may vary with the activation/differentiation stage of the T cell. The effects of CS described above may further explain some of their beneficial activities in the treatment of acute inflammation and chronic allergic/asthmatic disease.

5.2.4 Kinetics of IL-4 and IL-13 Production by T Cells

The kinetics of IL-13 mRNA expression in activated human CD4$^+$ and CD8$^+$ T cells is markedly different from that of IL-4, which is transient. In human peripheral

T cells, both IL-4 and IL-13 mRNA are induced 4 h after activation by ionomycin and PMA. However, IL-13 mRNA is still present after 48 h, whereas IL-4 mRNA is strongly decreased after 8 h and absent after 24 h of stimulation (5). Accordingly, we found that human CD4$^+$ T cells activated via the TCR by anti-CD3 mAb secrete low amounts of IL-4 only during the initial 24 h of stimulation, whereas IL-13 (and IFN-γ) is produced in large amounts for at least 6 days (38, 39). However, the mechanisms that repress the IL-4 gene may be gradually reduced during Th2 cell differentiation, since PKC activation suppresses IL-4 production by ionomycin-stimulated primary T cells but not by long-term Th2 clones (54). Therefore, in allergic disease, persistently (re)stimulated Th2 effector cells may produce both IL-4 and IL-13. The significance of these findings in respect to the IgE helper potential of such IL-13-producers is discussed in Section 5.4.

5.2.5 Production of IL-4 and IL-13 by Mast Cells and Basophils

Besides T cells, activated human and murine mast cells/basophils can produce IL-4 and IL-13 (8–11), and human eosinophils can produce IL-4 (12). In human inflamed airway tissues, IL-4 production has been localized to eosinophils (12) and mast cells (11), but also to mononuclear cells/CD3$^+$ T lymphocytes (75, 76). Like T cells, mast cells (77) and eosinophils (78) express functional CD40 ligand (CD40L), and as a consequence can activate B cells via surface CD40 (77). It is therefore possible that, in chronic disease situations, mast cells and eosinophils may drive allergic immune reactions and promote IgE synthesis independent of T cells (see also Chapter 2).

5.3 FUNCTION OF IL-4 AND IL-13

5.3.1 Structure of IL-4 and IL-13 Receptors

The overlapping biological properties of IL-4 and IL-13 relate to the fact that their receptors share a common component (33-35). The IL-4R is a heterodimer comprising an α chain (p140) and a γ chain. The fact that anti-human α chain mAbs blocked the biological function of both IL-4 and IL-13 indicated that the α chain is a component of both the IL-4R and the IL-13R (79, 80). However, IL-13 does not bind to the IL-4R or the IL-4R α chain (34, 81), but binds to a novel p60–70 protein now believed to be the second chain of the IL-13R (82, 83). From these data it may be concluded that the IL-4R α chain can associate either with the γ chain to form an IL-4R that does not bind IL-13, or with an IL-13 binding chain to form an IL-13R (35).

Initially it was speculated that also the IL-2R γ chain would be a common component of the IL-4R and IL-13R, since this chain had already been found to associate with the receptors for IL-2, IL-4, IL-7, IL-9, and IL-15. However, studies with MC/9 mast cells (which constitutively express γ chain and respond to IL-4 and IL-13) showed that proliferation in response to IL-4 but not IL-13 can be blocked by anti-γ chain mAbs (84). Furthermore, B9 plasmacytoma cells proliferating in response to IL-4 and IL-13 do not express γ chain, and transfection of γ chain-negative B9 cells with the respective cDNA affected the proliferative response to IL-4 but not IL-13 (84). These data suggested that the γ chain contributes to the IL-4R, but not to the IL-13R in lymphoid cells. However, renal carcinoma cells that do not express γ chain respond to both IL-4 and IL-13 (85). These data suggest that the γ chain may be a functional component of the IL-4R in lymphoid cells, but not in renal carcinoma cells. It is tempting to speculate that in renal carcinoma cells, IL-4 may signal through an IL-13R comprised of the IL-4R α chain and the novel p60–70 protein component. Therefore, the failure of murine B cells and human and murine T cells to respond to IL-13 may relate to the lack of expression of this p60–70 subunit. In the future it will be important to distinguish between responses mediated by the IL-4R and the IL-13R.

5.3.2 Signalling via IL-4 and IL-13 Receptors: The JAK–STAT Pathway

Signalling via cytokine receptors on the cell surface is initiated when the cytokine interacts with two independent receptor chains, thereby promoting receptor dimerization (86). Once dimerized, this brings receptor-associated Janus kinases (JAK) into apposition, enabling them to transphosphorylate each other. The kinases, now activated, phosphorylate a distal tyrosine on the IL-4R α chain. This phosphotyrosyl residue is subsequently recognized by the Src homology 2 (SH2) domain of a defined STAT (signal transducer and activator of transcription) protein. To date, six STAT proteins have been described. As depicted in Figure 5.2, IL-4 binds to the α chain of the IL-4R, and the α chain specifically associates with Jak1, while the γ chain associates with Jak3 (80, 87). Interestingly, Jak1 but not Jak3 is also activated by IL-13 (88). However, both IL-4 and IL-13 specifically induce tyrosine phosphorylation of Stat6 (80, 87-89), a molecule also designated NF-IL-4 (90) or STF-IL-4 (89). This suggests that the specificity of Stat6 activation is due to Stat6 docking on the IL-4R α chain rather than to activation of Jak3. After homodimerization, Stat6 translocates to the nucleus, binds to an IL-4 responsive element (IL-4RE) in the promoter regions of IL-4/IL-13-dependent genes, and initiates transcription. The IL-4-dependent amplification of IL-4 transcription may be less affected by the IL-4 repressor RelA/NF-κB (57), since exogenous IL-4 can induce IL-4 production in naive murine T cells stimulated by a combination of PMA plus ionomycin (91). Alternatively, IL-4 signalling may actively suppress the NF-κB pathway, and this may explain the antagonistic effect of IL-4 on IL-2-dependent proliferation of activated T cells (39, 40). The frequently observed functional antagonism between IL-4/IL-13 and IFN-γ may relate to the fact that the IL-4RE is also recognized by an IFN-γ-induced DNA binding protein (92, 93). It is of interest that, like Stat6, the PKA-induced NF-κB subunit NFKB1 binds to the Ig heavy chain germline ε promoter and supports IgE expression (90). It remains to be determined whether NFKB1 may also be involved in the positive regulation of the IL-4 gene, and whether RelA, the IL-4-repressive subunit of NF-κB (57) also represses IgE. Taken all together there is a great likelihood for the JAK–STAT pathway to provide

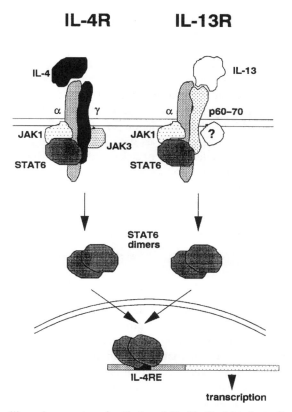

Figure 5.2. Signalling via receptors for IL-4 and IL-13. IL-4 binds to the IL-4R α chain (which is contained in both the IL-4R and the IL-13R) with low affinity, and the γ chain is then recruited to give high affinity IL-4 binding. IL-13 binds to the IL-13R p60–70 chain. The α chain specifically associates with the Janus kinase Jak1, and the γ chain associates with Jak3. Jak1, but not Jak3, is activated by IL-13. However, both IL-4 and IL-13 specifically induce tyrosine phosphorylation of Stat6. After homodimerization, Stat6 translocates to the nucleus, binds to an IL-4 responsive element (IL-4RE) in the promoter regions of IL-4/IL-13-dependent genes, and initiates transcription

specificity in the ligand-dependent activation of cytokine genes. The specificity of this pathway is convincingly demonstrated by the fact that IFN-γ and IFN-α (which antagonize production of IL-4 and IgE) specifically activate Stat1, and that targeted disruption of the Stat1 gene results in specific lack of responsiveness to these cytokines (94). Furthermore it was found that the Th1-inducing cytokine IL-12 uniquely phosphorylates Stat4 (95, 96). The observed specificity may occur at the level of the receptor–kinase complex, the STAT proteins and their interactions, and the DNA binding sites (see also Chapter 7).

Of high interest is the recent observation that murine pre-B cells transformed with the v-abl oncogene of the Abelson murine leukaemia virus display a constitutive activation of Jak1, Jak3, and Stat6, in the absence of IL-4 and IL-13 (97). Therefore, a direct link may exist between transformation of cells with certain viruses and cytokine signal transduction, and this may cause abnormal cytokine regulation in disease.

Besides activating JAKs and STATs, IL-4 (98) and IL-13 (99) induce tyrosine phosphorylation of IL-4-induced phosphotyrosine-substrate (4PS), also designated insulin receptor substrate-2 (IRS-2) because of its resemblance to IRS-1 (100). Furthermore, IL-4 induces phosphorylation of IRS-1 itself (97). It was found recently that 4PS/IRS-2 forms complexes with Jak1 and the IL-4R α chain (101), and may thereby facilitate interaction of Jak1 and Stat6. Both IRS-1 and IRS-2 possess a number of tyrosine phosphorylation sites that are within motifs that bind specific SH2-containing molecules known to be involved in mitogenic signalling, such as PI$_3$-kinase and Grb-2 (102). Interestingly, PI$_3$-kinase and Grb-2 are also recruited by CD28 (103), a costimulatory surface molecule on T cells, and this may provide a link between CD28 stimulation and the activation of Th2 cytokine genes (40).

5.3.3 Differential Role of IL-4 and IL-13 in B Cell Proliferation

Although IL-4 and IL-13 share many of their effects on the immune system (6, 7), they may differentially modulate B-cell proliferation in costimulation via surface IgM or CD40 antigen. It has been demonstrated earlier that B-cell activation via surface IgM or CD40 involves alternative signalling pathways and results in different B cell phenotypes (104). Human B cells proliferate well upon costimulation by IL-13 and anti-CD40 mAb, but not upon costimulation by IL-13 and anti-IgM antibody (35, 105). In contrast, IL-4 stimulates proliferation with either anti-IgM or anti-CD40 costimulation (35, 105, 106). Furthermore, costimulation of B cells with IL-2 and anti-IgM or anti-IgG antibody (but not IL-2 and anti-CD40 mAb) induces a good proliferative response (35, 106, and Brinkmann, unpublished). It has therefore been suggested that the common γ chain shared by the IL-2R and IL-4R may contribute preferentially to signals generated via surface Ig, whereas the IL-13R may costimulate more efficiently with CD40-generated signals (35). Given that surface Ig function as the specific antigen-receptor for B cells and that stimulation via CD40 provides a polyclonal signal for B-cell activation and Ig(E) switching, this may have consequences for the role of IL-4 and IL-13 in the production of antigen-specific versus polyclonal IgE.

5.3.4 Role of IL-4 and IL-13 in B Cell Differentiation and IgE Switching

Several recent reports have shown that IL-13 displays IL-4-like effects on human, but not on murine, B cells (Table 5.1). Both IL-4 and IL-13 induce Ig isotype switch of human mature IgM$^+$/IgD$^+$ B cells to IgG4 and IgE and increase IgM and total IgG production by B cells activated via CD40 (13–21). Functional studies (19) as well as molecular analysis (21) revealed that deletional switch recombination with

Table 5.1. Production and function of IL-4 and IL-13

Cells	Production by	Human		Mouse	
		IL-4	IL-13	IL-4	IL-13
T cells	CD4 T	+*	+	+	+
	CD8 T	+	+	+	nd†
	TH0	+	+	+	nd
	TH1	−	+	−	nd
	TH2	+	+	+	+
Mast cells/Basophils		+	+	+	+
Eosinophils		+	nd	nd	nd

Cells	Action on	Human		Mouse	
		IL-4	IL-13	IL-4	IL-13
T cells	proliferation	↑‡	−¶	↑	−
	TH2 cell differentiation	↑	(↑)**	↑	−
	TH1 cell differentiation	↓§	−	↓	−
B cells	MHC class II	↑	↑	↑	−
	CD23 (FcεRII)	↑	↑	↑	−
	proliferation	↑	↑	↑	−
	differentiation (Ig switch)	↑	↑	↑	−
B9 (mouse)	proliferation	−	↑	↑	↑
Monocytes/Macro-phages	APC function	↑	↑	↑	−
	MHC class II	↑	↑	↑	↑
	Selectins (CD11b, CD11c, CD18, CD29, CD49e/VLA5)	↑	↑	nd	nd
	CD23 (FcεRII)	↑	↑	↑	−
	FcγR	↓	↓	↓	↓
	Proinflammatory cytokines (IL-1α/β, IL-6, IL-8, Mip-1α, TNFα, IL-10, GM-CSF, G-CSF)	↓	↓	nd	nd
	IL-12, IFN-α	↓	↓	nd	nd
	IL-1 receptor antagonist	↑	↑	nd	nd
	Chemokines (IL-8, MIP-1α)	↓	↓	↓	↓
	ADCC	↓	↓	nd	nd
	NO production	nd	nd	↓	↓
Mast cells	CD54 (ICAM-1)	↑	↑	nd	nd
MC/9 (mouse)	proliferation	−	↑	↑	↑
Endothelial cells (HUVEC)	VCAM1 (eosinophil adhesion)	↑	↑	nd	nd

* + = cytokine mRNA or secreted protein detected; † nd = not determined; ‡ ↑ = up-regulation; § ↓ = down-regulation; ¶ − = no effect; ** = indirect effect via other cells.

direct $S\mu/S\epsilon$ joining represents the predominant mode of IgE switching. Compared to IL-4, IL-13 is generally 2- to 4-fold less potent in inducing IgE switching, but the ratios of the different isotypes produced in response to IL-13 are similar to those induced by IL-4 (6, 7) (see also Chapter 1).

IgE switching of human B cells in response to IL-4 or IL-13 is preceded by the induction of germline ϵ mRNA synthesis (6, 14, 107, 108), and costimulation of B cells via surface CD40 antigen provides a second signal that is required for the induction of productive ϵ mRNA transcripts and IgE synthesis (6, 13, 21, 109). *In vivo*, this second signal is delivered by binding of CD40L transiently expressed on activated CD4$^+$ T cells to CD40 constitutively expressed on B cells (110), and CD40L deficiency leads to the absence of Ig switching and the development of hyper-IgM syndrome (111). However, under certain conditions, other signals may bypass the requirement for CD40 stimulation, since activated T-cell clones from a patient with X-linked hyper-IgM syndrome induce IgE switching *in vitro* despite the expression of non-functional CD40L (112). Such signals may be provided by membrane tumour necrosis factor (TNF)-α (113), but also by other undefined molecules (112).

IL-4 strongly induces expression of CD23 (the low affinity receptor for IgE, FcϵRII), CD40, and major histocompatibility complex (MHC) class II antigens on a subset of human surface IgM$^-$ CD19$^+$ pre-B cells, whereas IL-13 does not act on these cells (14). In contrast, both IL-4 and IL-13 act on the majority of mature adult B cells and upregulate expression of MHC class II, surface IgM, CD23, the transferrin receptor CD71, and CD72, the counter-receptor for CD5 on T cells (6, 14, 18, 114). In contrast, the expression of MHC class I, CD25 (IL-2R), CD40, CD80 (B7-1), CD54 (intracellular adhesion molecule 1; ICAM-1), CD11a (leukocyte-function associated antigen; LFA-1), or CD58 (LFA-3) is unaffected. These data show that both IL-4 and IL-13 directly modulate the surface phenotype of human B cells. However, unlike IL-4, IL-13 activates B cells only after they are past the pre-B cell stage. Indeed, if pre-B cell maturation is induced *in vitro* by activated CD4$^+$ T cells and IL-7, B cells respond to IL-13 with proliferation, isotype switching, and Ig synthesis (14).

To date, IL-13 action on murine primary B cells has not been demonstrated. However, the mouse plasmacytoma cell line B9 expresses functional IL-13R and proliferates in response to IL-13 (6, 7). Furthermore, activated murine T cells produce IL-13 (36), and IL-4-independent IgE production can occur in parasite-infected IL-4-deficient mice (115) and in IL-4R transgenic mice, which produce up to 3 μg/ml of soluble receptor in the serum (116). It is tempting to speculate that *in vivo* primary murine B cells may acquire additional activation signals that enable them to respond to IL-13.

5.3.5 Role of IL-4 and IL-13 in Th2 Cell Differentiation

5.3.5.1 IL-4-dependent Amplification of Th2 Immunity

It is well established that IL-4 promotes Th2 immunity and IL-4 production in an autocrine fashion (1–4). Experiments using TCR transgenic mice (1) or human neonatal T cells (42) proved that Th2 cell-derived IL-4 can act on immunologically naive uncommitted T cells. Furthermore, in concert with IL-1, IL-4 supports clonal expansion of established murine Th2 clones, but not of Th1 clones, which lack IL-1R (1). Recent data from our laboratory show that IL-4 coregulates IL-4 and IL-13 production by T cells. IL-4 added during anti-CD3-induced activation of human CD4$^+$ T cells strongly increases their potential to produce IL-4, IL-13 and IL-5 upon restimulation, but blocks their potential to produce IFN-γ (38, 40). Under similar conditions, CD8$^+$ T cells secrete even larger amounts of IL-13 and IL-5, but lower levels of IL-4, and no IFN-γ (38). These data demonstrate that IL-4 supports IL-4 and IL-13 production in both CD4$^+$ and CD8$^+$ T cells. Indeed, it has been previously demonstrated that CD8$^+$ cells can differentiate into Th2-like cells, which display a reduced cytolytic potential (91), express CD40L, and provide helper activity for IgE synthesis, e.g. in AIDS patients with CD4$^+$ T cell-deficiency and hyper-IgE syndrome (117). These data suggest that CD8 effector functions are potentially diverse and could be exploited by viruses that switch off host protective cytolytic responses.

These data altogether show that the genes for IL-4, IL-5, and IL-13 are positively regulated by IL-4 in both CD4$^+$ and CD8$^+$ T cell populations. The results are consistent with the observation that IL-4-deficient mice are impaired in their ability to produce IL-5, IL-6, IL-10, and IL-13 (118). However, as described above, the genes for IL-4 and IL-13 can be differentially modulated, e.g. by PKC activators. This is consistent with the suggestion that the expression of each cytokine in individual cells can be independently regulated (118, 119), and that the fine tuning of cytokine gene expression may differ depending on the activation/differentiation stage of the T cell (74). Some degree of caution is therefore warranted, since the concept of distinct Th1 and Th2 subsets and cytokines may not accurately reflect more complex *in vivo* biology.

5.3.5.2 CD28/IL-2-dependent Th2 Differentiation

Recent reports suggested that binding of the T cell surface antigen CD28 (120) to its counter-receptor B7-2 (rather than B7-1) on accessory cells favours Th2 commitment (121, 122). Interestingly, we observed that ligation of CD28 may support either Th1 or Th2 commitment, depending on the quality of the TCR signal (40). This is suggested by the finding that > 99% of uncommitted naive human CD4$^+$ CD45R0$^-$ T cells differentiate into Th1 cells, if they are costimulated by anti-CD3 and anti-CD28 mAbs. In contrast, 5–10% of uncommitted T cells differentiate into Th2 'precursor' cells, if they are activated by anti-CD28 plus IL-2 in the complete absence of TCR/CD3 signals. Upon restimulation via the TCR by anti-CD3 or the superantigen *Staphylococcus* enterotoxin B (SEB), such Th2 'precursors' produce extremely large amounts of IL-4, IL-5 and IL-13 (40). It is possible that antigen/TCR-independent activation of T cells occurs in highly inflamed tissues, if uncommitted T cells (which constitutively express high levels of CD28) interact with accessory cells bearing the natural CD28 ligands B7-1 and B7-2 (120–122), and if these T cells are simultaneously exposed to high concentrations of IL-2 secreted by Th1 cells. The priming of as yet uncommitted cells for a Th2 phenotype may help limit the overshooting of Th1/IFN-γ-driven immune responses.

Interestingly, the CD28-dependent proliferation and differentiation of Th2 'precursors' is not affected by neutralizing anti-IL-4 mAb, but is extremely sensitive to suppression by IL-4, since addition of 0.1 U of IL-4 completely blocks CD28/IL-2-induced proliferation (40). In contrast, IL-4 does not block the effector phase of Th2 precursors if they are restimulated via the TCR. It is tempting to speculate that the human Th2 cell subset is homologous to murine CD4$^+$/NK1.1$^+$ T cells, which are present at low frequency in mice, and require costimulatory signals (but not IL-4) to become IL-4 producers (123). This is also suggested by the fact that murine CD4$^+$/NK1.1$^+$ T cells display a skewed expression of TCR-β chains (with Vβ8, Vβ7 and Vβ2 dominating), and therefore these cells (like the human Th2 'precursors') secrete IL-4 upon stimulation by SEB (123). These T-cell subsets may be crucial in the induction phase of Th2 immune responses, since defective IgE production in SJL mice has been linked to the absence of CD4$^+$/NK1.1$^+$ T cells (124).

It should be stressed again that > 99% of naive CD4$^+$ CD45RO$^-$ T cells follow the Th1 pathway by default, if they are costimulated via CD28 and CD3 (40). Under these conditions, the CD28 costimulus strongly increases clonal expansion of the Th1 cells but does not promote Th2 switch. Interestingly, addition of exogenous IL-4 does not affect proliferation, but completely blocks differentiation towards IFN-γ production, and induces massive production of IL-13 and IL-5, but not IL-4 (40). Preliminary data from our lab indicate that, in the presence of IL-4, another signal, unrelated to CD28 and IL-4, has to be provided by accessory cells to induce differentiation of immunologically naive T cells towards IL-4 production. This signal, rather than the one given by binding of B7-2 to CD28 (121, 122), may be responsible for the initiation of IL-4 production (40). Interestingly, this accessory signal is not required to induce IL-4-dependent production of IL-13 and IL-5 (39, 40).

5.3.5.3 CD23/IgE-facilitated Allergen Presentation and Th2 Differentiation

The stimulatory effect of both IL-4 and IL-13 on CD23 expression may have profound effects on the presentation of antigen/allergen via IgE-mediated mechanisms (125). Binding of IgE to CD23 allows non-specific B cells to bind antigen specifically, and to present very low amounts of antigen to antigen-specific T cells. A very recent study has suggested a direct role of IgE-mediated allergen presentation in the induction of lung eosinophilia and Th2 cytokine production (126). Mice immunized and challenged with house dust mite antigen develop lung eosinophilia, associated with the production of IL-4 and IL-5 from lung-purified T cells. Administration of a non-anaphylactogenic anti-IgE mAb (which does not recognize mast cell-bound IgE) before antigen challenge neutralizes serum IgE, but not IgG. Interestingly, the anti-IgE mAb inhibited the recruitment of eosinophils into the lungs and the production of the Th2 cytokines IL-4 and IL-5, but not of the Th1 cytokine IFN-γ, by lung T cells. Studies performed using an anti-CD23 mAb, CD23-deficient or mast cell-deficient mice further suggest that the anti-IgE mAb suppresses eosinophil infiltration and Th2 cytokine production by inhibiting IgE/CD23-facilitated antigen presentation to T cells. Therefore, both IL-4 and IL-13 could indirectly induce Th2 development by increasing CD23 expression and IgE production by B cells, thereby facilitating CD23/IgE-dependent antigen presentation (see also Chapter 3).

5.3.6 Anti-inflammatory Effects of IL-4 and IL-13 on Monocytes

IL-4 and IL-13 play an important role in suppressing inflammatory immune responses by regulating effector functions of monocytes/macrophages (Table 5.1). Both IL-4 and IL-13 strongly inhibit the production of pro-inflammatory cytokines, hematopoietic growth factors and chemokines, including IFN-α, IL-12, IL-1α, IL-1β, IL-6, IL-8, MIP-1α, TNF-α, GM-CSF, G-CSF (6, 7, 30). In contrast, IL-4 and IL-13 increase production of the anti-inflammatory IL-1 receptor antagonist (30, 127). Additional anti-inflammatory effects of IL-4 and IL-13 may relate to their ability to suppress expression of CD14, the receptor for lipopolysaccharide on monocytes (128, 129). The striking suppressive effects of IL-4 and IL-13 on the expression of IL-12 and IFN-α (which reportedly induce Th1 cell differentiation) imply that both cytokines indirectly support Th2 commitment (42–45).

On human monocytes, both IL-4 and IL-13 enhance expression of MHC class II antigens and of several members of the integrin superfamily, including CD11b (Mac1), CD11c, CD18, CD29, and CD49e (very late activation antigen 5; VLA-5), but not of CD11a (LFA-1), CD49b (VLA-2), CD49c (VLA-3), CD49d (VLA-4), and CD49f (VLA-6) (30). The upregulation of adhesion molecules and MHC class II antigens may account for the enhanced antigen presenting capacity of IL-4/IL-13-treated human monocytes (7) and IL-4-treated murine macrophages (130).

IL-4 and IL-13 upregulate CD23 expression on monocytes, whereas they downregulate the expression of CD64 (FcγRI), CD32 (FcγRII), and CD16 (FcγRIII) (30). On murine macrophages, both IL-4 and IL-13 downregulate FcγRs, and IL-4 upregulates CD23 (28). The increased CD23 expression by phagocytes may facilitate presentation of allergen via CD23/IgE-mediated mechanisms as described above for B cells (125).

IL-13, like IL-4, reduces production of nitric oxide (NO) by activated murine macrophages, which correlates with the enhanced *in vitro* survival of the intracellular parasite *Leishmania major* (28, 29). The inhibitory effect may be indirectly mediated through blocking of endogenous TNF-α production, which is required for triggering NO production and cytotoxic function. However, the phagocytic function of activated macrophages appears not to be affected.

In conclusion, both IL-4 and IL-13 suppress the cytotoxic and inflammatory functions of monocytes/macrophages, but do not inhibit their phagocytic potential, and through induction of MHC class II expression they upregulate their potential to present antigen. Furthermore, both IL-4 and IL-13 may indirectly favour Th2 commitment by inhibiting IL-12 and IFN-α production in monocytes.

5.3.7 Modulation of Adhesion Molecules on Mast Cells and Endothelial Cells by IL-4 and IL-13

IL-4 and IL-13 are secreted by activated mast cells and basophils (8, 10), and both cytokines increase expression of the adhesion molecule CD54 (ICAM-1) and decrease expression of CD117 (c-kit), the receptor for stem cell factor (131), on these cells. It is possible that an increased expression of ICAM-1 facilitates inter-action of mast cells with activated leukocytes expressing the CD54 ligand CD11a (LFA-1). Recent data also show that both IL-4 and IL-13 induce adherence of human eosinophils, but not neutrophils, to human umbilical vein endothelial cells (HUVEC) (31, 32). This phenomenon may relate in large part to the ability of IL-4 and IL-13 to selectively induce surface expression of vascular cell adhesion molecule-1 (VCAM-1) on HUVEC, since IL-4/IL-13-induced adhesion can be blocked completely by an anti-VCAM-1 mAb (32). It is possible that IL-4 and IL-13 promote highly selective VCAM-1-dependent accumulation of eosinophils in allergic inflammatory tissues.

5.4 ROLE OF IL-4 AND IL-13 IN ATOPY

There is now increasing evidence that both IL-4 and IL-13 play an important role in IgE-related allergic diseases. *In vivo*, the relative contribution of these cytokines to IgE switching may critically depend on whether the transient expression of CD40L on T cells, and the resulting physical interaction of CD40L-expressing T cells with CD40-expressing B cells coincides with IL-4 or IL-13 production. We have recently shown that uncommitted naive human CD4$^+$ CD45RO$^-$ T cells can differentiate *in vitro* into effector cells secreting large amounts of IL-13 but no IL-4, and that these effectors induce efficient IgE switching of surface IgM$^+$ B cells exclusively via IL-13 (39), suggesting that IL-13 production can have functional consequences. We further observed that human CD4$^+$ CD45RO$^+$ T cells, which contain *in vivo* pre-activated memory T cells capable of producing IL-4, require prolonged activation *in vitro* to develop optimal IgE helper potential (39), and optimal B-cell help coincides with production of IL-13 rather than IL-4 (38, 39). Interestingly, addition of exo-genous IL-4 to CD4$^+$ CD45RO$^+$ T cells increases production of IL-4 and IL-13 to a similar extent, but the total amounts of secreted IL-13 always exceed those of IL-4 (38, 40). These *in vitro* results suggest that IgE switching in response to IL-13 may be a frequent event (see also Chapter 1).

Indeed, it was found that in patients infected with filarial parasites, both polyclonal and antigen-specific IgE and IgG4 responses depend to a similar degree on IL-4 and IL-13 (132). Recombinant filarial parasite proteins recognized by sera from indivi-duals with tissue-invasive filarial infections stimulate the secretion of Th2 rather than Th1 cytokines *in vitro* and induce both polyclonal and antigen-specific IgE/IgG4 responses that can be blocked by a combination of Abs to IL-4 and IL-13. Another study showed that the increased IgE and IgG4 production in patients with nephrotic syndrome is related exclusively to IL-13, since spontaneous IgE and IgG4 production by their peripheral blood mononuclear cells (PBMC) is specifically blocked by anti-IL-13 Abs (133). It is therefore tempting to speculate that the previously described spontaneous, IL-4-independent IgE production by PBMC from atopic individuals also depends on IL-13, rather than on *in vivo* pre-switched IgE memory B cells. Indeed, recent studies demonstrated an increased expression of IL-13 mRNA in the nasal mucosa of patients with perennial allergic rhinitis, but not in chronic infectious rhinitis or in healthy subjects (134). Similarly, a significant enhancement of both IL-13 transcripts and secreted protein can be demonstrated in allergen-challenged bronchoalveolar lavage of asthmatics, but not in saline-challenged asthmatics or allergen-challenged non-asthmatics, and production of IL-13 is higher compared to IL-4 and IL-5 (75). These results altogether suggest that IL-13 may indeed play a role in the regulation of allergen-induced late phase inflammatory responses.

The fact that both Th1 and Th2 cells produce IL-13 and express CD40L (5 and Brinkmann, unpublished) raises the question of how IgE switching in response to IL-13 is controlled *in vivo*. One possibility would be that atopic individuals lack suppressive mechanisms that control IgE switching in non-atopic individuals. Indeed we observed that PBMC from atopic subjects (but not from non-atopics) secrete large amounts of IgE *in vitro* without addition of exogenous IL-4 or IL-13, if both the T- and the B-cell compartment is activated by anti-CD3 and soluble CD40L, respectively (38). Under these conditions, IgE is not produced by *in vivo* pre-switched IgE memory B cells, since IgE production can be blocked by a combination of neutralizing anti-IL-4 plus anti-IL-13 mAbs. Although PBMC from non-atopics do not secrete IgE under these conditions, they produce IL-4, IL-13, and the IgE switching inhibitor IFN-γ with kinetics and at concentrations comparable to PBMC from atopic individuals. Moreover, purified B cells from both donor populations respond comparably to exogenous IL-4 and IL-13 if they are activated by soluble CD40L in the absence of activated T cells. These data imply that in non-atopics IgE switching may be suppressed by an IFN-γ-independent mechanism. It is therefore possible that excessive IgE switching in atopy may result at least in part from a lack of suppression of IL-4/IL-13 action, rather than from an overproduction of these cytokines.

Taken together, our data indicate that activated human CD4$^+$ effector T cells may induce IgE switching largely via IL-13. This implies that the use of antagonists specific for IL-4 will not be sufficient to intervene in IgE-mediated allergic disease. Since IL-4 and IL-13 signal via a common pathway, a drug which abrogates this pathway may provide the most efficient way to block IgE production and therefore may be of therapeutic benefit.

5.5 CONCLUSIONS

The cytokines IL-4 and IL-13 are produced by activated T cells and mast cells/basophils, and display multiple common effects on the immune system. Both IL-4 and IL-13 exert anti-inflammatory actions by inhibiting the production of pro-inflammatory cytokines and chemokines by monocytes/macrophages. Moreover, both cytokines may be crucial to the pathophysiology of allergy and asthma, since they induce IgE switching of B cells, and selectively recruit eosinophils to inflam-matory tissues by inducing the appropriate adhesion molecules on endothelial cells. In striking contrast to IL-4, IL-13 does not act directly on T cells, and therefore may not amplify established Th2 immunity in an autocrine fashion. However, both IL-4 and IL-13 may indirectly drive Th2 cell development by inhibiting macrophage production of IL-12 and IFN-α, cytokines which reportedly induce Th1 cell differ-entiation, and by supporting IgE/CD23-facilitated allergen presentation.

Although both IL-4 and IL-13 were initially classified as Th2 cytokines, it is now clear that their genes can be independently expressed, and that IL-13 is also pro-duced by Th1 cells. Compared to IL-4, IL-13 is produced by activated T cells in larger quantities and for longer periods of time, and effector T cells exist which induce IgE isotype switching of human B cells exclusively via IL-13. The over-lapping biological properties of IL-4 and IL-13 relate to the fact that their receptors share a common component. The IL-4R consists of the IL-4 binding α chain and the common IL-2R γ chain, whereas the IL-13R consists of the IL-4R α chain and a novel IL-13 binding p60–70 subunit. Therefore, IL-4 may signal through both the classical IL-4R (α/γ chain) as well as the IL-13R (α chain/p60–70).

Both IL-4 and IL-13 are involved in IgE-related diseases. An increased expression of IL-13 mRNA has been demonstrated in the nasal mucosa of allergic rhinitis patients and at the sites of allergen challenge in asthmatics. Accordingly, the secretion of IgE by PBMC from atopic individuals has been related to both IL-4 and IL-13. Furthermore, the polyclonal and antigen-specific IgE and IgG4 responses in individuals with tissue-invasive filarial infections depend on IL-4 and IL-13, and the spontaneous IgE production in nephrotic syndrome exclusively depends on IL-13. Altogether these results suggest that IL-13 may play a key role in the regulation of allergen-induced late phase inflammatory responses.

A better understanding of how naive uncommitted T cells differentiate into IL-4 and IL-13-producing T effector cells could help us to design better, perhaps pre-ventive, therapies for IgE-dependent allergic diseases. Future drugs preventing induction of Th2 immunity may target molecules in the cAMP/PKA-dependent signalling pathways. However, suppression of already committed Th2 cells may be achieved best by targeting members of the JAK–STAT signalling pathway (e.g. Stat6), which transduce signals from IL-4/IL-13 receptors on the cell surface to the respective genes in the nucleus.

ACKNOWLEDGEMENTS

We are grateful to P. Lane, Basel Institute for Immunology, Basel, Switzerland, for providing the recombinant CD40L–CD8a fusion protein, and to L. Aarden, Central Laboratory of the Netherlands Red Cross Blood Transfusion Service (CLB),

Amsterdam, The Netherlands, for the monoclonal anti-CD28 Ab CLB-CD28/1. Furthermore we thank our collegues, S. Alkan, J. Bews, G. Bilbe, K. Einsle, C. Heusser, E. Kilchherr, V. Mandak, G. McMaster, and K. Wagner, for providing several mAbs and recombinant cytokines, C. Kristofic and M. Noorani for their excellent technical assistance, and A. Kiefer and M. Wesp for FACS analysis. Furthermore we are grateful to A. Coyle, F. Erard, C. Heusser, and M. Mercep for helpful discussions, and to G. Anderson and G. Bilbe for their comments on the manuscript.

REFERENCES

1. Seder RA and Paul WE (1994) Acquisition of lymphokine-producing phenotype by CD4$^+$ T cells. *Annu Rev Immunol* **12:**635–673.
2. Mosmann TR (1991) Cytokine secretion patterns and cross-regulation of T cell subsets. *Immunol Res* **10:**183–188.
3. Romagnani S (1992) Induction of Th1 and Th2 responses: A key role for natural immune response? *Immunol Today* **13:**379–381.
4. Romagnani S (1994) Lymphokine production by human T cells in disease states. *Annu Rev Immunol* **12:**227–257.
5. De Waal Malefyt R, Abrams JS, Zurawski SM *et al* (1995) Differential regulation of IL-13 and IL-4 production by human CD8$^+$ and CD4$^+$ Th0, Th1, and Th2 cell clones and EBV-transformed B cells. *Int Immunol* **7:**1405–1416.
6. Zurawski G and de Vries JE (1994) Interleukin 13, an interleukin 4-like cytokine that acts on monocytes and B cells, but not on T cells. *Immunol Today* **15:**19–26.
7. De Vries JE and Zurawski G (1995) Immunoregulatory properties of IL-13: its potential role in atopic disease. *Int Arch Allergy Immunol* **106:**175–179.
8. Gordon JR, Burd PR and Galli SJ (1990) Mast cells as a source of multifunctional cytokines. *Immunol Today* **11:**458–464.
9. Aoki I, Kinzer C, Shirai A, Paul WE and Klinman DM (1995) IgE receptor-positive non-B/non-T cells dominate the production of interleukin 4 and interleukin 6 in immunized mice. *Proc Natl Acad Sci USA* **92:**2534–2538.
10. Burd PR, Thompson WC, Max EE and Mills FC (1995) Activated mast cells produce interleukin 13. *J Exp Med* **181:**1373–1380.
11. Bradding P, Roberts JA, Britten KM *et al* (1994) Interleukin-4, -5, and -6 and tumor necrosis factor alpha in normal and asthmatic airways: evidence for the human mast cell as a source of these cytokines. *Am J Respir Cell Mol Biol* **10:**471–480.
12. Nonaka M, Nonaka R, Woolley K *et al* (1995) Distinct immunohistochemical localization of IL-4 in human inflamed airway tissues. IL-4 is localized to eosinophils *in vivo* and is released by peripheral blood eosinophils. *J Immunol* **155:**3234–3244.
13. Cocks BG, de Waal Malefyt R, Galizzi JP, de Vries JE and Aversa G (1993) IL-13 induces proliferation and differentiation of human B cells activated by CD40L. *Int Immunol* **5:**657–663.
14. Punnonen J and de Vries JE (1994) IL-13 induces proliferation, Ig isotype switching, and Ig synthesis by immature human fetal B cells. *J Immunol* **152:**1094–1102.
15. Coffman RL, Ohara J, Bond MW, Carty J, Zlotnik A and Paul WE (1986) B cell stimulatory factor-1 enhances the IgE response of lipopolysaccharide-activated B cells. *J Immunol* **136:**4538-4541.
16. Schultz C and Coffman RL (1991) Control of isotype switching by T cells and cytokines. *Curr Opin Immunol* **3:**350–355.

17. Finkelman FD, Holmes J, Katona IM *et al* (1990) Lymphokine control of *in vivo* immunoglobulin isotype selection. *Annu Rev Immunol* **8**:303–333.

18. Punnonen J, Aversa G, Cocks BG *et al* (1993) Interleukin 13 induces interleukin 4-independent IgG4 and IgE synthesis and CD23 expression by human B cells. *Proc Natl Acad Sci USA* **90**:3730–3735.

19. Brinkmann V and Heusser C (1992) T cell dependent differentiation of human B cells: Direct switch from IgM to IgE, and sequential switch from IgM via IgG to IgA production. *Mol Immunol* **29**:1159–1164.

20. Brinkmann V and Heusser C (1993) T cell dependent differentiation of human B cells into IgM-, IgG-, IgA-, or IgE-plasma cells: high rate of antibody production by IgE plasma cells, but limited clonal expansion of IgE precursors. *Cell Immunol* **152**:323–332.

21. Vercelli D (1993) Regulation of IgE synthesis. *Allergy Proc* **14**:413–416.

22. Powrie F and Coffman RS (1993) Cytokine regulation of T-cell function: potential for therapeutic intervention. *Immunol Today* **14**:270–275.

23. Mosmann TR (1991) Cytokines: is there biological meaning? *Curr Opin Immunol* **3**:311–314.

24. Anderson GP and Brinkmann V (1995) Innovative therapies for asthma: cytokines. In: Leff R (Ed.) *Pulmonary Pharmacology and Therapeutics*. London, New York (in press).

25. Marsh DG, Neely JD, Breazeale DR *et al* (1994) Linkage analysis of IL4 and other chromosome 5q31.1 markers and total serum immunoglobulin E concentrations. *Science* **264**:1152–1156.

26. Levitt RC and Holroyd KL (1995) Fine-structure mapping of the genes providing susceptibility to asthma on chromosome 5q31–q33. *Clin Exp Allergy* **25(Suppl 2)**:119–123.

27. Meyers DA, Xu J, Postma DS, Levitt RC and Bleecker ER (1995) Two locus segregation and linkage analysis for total serum IgE levels. *Clin Exp Allergy* **25(Suppl 2)**:113–115.

28. Doherty TM, Kastelein R, Menon S, Andrade S and Coffman RL (1993) Modulation of murine macrophage function by IL-13. *J Immunol* **150**:5476–5483.

29. Doyle AG, Herbein G, Montaner LJ *et al* (1994) Interleukin-13 alters the activation stage of murine macrophages *in vitro*: comparison with interleukin-4 and interferon-gamma. *Eur J Immunol* **24**:1441–1445.

30. De Waal Malefyt R, Figdor CG, Huijbens R *et al* (1993) Effects of IL-13 on phenotype, cytokine production and cytotoxic function of human monocytes. Comparison with IL-4 and modulation by IFN-γ or IL-10. *J Immunol* **151**:6370–6381.

31. Wardlaw AJ (1993) Eosinophil adhesion receptors. *Behring Inst Mitt* **92**:178–183.

32. Bochner BS, Klunk DA, Sterbinski SA, Coffman RL and Schleimer RP (1995) IL-13 selectively induces vascular cell adhesion molecule-1 expression in human endothelial cells. *J Immunol* **154**:799–803.

33. Lefort S, Vita N, Reeb R, Caput D and Ferrara P (1995) IL-13 and IL-4 share signal transduction elements as well as receptor components in TF1 cells. *FEBS Letters* **336**:122–126.

34. Zurawski SM, Chomarat P, Djossou O *et al* (1995) The primary binding subunit of the human interleukin-4 receptor is also a component of the interleukin-13 receptor. *J Biol Chem* **270**:13869–13878.

35. Callard RE, Matthews DJ and Hibbert L (1996) IL-4 and IL-13 receptors: are they one and the same? *Immunol Today* **17**:108–110.

36. Cherwinski HM, Schumacher JH, Brown KD and Mosmann TR (1987) Two types of mouse T cell clone. III. Further differences in lymphokine synthesis between Th1 and Th2 clones revealed by RNA hybridization, functionally monospecific bioassays, and monoclonal antibodies. *J Exp Med* **166**:1229–1244.

37. Brown KD, Zurawski SM, Mosmann TR and Zurawski G (1989) A family of small inducible proteins secreted by leukocytes are members of a new superfamily that induces

leukocyte and fibroblast-derived inflammatory agents, growth factors, and indicators of various activation processes. *J Immunol* **142**:679–685.

38. Levy F, Kristofic C, Heusser C and Brinkmann V (1997) Role of IL-13 in CD4 T cell-dependent IgE production in atopy. *Int Arch Allergy Immunol* 112:49–58.

39. Brinkmann V and Kristofic C (1995) TCR-stimulated naive human CD4$^+$ 45RO$^-$ T cells develop into effector cells that secrete IL-13, IL-5, and IFN-γ, but not IL-4, and help efficient IgE production by B cells. *J Immunol* **154**:3078–3087.

40. Brinkmann V, Kinzel B and Kristofic C (1996) TCR-independent activation of human CD4$^+$ CD45RO$^-$ T cells by anti-CD28 plus IL-2: induction of clonal expansion and priming for a Th2 phenotype. *J Immunol* **156**:4100–4106.

41. Le Gros G, Ben Sasson SZ, Seder R, Finkelman FD and Paul WE (1990) Generation of IL-4-producing cells *in vivo* and *in vitro*: IL-2 and IL-4 are required for the *in vitro* generation of IL-4 producing cells. *J Exp Med* **172**:921–929.

42. Demeure CE, Wu CY, Shu U *et al* (1994) *In vitro* maturation of human neonatal CD4 T lymphocytes. II. Cytokines present at priming modulate the development of lymphokine production. *J Immunol* **152**:4775–4782.

43. Peleman R, Wu J, Fargeas C and Delespesse G (1989) Recombinant interleukin 4 suppresses the production of interferon γ by human mononuclear cells. *J Exp Med* **170**:1751–1756.

44. Trinchieri G (1993) Interleukin-12 and its role in the generation of Th1 cells. *Immunol Today* **14**:335–339.

45. Brinkmann V, Geiger T, Alkan S and Heusser C (1993) IFN-α increases the frequency of IFN-γ-producing human CD4-positive T cells. *J Exp Med* **178**:1655–1663.

46. Levitt RC, Eleff SM, Zhang LY, Kleeberger SR and Ewart SL (1995) Linkage homology for bronchial hyperresponsiveness between DNA markers on human chromosome 5q31–q33 and mouse chromosome 13. *Clin Exp Allergy* **25(Suppl 2)**:61–63.

47. Arai N, Nomura D, Villaret D *et al* (1989) Complete nucleotide sequence of the chromosomal gene for human IL-4 and its expression. *J Immunol* **142**:274–282.

48. Smirnov DV, Smirnova MG, Korobko VG and Frolova EI (1995) Tandem arrangement of human genes for interleukin-4 and interleukin-13: resemblance in their organization. *Gene* **155**:277–281.

49. Seger R and Krebs EG (1995) The MAPK signalling cascade. *FASEB J* **9**:726–735.

50. Abe E, de Waal Malefyt R, Matsuda I, Arai K and Arai N (1992) An 11-base-pair DNA sequence motif apparently unique to the human interleukin 4 gene confers responsiveness to T-cell activation signals. *Proc Natl Acad Sci USA* **89**:2864–2868.

51. Szabo SJ, Gold JS, Murphy TL and Murphy KM (1993) Identification of *cis* regulatory elements controlling interleukin-4 gene expression in T cells: roles for NF-Y and NF-ATc. *Mol Cell Biol* **13**:4793–4805.

52. Rao A (1994) NF-ATp: a transcription factor required for the coordinate induction of several cytokine genes. *Immunol Today* **15**:274–281.

53. Rooney JW, Hodge MR, McCaffrey PG, Rao A and Glimcher LH (1994) A common factor regulates both Th1- and Th2-specific cytokine gene expression. *EMBO J* **13**:625–633.

54. Naora H, Altin JG and Young IG (1994) TCR-dependent and -independent signaling mechanisms differentially regulate lymphokine gene expression in the murine T helper clone D10.G4.1. *J Immunol* **152**:5691–5702.

55. Hama N, Paliogianni F, Fessler BJ and Boumpas DT (1995) Calcium/calmodulin-dependent protein kinase II downregulates both calcineurin and protein kinase C-mediated pathways for cytokine gene transcription in human T cells. *J Exp Med* **181**:1217–1222.

56. Cook SJ and McCormick F (1993) Two major signal pathways linked. *Science* **262**:988–990.

57. Casolaro V, Georas SN, Song Z et al (1995) Inhibition of NF-AT-dependent transcription by NF-κB: Implications for differential gene expression in T helper cell subsets. Proc Natl Acad Sci 92:11623–11627.

58. Ito CY, Kazantsev AG and Baldwin AS (1994) Three NF-κB sites in the IκB-α promoter are required for induction of gene expression by TNF-α. Nucleic Acids Res 22:3787–3792.

59. Diaz-Meco MT, Dominguez I, Sanz L et al (1994) ζ PKC induces phosphorylation and inactivation of IκB-α in vitro. EMBO J 13:2842-2848.

60. Hoyos B, Ballard DW, Bohnlein E, Siekevitz M and Greene W (1989) κ-specific DNA binding proteins: role in the regulation of human interleukin-2 gene expression. Science 244:457–460.

61. Lederer JA, Liou JS, Todd MD, Glimcher LH and Lichtman AH (1994) Regulation of cytokine gene expression in T helper cell subsets. J Immunol 152:77–86.

62. Cook SJ and McCormick F (1993) Inhibition by cAMP of Ras-dependent activation of Raf. Science 262:1069–1072.

63. Neumann M, Grieshammer T, Chuvpilo S et al (1995) RelA/p65 is a molecular target for the immunosuppressive action of protein kinase A. EMBO J 14:1991–2004.

64. Kang SM, Tran AC, Grilli M and Lenardo MJ (1992) NF-κB subunit regulation in nontransformed CD4+ T lymphocytes. Science 256:1452–1456.

65. Munoz E, Zubiaga AM, Merrow M, Sauter NP and Huber BT (1990) Cholera toxin discriminates between T helper 1 and 2 cells in T cell receptor-mediated activation: role of cAMP in T cell proliferation. J Exp Med 172:95–103.

66. Munoz E, Zubiaga AM, Munoz J and Huber BT (1990) Regulation of IL-4 lymphokine gene expression and cellular proliferation in murine T helper type II cells. Cell Regul 1:425–434.

67. Watanabe S, Yssel H, Harada Y and Arai K (1994) Effects of prostaglandin E2 on Th0-type human T cell clones: modulation of functions of nuclear proteins involved in cytokine production. Int Immunol 6:523–532.

68. Garrone P, Galibert L, Rousset F, Fu SM and Banchereau J (1994) Regulatory effects of prostaglandin E2 on the growth and differentiation of human B lymphocytes activated through their CD40 antigen. J Immunol 152:4282–4290.

69. Davydov IV, Bohmann D, Krammer PH and Li-Weber M (1995) Cloning of the cDNA encoding C/EBPγ, a protein binding to the PRE-I enhancer of the human interleukin-4 promoter. Gene 161:271–275.

70. Li-Weber M, Eder A, Krafft-Czepa H and Krammer PH (1992) T-cell specific negative regulation of transcription of the human cytokine IL-4. J Immunol 148:1913–1918.

71. Hodge MR, Rooney JW and Glimcher LH (1995) The proximal promoter of the IL-4 gene is composed of multiple essential regulatory sites that bind at least two distinct factors. J Immunol 154:6397–6405.

72. Staynov DZ, Cousins DJ and Lee TH (1995) A regulatory element in the promoter of the human granulocyte–macrophage colony-stimulating factor gene that has related sequences in other T-cell-expressed cytokine genes. Proc Natl Acad Sci USA 92:3606–3610.

73. Henkel G, Weiss DL, McCoy R, Deloughery T, Tara D and Brown MA (1992) A DNase I hypersensitive site in the second intron of the murine IL-4 gene defines a mast cell-specific enhancer. J Immunol 149:3239–3246.

74. Brinkmann V and Kristofic C (1995) Regulation by corticosteroids of Th1 and Th2 cytokine production in human CD4+ effector T cells generated from CD45RO− and CD45RO+ subsets. J Immunol 155:3322–3328.

75. Huang SK, Xiao HQ, Kleine-Tebbe J et al (1995) IL-13 expression at the sites of allergen challenge in patients with asthma. J Immunol 155:2688–2694.

76. Kay AB, Ying S and Durham SR (1995) Phenotype of cells positive for interleukin-4 and interleukin-5 mRNA in allergic tissue reactions. Int Arch Allergy Immunol 107:208–210.

77. Gauchat JF, Henchoz S, Mazzei G et al (1993) Induction of human IgE synthesis in B cells by mast cells and basophils. *Nature* **365**:340–343.
78. Gauchat JF, Henchoz S, Fattah D et al (1995) CD40 ligand is functionally expressed on human eosinophils. *Eur J Immunol* **25**:863–868.
79. Renard N, Duvert V, Banchereau J and Saeland S (1994) Interleukin-13 inhibits the proliferation of normal and leukemic human B-cell precursors. *Blood* **84**:2253–2260.
80. Lin JX, Migone TS, Tsang M et al (1995) The role of shared receptor motifs and common Stat proteins in the generation of cytokine pleiotropy and redundancy by IL-2, IL-4, IL-7, IL-13, and IL-15. *Immunity* **2**:331–339.
81. Zurawski SM, Vega F, Huyghe B and Zurawski G (1993) Receptors for interleukin-13 and interleukin-4 are complex and share a novel component that functions in signal transduction. *EMBO J* **12**:2663–2670.
82. Vita N, Lefort S, Laurent P, Caput D and Ferrara P (1995) Characterization and comparison of the interleukin 13 receptor with the interleukin 4 receptor on several cell types. *J Biol Chem* **270**:3512–3517.
83. Obiri NI, Debinski W, Leonard WJ and Puri RK (1995) Receptor for interleukin 13. Interaction with interleukin 4 by a mechanism that does not involve the common γ chain shared by receptors for interleukins 2, 4, 7, 9, and 15. *J Biol Chem* **270**:8797–8804.
84. He YW and Malek TR (1995) The IL-2 receptor γ chain does not function as a subunit shared by the IL-4 and IL-13 receptors. Implication for the structure of the IL-4 receptor. *J Immunol* **155**:9–12.
85. Obiri NI and Puri RK (1994) Characterization of interleukin-4 receptors expressed on human renal cell carcinoma cells. *Oncol Res* **6**:419–427.
86. Schindler, C (1995) Transcriptional responses to polypeptide ligands: The JAK–STAT pathway. *Annu Rev Biochem* **64**:621–651.
87. Hou J, Schindler U, Henzel WJ, Ho TC, Brasseur M and McKnight SL (1994) An interleukin-4-induced transcription factor: IL-4 Stat. *Science* **265**:1701–1706.
88. Welham MJ, Learmonth L, Bone H and Schrader JW (1995) Interleukin-13 signal transduction in lymphohemopoietic cells. Similarities and differences in signal transduction with interleukin-4 and insulin. *J Biol Chem* **270**:12286–12296.
89. Schindler C, Kashleva H, Pernis A, Pine R and Rothman P (1994) STF-IL-4: a novel IL-4-induced signal transducing factor. *EMBO J* **13**:1350–1356.
90. Delphin S and Stavnezer J (1995) Characterization of an interleukin 4 (IL-4) responsive region in the immunoglobulin heavy chain germline ε promoter: regulation by NF-IL-4, a C/EBP family member and NF-κB/p50. *J Exp Med* **181**:181–192.
91. Erard F, Wild MT, Garcia-Sanz JA and Le Gros G (1993) Switch of CD8 T cells to noncytolytic CD8$^-$ CD4$^-$ cells that make Th2 cytokines and help B cells. *Science* **260**:1802–1805.
92. Kohler I, Alliger P, Minty A et al (1994) Human interleukin-13 activates the interleukin-4-dependent transcription factor NF-IL4 sharing a DNA binding motif with an interferon-γ-induced nuclear binding factor. *FEBS Letters* **345**:187–192.
93. Fenghao X, Saxon A, Nguyen A, Ke Z, Diaz-Sanchez D and Nel A (1995) Interleukin 4 activates a signal transducer and activator of transcription (Stat) protein which interacts with an interferon-γ activation site-like sequence upstream of the Iε exon in a human B cell line. Evidence for the involvement of Janus kinase 3 and interleukin-4 Stat. *J Clin Invest* **96**:907–914.
94. Meraz MA, White M, Sheelan CF et al (1996) Targeted disruption of the STAT1 gene in mice reveals unexpected physiologic specificity in the JAK–STAT pathway. *Cell* **84**:431–442.
95. Bacon CM, Petricoin EF, Ortaldo JR et al (1995) Interleukin 12 induces tyrosine phosphorylation and activation of STAT4 in human lymphocytes. *Proc Natl Acad Sci USA* **92**:7307–7311.

96. Quelle FW, Shimoda K, Thierfelder W *et al* (1995) Cloning of murine Stat6 and human Stat6, Stat proteins that are tyrosine phosphorylated in responses to IL-4 and IL-3 but are not required for mitogenesis. *Mol Cell Biol* **15**:3336–3343.

97. Danial NN, Pernis A and Rothman PB (1995) Jak–STAT signaling induced by the v-abl oncogene. *Science* **269**:1875–1877.

98. Pernis A, Witthuhn B, Keegan AD *et al* (1995) Interleukin 4 signals through two related pathways. *Proc Natl Acad Sci USA* **92**:7971–7975.

99. Keegan AD, Johnston JA, Tortolani PJ *et al* (1995) Similarities and differences in signal transduction by interleukin 4 and interleukin 13: analysis of Janus kinase activation. *Proc Natl Acad Sci USA* **92**:7681–7685.

100. Sun XJ, Wang L-M, Zhang Y *et al* (1995) Role of IRS-2 in insulin and cytokine signalling. *Nature* **377**:173–177.

101. Yin T, Tsang MLS and Yang YC (1994) JAK1 kinase forms complexes with interleukin-4 receptor and 4PS/insulin receptor substrate-1-like protein and is activated by interleukin-4 and interleukin-9 in T lymphocytes. *J Biol Chem* **269**:26614–26617.

102. Wang LM, Keegan AD, Paul WE, Heidaran MA, Gutkind JS and Pierce JH (1992) IL-4 activates a distinct signal transduction cascade from IL-3 in factor-dependent myeloid cells. *EMBO J* **11**:4899–4908.

103. Schneider H, Cai Y-C, Prasad KVS, Shoelson SE and Rudd CE (1995) T cell antigen CD28 binds to the GRB-2-SOS complex, regulators of p21(ras). *Eur J Immunol* **25**:1044–1050.

104. Wortis HH, Teutsch M, Higer M, Zheng J and Parker DC (1995) B-cell activation by crosslinking of surface IgM or ligation of CD40 involves alternative signal pathways and results in different B-cell phenotypes. *Proc Natl Acad Sci USA* **92**:3348–3352.

105. McKenzie ANJ, Culpepper JA, de Waal Malefyt R *et al* (1993) Interleukin 13, a T-cell-derived cytokine that regulates human monocyte and B cell function. *Proc Natl Acad Sci USA* **90**:3735–3739.

106. Defrance T, Carayon P, Billian G *et al* (1994) Interleukin 13 is a B cell stimulating factor. *J Exp Med* **179**:135–143.

107. Shapira SK, Vercelli D, Jabara HH, Fu SM and Geha RS (1992) Molecular analysis of the induction of immunoglobulin E synthesis in human B cells by interleukin 4 and engagement of CD40 antigen. *J Exp Med* **175**:289–292.

108. Punnonen J, Cocks BG and de Vries JE (1995) IL-4 induces germline IgE heavy chain gene transcription in human fetal pre-B cells. *J Immunol* **155**:4248–4254.

109. Fuleihan R, Ramesh N and Geha RS (1993) Role of CD40–CD40L interaction in Ig isotype switching. *Curr Opin Immunol* **5**:963–967.

110. Roy M, Waldschmidt T, Aruffo A, Ledbetter JA and Noelle RJ (1993) The regulation of the expression of gp39, the CD40 ligand, on normal and cloned CD4$^+$ T cells. *J Immunol* **151**:2497–2510.

111. Callard RE, Armitage RJ, Fanslow WC and Spriggs MK (1993) CD40L and its role in X-linked hyper IgM syndrome. *Immunol Today* **14**:559–564.

112. Life P, Gauchat JF, Schnuringer V *et al* (1994) T cell clones from an X-linked hyper-IgM patient induce IgE synthesis *in vitro* despite expression of nonfunctional CD40 ligand. *J Exp Med* **180**:1775–1784.

113. Del Prete G, De Carli M, D'Elios MM *et al* (1994) Polyclonal B cell activation induced by herpesvirus saimiri-transformed human CD4$^+$ T cell clones. Role of membrane TNF-α/TNF-α receptors and CD2/CD58 interactions. *J Immunol* **153**:4872–4879.

114. Defrance T, Aubry JP, Rousset F *et al* (1987) Human recombinant interleukin 4 induces Fcε receptors (CD23) on normal human B lymphocytes. *J Exp Med* **165**:1459–1465.

115. Von der Weid T, Kopf M, Kohler G and Langhorne J (1994) The immune response to *Plasmodium chabaudi* malaria in interleukin-4-deficient mice. *Eur J Immunol* **24**:2285–2293.

116. Maliszewski CR, Sato TA, Davison B, Jacobs CA, Finkelman FD and Fanslow WC (1994) *in vivo* biological effects of recombinant soluble interleukin-4 receptor. *Proc Soc Exp Biol Med* **206**:233–237.

117. Paganelli R, Scala E, Ansotegui IJ *et al* (1995) CD8$^+$ T lymphocytes provide helper activity for IgE synthesis in human immunodeficiency virus-infected patients with hyper-IgE. *J Exp Med* **181**:423–428.

118. Kopf M, Le Gros G, Coyle AJ, Kosco Vilbois M and Brombacher F (1995) Immune responses of IL-4, IL-5, IL-6 deficient mice. *Immunol Rev* **148**:45–69.

119. Kelso A (1995) Th1 and Th2 subsets: Paradigm lost? *Immunol Today* **16**:374–379.

120. June CH, Bluestone JA, Nadler JM and Thompson CB (1994) The B7 and CD28 receptor families. *Immunol Today* **15**:321–324.

121. Freeman GJ, Boussiotis VA, Anumanthan A *et al* (1995) B7-1 and B7-2 do not deliver identical co-stimulatory signals, since B7-2 but not B7-1 preferentially co-stimulates the initial production of IL-4. *Immunity* **2**:523–528.

122. Kuchroo VK, Das MP, Brown JA *et al* (1995) B7-1 and B7-2 co-stimulatory molecules activate differentially the Th1/Th2 developmental pathways: application to autoimmune disease therapy. *Cell* **80**:707–712.

123. Yoshimoto T and Paul WE (1994) CD4$^+$, NK1.1 + T cells promptly produce interleukin 4 in response to *in vivo* challenge with anti-CD3. *J Exp Med* **179**:1285–1290.

124. Yoshimoto T, Bendelac A, Hu-Li J and Paul WE (1995) Defective IgE production by SJL mice is linked to the absence of CD4$^+$ NK1.1 + T cells that promptly produce interleukin 4. *Proc Natl Acad Sci USA* **92**:11931–11934.

125. Mudde GC, Bheekha R and Bruijnzeel-Koomen CAFM (1995) Consequences of IgE/CD23-mediated antigen presentation in allergy. *Immunol Today* **16**:380–383.

126. Coyle AJ, Wagner K, Bertrand C, Tsuyuki S, Bews J and Heusser C (1996) Central role of IgE in the induction of lung eosinophil infiltration and Th2 cytokine production: Inhibition of a non-anaphylactogenic anti-IgE antibody. *J Exp Med* **183**:1303–1310.

127. Minty A, Chalon P, Derocq JM *et al* (1993) Interleukin-13 is a new human lymphokine regulating inflammatory and immune responses. *Nature* **362**:248–250.

128. Viale G and Vercelli D (1995) Interleukin-13 regulates the phenotype and function of human monocytes. *Int Arch Allergy Immunol* **107**:176–178.

129. Cosentino G, Soprana E, Thienes CP, Siccardi AG, Viale G and Vercelli D (1995) IL-13 down-regulates CD14 expression and TNF-α secretion in normal human monocytes. *J Immunol* **155**:3145–3151.

130. Zlotnik A, Fischer M, Roehm N and Zipori D (1987) Evidence for effects of interleukin 4 (B cell stimulatory factor 1) on macrophages: enhancement of antigen presenting ability of bone marrow-derived macrophages. *J Immunol* **138**:4275–4279.

131. Nilsson G and Nilsson K (1995) Effects of interleukin (IL)-13 on immediate–early response gene expression, phenotype and differentiation of human mast cells. Comparison with IL-4. *Eur J Immunol* **25**:870–873.

132. Garraud O, Nkenfou C, Bradley JE, Perler FB and Nutman TB (1995) Identification of recombinant filarial proteins capable of inducing polyclonal and antigen-specific IgE and IgG4 antibodies. *J Immunol* **155**:1316–1325.

133. Kimata H, Fujimoto M and Furusho K (1995) Involvement of IL-13, but not IL- 4, in spontaneous IgE and IgG4 production in nephrotic syndrome. *Eur J Immunol* **25**:1497–1501.

134. Pawankar RU, Okuda M, Hasegawa S *et al* (1995) Interleukin 13 expression in the nasal mucosa of perennial allergic rhinitis. *Am J Respir Med* **152**:2059–2067.

6 The IL-4 Promoter in Mast Cells and T Cells

MELISSA A. BROWN

Department of Experimental Pathology, Emory University School of Medicine, Atlanta GA, USA

6.1 INTRODUCTION

Interleukin (IL)-4 is a multifunctional cytokine that has been implicated in a variety of immune and developmental processes (1, 2). Among the myriad of activities ascribed to IL-4 based on *in vitro* functional assays, the regulation of T helper (Th) cell development and immunoglobulin (Ig) E production are examples of those that have been confirmed in *in vivo* studies. Because IL-4 plays an important immunoregulatory role, dysregulation in the production of this cytokine has pathological consequences resulting in the inability to resolve certain types of infections, autoimmune responses and allergic reactions. Not surprisingly, the production of IL-4 is very restricted and highly regulated. Only a subset of T cells, cells of the mast cell/ basophil lineage and most recently, eosinophils, have been demonstrated to express IL-4 (reviewed in (1)). Due to differences in tissue distribution, IL-4 produced by T cells or mast cells may act locally upon different subsets of target cells. Thus T-cell derived and mast-cell derived IL-4 may lead to entirely distinct or only partially overlapping physiological responses.

All IL-4-producing cell types require activation to produce easily detectable amounts of this cytokine. Stimulation-dependent expression is transient: peak levels are detected in normal peripheral blood T cells 6 hours post-activation and quickly diminish (3). In T- and mast-cell lines, the kinetics of mRNA appearance vary, but the increase is due in part to the initiation of new transcription in stimulated cells (4, 5). In mast cells and basophils there is low level constitutive production of IL-4 mRNA and protein. Cell activation increases the transcriptional activity of the IL-4 gene and stimulates the release of preformed IL-4 which is stored in granules (6–9).

6.2 CELL SURFACE SIGNALS THAT MODULATE IL-4 EXPRESSION

The identification of signaling intermediates that lead to IL-4 expression will allow the development of strategies to manipulate its expression in a cell-specific way. The

IgE Regulation: Molecular Mechanisms. Edited by D. Vercelli. © 1997 John Wiley & Sons Ltd.

challenge in studies of IL-4 gene regulation is to define the signals that regulate IL-4 production in different cell populations. Towards that end, there has been an intensive study of the cell surface signals that lead to IL-4 production in T cells, mast cells and basophils. In several T cell clones/lines, cross-linkage of the T-cell antigen receptor (TCR) or treatment with calcium ionophore is sufficient to initiate transcription. Costimulatory signals such as those delivered through the interaction of CD28 on T cells with B7 molecules expressed on antigen presenting cells (or CD40/CD40 ligand (CD40L), as discussed below) also influence IL-4 gene expression. These signals, which can be replaced by phorbol ester treatment, appear to be required for expression in *in vivo*-derived cell populations (10, 11). Mast cells and basophils are activated through the interaction of IgE-antigen complexes with high affinity Fcε receptors (FcεRI). Interaction of the complement component, C5a, or the bacterially-derived peptide, *N*-formyl-Met-Leu-Phe (FMLP), with basophils also induces secretion of this cytokine, indicating an antigen-independent mechanism for IL-4 production (13). An absolute requirement for costimulatory signals does not appear to be necessary in FcεRI$^+$ cells.

The interaction of CD40L on T cells with the CD40 counter-receptor on B cells can generate critical signals in addition to those delivered by IL-4, resulting in IgE isotype switching (reviewed in (14, 15)). It was recently demonstrated that antigen presentation by B cells preferentially induces a Th2 response. This response was blocked by addition of anti-CD40 antibodies to the culture (16). The implications of these data are two-fold. First, they suggest that CD40–CD40L interaction can signal a cell to express IL-4. Furthermore, they highlight the importance of signals delivered to the T cell in cognate B and T cell interaction, signals favoring a T-cell response that augments antibody production by B cells. Mast cells and basophils also express CD40L and can induce IgE production *in vitro* (17). It has been speculated that although most Ig isotype switching occurs in lymph node germinal centers, FcεRI$^+$ cells can influence IgE antibody production in sites such as the skin and lung where mast cells are prevalent. The potential role of CD40–CD40L in directly influencing IL-4 production by both T cells and FcεRI$^+$ cells *in vivo* is one of extreme interest that deserves further study (see also Chapters 2 and 5).

6.2.1 Early Cytoplasmic Signals Delivered by the TCR and FcεRI: Similarities and Differences

The T-cell antigen receptor and FcεRI recognize very different molecular complexes and thus are distinct with respect to their extracellular structure and function. However, there are striking similarities in their cytoplasmic domains and many of the early signaling events that occur in response to FcεRI cross-linking resemble those triggered by antigen–major histocompatibility complex (MHC) interaction with the T-cell receptor (reviewed in (18, 19)). These include activation of src family kinases (lck and fyn in T cells versus lyn in mast cells), phosphorylation of conserved ARAM (Immunoreceptor Tyrosine-based Activation Motif, ITAM) motifs within the cytoplasmic domains of both receptors, involvement of ZAP 70 family kinases

(ZAP70 in T cells and syk in mast cells), activation of PLCγ1, and increase in free Ca^{2+} due to release from intracellular stores as well as an extracellular Ca^{2+} influx. The increase in intracellular calcium concentration in T cells activates the Ca^{2+}-dependent phosphatase, calcineurin. Calcineurin regulates the DNA-binding activity of transcription factors involved in IL-2 gene regulation and thus provides a link to nuclear regulatory events (20, 21). Calcineurin likely has a role in regulating transcription factors involved in IL-4 gene transcription as well (22, 23).

6.2.2 Nuclear Events that Regulate Transcription

The nuclear proteins that associate with specific DNA sequences are the final targets of signals that initiate at the cell surface leading to IL-4 transcription. Studies of transcriptional regulation, though minimized by some as mere 'promoter bashing', are key to delineating the signals that control the cell-specific and transient expression of IL-4 and provide the necessary link with more membrane proximal signals. Many of the earlier signaling events occur within seconds or minutes, thus providing only a small window through which to examine them. In contrast, indicators of nuclear activation are relatively stable and methods to assay them are fairly straightforward. If one is aware of the constraints of reporter gene assays and *in vitro* binding assays (where influences conferred by chromatin context are removed), much information can be gained to initially delineate *cis*- and *trans*-acting regulatory elements.

The regulation of a gene at the transcriptional level is generally mediated by the interplay of multiple *trans*-acting factors that interact with specific *cis*-acting DNA elements (reviewed in (24)). It is the unique combination of ubiquitous and relatively cell-restricted factors that confer cell type-specific transcriptional activity (25). These factors can be either synthesized *de novo* or modulated to an 'active' form by intracellular signal transduction pathways. It has been demonstrated that interactions of several positive *cis*- and *trans*-acting elements are necessary to provide sufficient stability to the basal transcription complex to mediate transcription. Conversely, negative elements may destabilize a complex and reduce activity (26, 27). The goals of transcriptional analysis of a regulated gene are to: (1) define the DNA sequences that serve as specific binding sites for transcription factors; (2) identify the transcription factors, including those that directly bind DNA and those that associate with other proteins solely through protein–protein interactions; and (3) determine the mechanism through which these transcription factors are activated by cell stimulation to initiate or increase transcription. In the case of polarized Th cytokine responses, for example, the ultimate challenge is to understand how very similar cytoplasmic signaling events initiated at the cell surface through the TCR can lead to distinct patterns of gene expression.

Studies to date have indicated that regulation of the IL-4 gene can serve as a paradigm for transcriptional regulation: the gene contains positive and negative elements that associate with both cell-restricted and ubiquitous factors to regulate transcriptional activity.

6.3 REGULATORY ELEMENTS OF THE IL-4 GENE DEFINED IN T CELLS

The majority of information regarding IL-4 transcriptional control elements has come from studies of T cells. An analysis of tissues from transgenic mice containing IL-4 5′ sequences fused to the herpes thymidine kinase (tk) gene revealed that sequences within 3 kb of the transcription initiation site (TIS, conventionally designated + 1) are sufficient to promote T cell-specific and activation-dependent transcription in a manner that parallels IL-4 gene expression *in vivo* (28). Studies in both human and murine T cell lines using reporter gene constructs in transient transfection assays have defined some of the elements involved (5, 28–35). In these assays, the ability of defined segments of putative IL-4 regulatory regions to drive expression of a linked reporter gene such as chloramphenicol acetyltransferase (CAT) or luciferase is assayed. Multiple elements are active in such assays demonstrating the complexity of IL-4 regulation (Figure 6.1). Those most critical for activation- and cell-specific expression are located quite proximal to the IL-4 promoter. A negative regulatory element defined in the human gene and a distal element located over 5 kb from the TIS, likely modulate the rate of transcription.

Several laboratories, including our own, have concentrated on the analysis of sequences within − 87 base pairs of the TIS (3, 31, 32, 36, 37). There are several reasons why this region is of interest. First, these sequences are sufficient to mediate cell-specific transcription of a linked reporter gene. Second, within this region is an element we have termed the ARE (activation responsive element) that is required for transcriptional activity in response to T-cell activation signals. This finding suggests that the ARE provides a critical nuclear link with the signals initiated through antigen interaction with the TCR (5, 29).

The murine sequences comprising the ARE were first defined in the EL-4 T-cell line (5, 30). Results were subsequently confirmed by us and others in antigen-specific T-cell lines (5, 31, 38). Using constructs containing progressive 5′ deletions of the IL-4 upstream regulatory region, it was observed that − 87 IL-4/CAT (− 87 to + 5), but not − 70 IL-4/CAT, drove reporter gene expression in EL-4 cells stimulated with phorbol esters. These results indicate that sequences between − 87 and − 70 are critical. Mutagenesis studies suggest that the most important nucleotides lie between − 79 and − 69, and comprise an element termed P1. These nucleotides conform to a consensus sequence, ATTTTCCNNTG, that is present in four additional locations within 250 base pairs of the murine IL-4 promoter (termed P0–P4: Figure 6.1). Although mutation of P0, P2, P3, or P4, in the context of a larger reporter gene construct, decreases the level of stimulation-dependent transcription, these elements cannot compensate for the loss of complete activity conferred by mutations within the P1 element. Thus, P1 plays an essential role. As discussed below, these sites also share identity with an element that regulates IL-2 gene transcription.

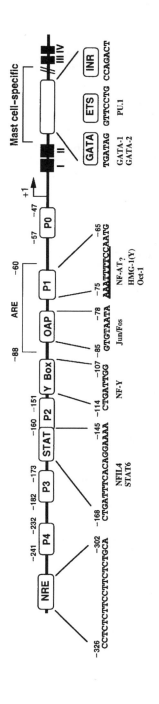

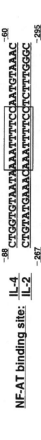

Figure 6.1. Multiple elements contribute to IL-4 gene transcription. (Top) DNA elements defined in the murine IL-4 gene are denoted by boxes [coordinates and sequences listed below are expressed relative to the TIS (+1)]. Previously described transcription factors that can bind to these regions *in vitro* are listed below. The NF-AT? designation reflects the uncertainty regarding the NF-AT family member involved in IL-4 transcription. (Bottom) Sequence comparison of the murine IL-4 ARE and the IL-2 distal NF-AT binding site

6.3.1 Identification of Protein Factors that Regulate ARE-mediated IL-4 Gene Transcription in T Cells

A model for transcriptional activation of the IL-4 gene was developed based on our studies of the proteins that bind to the ARE (Figure 6.2). Using electrophoretic mobility shift assays (EMSA), which assess the ability of transcription factors to specifically bind to a radiolabeled DNA probe and retard its mobility in a native gel, it was observed that proteins in the nucleus of both unstimulated and stimulated T cells could form specific DNA–protein complexes. Cell-activation signals result in a complex of reduced mobility, suggesting the association of 'stimulation-dependent' proteins with the pre-existing complex. UV cross-linking and mutagenesis studies support the idea that similar proteins are present in both the constitutive and inducible complexes. Thus some of the factors necessary for transcriptional activation are pre-existing and available for binding in unstimulated cells. Stimulation induces the binding of additional proteins either through new synthesis or activation via post-translational modification.

Most of the IL-4 ARE-associated proteins have not been identified. However, factors belonging to two well-studied transcription factor families, activator protein-1 (AP-1) and nuclear factor of activated T cells (NF-AT), appear to be involved. Surprisingly, these are also key components of the transcription of other cytokine genes, including IL-2, a hallmark Th1 cytokine. IL-2 and IL-4 are often expressed reciprocally in a polarized Th response. Thus, it was rather unexpected to find that the inducible expression of both genes may be regulated by the same transcription factors. As described below, the discovery of multiple NF-AT and AP-1 family members, all of which can bind with some affinity *in vitro*, raises the possibility that different gene-specific family members operate *in vivo*.

6.3.2 NF-AT: A Family of Transcription Factors with Gene-specific Roles in Cytokine Gene Regulation?

NF-AT was initially described as a transcription factor that binds to two separate sites within the IL-2 gene 5′ region (termed NF-AT binding sites) and regulates IL-2 gene expression (39). The first studies detected NF-AT only in the nucleus of activated T cells. Further analysis by several laboratories provided the initial framework for a model of NF-AT regulation and assembly of an active transcription complex leading to IL-2 gene transcription (20, 21). According to this model, NF-AT is a constitutive phosphoprotein that is sequestered in the cytoplasm of unstimulated cells. T-cell activation signals that trigger increases in intracellular calcium result in the activation of calcineurin, a calcium-dependent phosphatase. NF-AT is a direct substrate of calcineurin (40) and its dephosphorylation leads to translocation of this factor to the nucleus where it can bind DNA. In addition, these early TCR-mediated signals activate protein kinase C, initiating events which induce the *de novo* synthesis of transcription factors of the AP-1 family (20). It is this combination of AP-1 and NF-AT factors that form the minimal active NF-AT complex. Thus, the events leading to

109

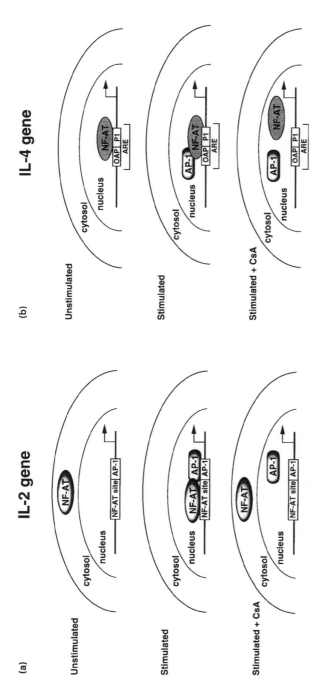

Figure 6.2. A comparative model of IL-4 and IL-2 gene regulation by NF-AT/AP-1 at the IL-4 ARE and IL-2 NF-AT binding sites. Unlike the IL-2 gene factor, IL-4 NF-AT is not sequestered in the cytoplasm of unstimulated cells and thus can bind the P1 site constitutively. Cell activation results in the association of proteins synthesized *de novo*, including members of the AP-1 family of transcription factors. As observed in studies of IL-2 gene regulation, it is this DNA–protein complex that forms the minimal active IL-4 gene transcription complex. The action of CSA on the IL-4 and IL-2 DNA–protein complexes is distinct. CSA inhibits binding of proteins to both complexes. However, CSA-induced inhibition of calcineurin results in return of IL-2 NF-AT to the cytosol. Because IL-4 NF-AT is constitutively in the nucleus, CSA must have a distinct mode of action to prevent DNA–protein complex formation in both unstimulated and stimulated cells

NF-AT-mediated transcription explain, on a molecular level, the inducible nature of IL-2 gene expression.

Subsequent to the development of this NF-AT regulation model, four NF-AT family members, human NF-ATc (41), murine NF-ATp (42), murine NF-ATc3 (43) and its human homologue, NF-AT4/NF-ATx (44, 45), and human NF-AT3 (44), were cloned and characterized. All four molecules have similar DNA-binding domains and are distantly related to the NF-κB (dorsal/rel) family of transcription factors. However, each factor differs in tissue distribution profile and in some details of their intracellular location and regulation. Another level of complexity is added when considering that several splice variants of NF-AT have also been described. These findings are consistent with the idea that NF-AT family members are not redundant and have gene-specific activities.

6.3.3 Comparison Between the IL-4 ARE and IL-2 NF-AT Transcription Complexes: Similarities, Yet Important Differences

Many similarities in the IL-2 NF-AT complex and the ARE have been defined in *in vitro* EMSA assays. Despite these similarities, there are also important differences that could be the key to differential regulation. Within the ARE, P1 shares 9 bp of identity with the murine IL-2 gene NF-AT binding site (Figure 6.2). Antibodies raised to NF-ATc and NF-ATp react with proteins in the ARE complex in EMSA supershift assays indicating that both are present in at least some IL-4-producing T cells and can associate *in vitro*. AP-1 proteins make up at least some of the inducible components as demonstrated using specific antibodies. Whether these proteins utilize a specific DNA-binding site or associate through protein–protein interactions is a question of some controversy (29, 35). ARE sequences between -85 and -78 are identical to the IL-2 gene OAP (octamer associated protein) element, a defined jun/fos (AP-1) binding site, suggesting a possible site of DNA interaction. However, mutation of the IL-4 OAP site clearly reduces, but does not abolish, ARE-mediated transcription. The ability to form the AP-1-containing ARE-stimulation-dependent complex *in vitro* is unaffected by such mutations (29). These data support the idea that AP-1 associates with the IL-4 ARE primarily through protein–protein interactions. Binding of AP-1 to the OAP site may confer stability to this NF-AT complex. Thus, this interaction is fundamentally different from that observed in the IL-2 gene which has an absolute requirement for a variant AP-1 site, proximal to the NF-AT binding site, for association.

The inhibition of IL-2 production in T cells by cyclosporin A (CSA), a clinically important immunosuppressive drug, involves this NF-AT pathway as well: CSA acts to prevent calcineurin activity, thus blocking dephosphorylation of NF-AT and its translocation (21). The delineation of the mechanism of CSA action in T cells was key to understanding stimulation-dependent IL-2 transcription through NF-AT. CSA also inhibits IL-4 production by T cells and one target of action is the ARE site: -87 to $+5$ IL-4/CAT gene reporter construct activity is inhibited in CSA-treated cells as is the ability to form the ARE stimulation-dependent complex *in vitro* (29).

However, there are important differences that imply the presence of gene-specific factors that may be targets of differential signals in a Th response. Proteins present in unstimulated nuclei can also associate with the ARE, but not the IL-2 gene NF-AT site. This constitutive complex lacks the inducible AP-1 components but, surprisingly, does contain NF-AT antibody reactive proteins. CSA inhibits the formation of this complex as well (Figure 6.2). Because these proteins are already in the nucleus, it is the binding and not the translocation of these proteins that is inhibited by CSA. These findings suggest a model of IL-4 gene regulation by NF-AT that is distinct from the IL-2 gene model: a constitutive nuclear form of NF-AT associates with factors from the AP-1 family of proteins to create an inducible complex that can influence the transcription rate of IL-4. This implies that the IL-4 NF-AT is distinct from that associated with the IL-2 gene: it is either the product of a unique gene or is an alternative form of a previously described NF-AT family member, perhaps generated through alternative splicing or post-translational processing, and is regulated uniquely.

These data also indicate a calcium-independent role for CSA inhibition. Consistent with our findings, a recent report has demonstrated a constitutively nuclear form of human NF-AT that is thought to be a homologue of NF-ATp (46). CSA treatment of cells inhibits its ability to bind DNA. *In vitro* phosphatase treatment completely restores this DNA binding activity. This further supports our contention that all NF-AT isoforms are not limited to the cytoplasmic compartment of unstimulated cells. It will be of interest to examine how the NF-AT phosphorylation state affects binding to the IL-4 ARE.

Because all currently described NF-AT family members can bind to an NF-AT site with some affinity in gel mobility shift assays, gene-specific activities have not been ascribed. Proteins expressed from partial clones of NF-ATc1, NF-ATc2 (NF-ATp) and NF-ATc3 show some ability to differentially bind to IL-4 and IL-2 gene NF-AT sites *in vitro*. However, this does not always correlate with *trans*-activating function. For example, when overexpressed, NF-ATc3 can activate transcription via the IL-2 distal promoter in co-transfection studies. This occurs despite the finding that NF-ATc binds only weakly to the site *in vitro* and is not a part of the endogenous IL-2 NF-AT complex. These studies illustrate the difficulties with trying to correlate *in vitro* binding activity and *trans*-activating capability with *in vivo* functions.

Two groups have analyzed the phenotype of a NF-ATp knockout mouse (47, 48). In one study, the mice show an early defect in IL-4, but not IL-2, gene expression in response to anti-CD3 treatment *in vivo* (48). Because this study did not assay IL-4 production more than one hour after immunization, it is unclear whether this reflects a shift in kinetics of IL-4 production or a true inability to make IL-4 at early times post-immunization. Importantly, two responses that require IL-4, Th2 development and IgE production, were actually enhanced in both *in vitro* and *in vivo* assays. In a similar investigation by A. Rao and colleagues, enhanced Th1 and Th2 type cytokine responses were observed in NF-ATp-deficient mice, suggesting the possibility that NF-ATp plays a role in suppressing the transcription of these cytokine genes (47). Many questions remain unanswered regarding the physiologic role of NF-AT family members. Our ability to assign gene-specific activities to individual family members may be limited by the current assays available, as well as the real possibility that these factors have redundant functions *in vivo*.

6.3.4 Other *cis*-Acting Elements can Influence IL-4 Gene Transcription

Other regions that contribute to IL-4 transcription have been identified in muta-genesis studies (Figure 6.1). As previously mentioned, there are five 'P' sites within 300 bp of the IL-4 TIS, all of which contribute to IL-4 transcription. Among these is the more promoter proximal sequence P0 (also termed CS1 and PuBa by other laboratories). Activation induces the binding of inducible factors, including NF-AT, to P0 *in vitro*, suggesting that this region is also a target of TCR-mediated signals (33). As discussed below, this region may also contribute to Th2-specific IL-4 gene expression.

Sequences with homology to the Y box, an element found in all MHC class II promoters, are located between -114 and -107 in the murine gene (30) and between -120 and -99 in the human gene (34). Specific antibodies to the tran-scription factor NFY react with proteins associated with this region in *in vitro* DNA binding assays. Furthermore, point mutations within this region reduce transcrip-tional activity of IL-4 reporter constructs by $\approx 85\%$ in murine T-cell lines. However, complete inducibility of this construct is not abrogated. NFY is expressed con-stitutively and may play a role in enhancing the stability of the inducible protein-DNA complexes and increasing transcription.

A distal element between -6.0 and -4.8 kb was defined in reporter gene assays and appears to confer enhancer activity in stimulated EL-4 T cells. The proteins that associate with this region have not been identified, but there are several elements that share identity with previously described transcription factor binding sites (D. Weiss, unpublished results).

Recently, two elements within the IL-4 promoter have been identified that appear to be the targets of selective signals contributing to distinct patterns of cytokine production in T helper responses. As previously noted, IL-4 is an essential factor for the development of an IL-4-producing T-helper cell subset (49, 50). Thus, IL-4 must have a role in inducing its own synthesis, either directly or indirectly. An upstream site that overlaps P2 (between -168 and -145) has similarity to previously described STAT (signal transducer and activator of transcription) binding sites. STAT factors were first described as components of the interferon (IFN)-γ signaling pathway (51). It is now known that IL-4 uses a similar signal transduction system. Upon IL-4 receptor cross-linking, member(s) of the Janus kinase (JAK) family of kinases activate Stat6 (also named IL-4 STAT and NF-IL-4) which leads to its translocation to the nucleus, binding to STAT DNA elements and transcriptional activation of a number of IL-4-inducible genes including FcγR1 and Cε (52–54). The presence of a Stat6 binding site within the IL-4 promoter (-167 to -153) raises the possibility that it is a target for IL-4-directed transcription and is important in Th development. Indeed, Lichtman and colleagues have formally demonstrated Stat6 binding to this site in IL-4 producing cells (55). Importantly, the presence of Stat6 binding activity correlates with Th2 cell differentiation.

Reporter gene constructs containing P0 exhibit Th2-specific expression in transient transfection assays, indicating that P0 makes an important contribution to selective IL-4 production in a T helper cell cytokine response (31). This region (-42 to -37) was recently shown by Ho et al to contain a c-Maf response element and bind c-Maf, a basic region/leucine zipper transcription factor (56). c-Maf is differentially expressed in Th2 lineage cells and interacts with NF-ATp. Its critical role in IL-4 transcription was demonstrated in experiments showing that ectopic expression of both c-Maf and NF-ATp is sufficient to initiate expression in non-IL-4 producing cells. Together, these data indicate that there are multiple factors that influence Th2-specific IL-4 transcription.

Although not as well-defined as positive-acting elements, negative regulatory elements (NREs) can suppress the transcription of a gene in a non-expressor cell or downregulate a transient transcriptional response (26, 27). A region between -326 and -302 in the murine gene (D. Weiss, unpublished results) and between -310 and -270 in the human gene has significant similarity to previously characterized silencer elements within the IL-2Rα chain gene and the chicken lysozyme gene regulatory regions (36). Deletion or mutation of this element in IL-4/CAT reporter gene constructs results in an increase in transcriptional activity in T cells. The protein factors that associate with this region have not been well characterized but appear to bind constitutively. Ho et al show that cytokine expression in a Th response is not due to the action of a dominant-acting repressor (56). However, we speculate that the activation of a negative-acting factor may be important in turning off antigen-induced IL-4 transcription.

6.4 REGULATORY ELEMENTS OF THE IL-4 GENE DEFINED IN MAST CELLS

It has long been appreciated that mast cells play an important role in immediate-type hypersensitivity responses through their ability to release histamine and other mediators of the allergic reactions upon cross-linking of the high affinity Fcε receptor (57, 58). It is now known that, analogous to T cells, mast cells are important cytokine-producing cells (58). Perhaps not surprisingly in view of the T-cell paradigm, the profile of cytokines produced by mast cells in vitro is dependent on the culture conditions. Murine bone-marrow derived mast cells cultured in IL-3 acquire a mucosal-like phenotype and are capable of producing IL-4 (7, 59). In contrast, these cells express IL-12 when cultured with stem cell factor (c-kit ligand) (59). It is likely that FcεRI$^+$ cells (which include both mast cells and basophils) that produce IL-4 and other cytokines play a role not only in the initiation and maintenance of both immediate and delayed-type allergic inflammatory responses in vivo, but also in directing the nature of the T helper immune response in local sites (12).

As discussed earlier, many of the early signaling events resemble those in T cells. Thus, we embarked on a study of mast cell transcriptional regulation for two reasons: (1) to understand the signaling pathways in a critical cell type of immediate- and delayed-type hypersensitivity; and (2) it was hoped that mucosal-type mast cells would provide a model for determining exactly what nuclear events dictate the selective expression of Th2 cytokines in T cells as well as mast cells and basophils. Much of our data to date, however, indicates that the cells of the mast cell lineage utilize at least a subset of unique transcriptional regulatory elements and do not represent a good model for studying the restricted T-cell expression. These differences, once completely defined, can be exploited to develop strategies for manipulation of IL-4 in a cell-specific manner.

As in T cells, there are multiple elements that contribute to activation-dependent transcription in mast cells. Our laboratory has focused on two of these. (i) The region between -88 and -60, which is essential for activation-dependent transcription in mast cells as well as T cells. Surprisingly, it appears to be the target of cell-specific transcription factors. (ii) A region in the second intron of the IL-4 gene was first described as having mast cell-specific enhancer activity in transformed mast cells. Recent data indicates that the enhancer is active in 'normal', activation-dependent mast cell lines as well.

6.4.1 The ARE Element is Essential for Inducible Mast Cell IL-4 Transcription

CFTL 12 and CFTL 15 cells have been used as models to study inducible IL-4 transcription in mast cells. These cells have many of the characteristics of mucosal mast cells based on their profile of granule mediators. They are derived from fetal liver, are growth factor-dependent (can utilize IL-4 or IL-3), express low levels of IL-4 mRNA constitutively, and initiate new transcription upon stimulation through the FcεRI or through use of calcium ionophore, ionomycin (7, 60). Similar to our studies in T cells, a series of CAT reporter gene constructs containing the IL-4 5' flanking region from -797 to $+5$ as well as progressive 5' deletions of this sequence were used in transient transfection assays in mast cells to assess the minimum sequence requirements for activation-dependent transcription. Again, the -87 to $+5$ IL-4 construct was active in stimulated cells, whereas -70 was not. This indicated that the region, first defined in T cells, mediates transcription in response to cell activation signals. Mutation of nucleotides within the core of the P1 element in the context of the -797 IL-4 construct completely abolishes CAT activity, confirming the importance of this region for mast cell IL-4 transcription. As observed in T cells, CSA inhibits IL-4 production and the activity of the -87 to $+5$ IL-4 CAT construct in transfected cells.

6.4.2 Mast Cells Exhibit Unique ARE Protein Binding Profiles When Compared to T Cells

Three lines of evidence support the idea that T cells and mast cells utilize the same IL-4 gene DNA regulatory element for mediating inducible transcription and that at least a subset of ARE-associated proteins are common to both cell types. First, the effect of individual mutations within the ARE on protein binding is identical to that observed in T-cell binding assays, suggesting that the same sub-sequences are important. Second, a constitutive and inducible complex of unique mobility is observed in EMSA analyses using unstimulated and stimulated mast cell nuclear proteins, respectively. Third, proteins in both complexes react with NF-ATp and NF-ATc-specific antibodies and their binding is CSA sensitive (60). These results support a model for the regulation of the assembly of the mast cell IL-4 transcription complex, similar to that proposed for T cells: pre-existing nuclear proteins, including an NF-AT-related family member, associate with newly activated or newly synthesized proteins to induce transcription.

Several differences imply that at least a subset of the mast cell ARE binding proteins are unique, however (60). The size of the complexes observed in EMSA are distinct. AP-1 family members do not readily associate with the inducible complex *in vitro*. DNA affinity purification and Western blot analysis with anti-NF-ATp antisera demonstrated that the predominant NF-AT-related, ARE binding protein in mast cells is ≈41 kDa in mass. This species is distinct from previously described NF-AT family members expressed in T cells which have molecular weights estimated to be between 97 and 130 kDa. Whether this protein species is the product of a unique gene or generated as an alternate splice form of one of the previously described NF-AT family members is still unclear. Efforts to resolve this question are currently under investigation in our laboratory.

6.4.3 An Intronic Regulatory Element Exhibits Mast-cell Specific Activity

The earliest studies of IL-4 gene regulation were initiated in a number of transformed mast cell lines (6). This special class of mast cells includes ABFTL3, an Abelson murine leukemia virus-transformed cell line, and the common T cytotoxic cell target P815, a methyl cholanthrene-induced tumor mast cell line. These cells express high levels of IL-4 mRNA constitutively and mRNA levels can be upregulated further upon stimulation. Because the non-transformed counterparts of these cells can utilize IL-4 as a growth factor and ABFTL3 and P815 cells are growth-factor independent in *in vitro* culture, it was hypothesized that IL-4 was an autocrine growth factor for these cells and the dysregulated production of this cytokine contributed to the transformed phenotype. Thus, it was of interest to understand the molecular basis of this unregulated expression.

Initial attempts to detect CAT gene activity in transformed mast cells transfected with the 5′ IL-4 reporter gene constructs were only marginally successful. Therefore DNAse I hypersensitivity site analysis was utilized to investigate the possibility that other regions were more active in these cells. This assay identifies regions of intact chromatin that are hypersensitive to exposure to limiting concentrations of DNAse I (61). These sites have been shown to correlate with transcriptional regulatory elements in many genes. A hypersensitive site was observed within the second intron of the murine IL-4 gene in ABFTL3 and P815 cell nuclei (4). Subsequent analysis showed that this site, contained within a 683 bp Bgl II fragment, defines an element that exhibits enhancer activity. The enhancer is also active in non-transformed mast cells, but not in the T-cell lines examined. It is composed of several functionally independent subregions including sequences that are similar to ets and GATA binding sites (62). The transcription factors that associate with these sites and appear to regulate the enhancer are expressed in mast cells and not T cells, explaining the apparent cell-restricted activity of this enhancer. The ets family member, PU.1, and GATA-1 and GATA-2 are expressed constitutively in both transformed and non-transformed mast cells and can bind to the respective IL-4 intron sites. An *in vivo* role for these proteins remains to be demonstrated. There is complete sequence identity with the equivalent region in the human gene. This conservation within an intron suggests there is a physiologic role for this element.

The role of this enhancer in IL-4 gene transcription is unclear. Its location in the middle of the IL-4 gene is puzzling. We have performed many studies to examine the interaction of the intronic sequence with 5' IL-4 sequences, but found it functions only marginally. In fact, the magnitude of the response is much higher with the SV40 enhancer than with the native IL-4 promoter (4). These results could be due to artifacts created by the artificial genetic constructs used in these studies. However, a recent report has made us aware of another potential role for this regulatory element (63). Using RNAse protection assays, it was observed that a number of embryonic mast cell lines and factor-dependent mast cell cultures express a truncated form of the IL-4 mRNA. RNAse protection assays demonstrated that this species is protected by probes containing IL-4 sequences encoding exons 3 and 4 but not exons 1 or 2. The fact that the intronic regulatory element is upstream of exon 3 and does not efficiently interact with 5' regulatory regions has led us to hypothesize that the intronic regulatory element is actually a promoter that drives the transcription of an alternative transcript. In support of this idea, we have identified a consensus initiator element (Inr) that is present within the 683 bp Bgl II intronic fragment originally analyzed (J. Hural and M. Brown, unpublished results; Figure 6.1). Inr elements were first described in 'TATA-less' promoters (64, 65). They bind basal transcription factors such as TFIID and are critical in the positioning of RNA polymerase II for correct transcription initiation. Inr-containing promoters have been shown to direct tissue specific expression of a variety of genes, including the immunologically relevant T- and B-cell restricted genes, *RAG-1* and *TdT* (25, 65, 66). It is intriguing to speculate that this alternative transcript has a role in regulating the production and/or activity of biologically active IL-4. This line of research is an area of intense investigation in our laboratory.

6.5 CONCLUSIONS

There has been significant progress in recent years towards defining nuclear events that regulate IL-4 transcription. It is clear that the IL-4 promoter is complex and while many factors have been implicated in transcription, their *in vivo* role must be confirmed and other factors and elements are still undefined. Clearly a goal of this research is to determine the molecular basis of cell-restricted IL-4 expression and many questions remain in this regard. The signals that lead to differential transcription of Th1 and Th2 cytokines such as IL-2, IFN-γ and IL-4 as well as expression in other IL-4-producing cell types, such as eosinophils, that may be regulated uniquely are unknown. How most of the nuclear targets are related to earlier TCR/FcεRI and costimulatory molecule-mediated signaling events is unclear and this information will be necessary in order to design drugs that selectively interfere or augment cell type-specific cytokine expression. It is assumed that IL-4 gene-associated nuclear signals in basophils are highly related to those in mast cells, but this has not been investigated. Furthermore, little is known about the signals, particularly the requirement for costimulatory signals, delivered to the TCR $\alpha\beta^+$, NK1.1$^+$ population of T cells that lead to IL-4 production. Unlike most T cells, NK1.1$^+$ T cells do not require priming to express IL-4. They are thought to be the earliest producers of IL-4 in an immune response, and it is likely that NK1.1$^+$ T cells initiate the development of Th2 responses. It has been hypothesized that these cells represent a more primitive stage of development than the bulk of the T-cell population. Thus, it will be interesting to examine whether they utilize more T-cell like or mast-cell like IL-4 gene-regulatory elements. Although IL-4 does not act alone to regulate the immune response, its central role in influencing IgE production, mast cell growth and activation state, as well as the cytokine producing phenotype of T cells, implicates it as a major player in the pathogenesis of allergic disease. Thus, it is of utmost importance to understand the details of its regulated, or dysregulated expression, in all IL-4-producing cell types.

REFERENCES

1. Brown MA and Hural J (1997) Functions of IL-4 and control of its expression. *Crit Rev Immunol* **17**:1–32.
2. Paul WE (1991) Interleukin 4: A prototypic immunoregulatory cytokine. *Blood* **77**:1859–1870.
3. Chan SC, Brown MA, Li S-H, Stevens SR and Hanifin JC (1996) Abnormal IL-4 production by atopic T cells is reflected in altered nuclear protein interactions with an IL-4 transcriptional regulatory element. *J Invest Dermatol* **106**:1131–1136.
4. Henkel G, Weiss DL, McCoy R, Deloughery T, Tara D and Brown MA (1992) A DNAse I hypersensitive site defines a mast cell enhancer. *J Immunol* **149**:323–330.
5. Tara D, Weiss DL and Brown MA (1993) An activation responsive element in the murine interleukin-4 gene is the site of an inducible DNA-protein interaction. *J Immunol* **151**:3617–3626.
6. Brown MA, Pierce JH, Watson CJ, Falco J, Ihle JN and Paul WE (1987) B cell stimulatory factor-1/interleukin-4 mRNA is expressed by normal and transformed mast cell lines. *Cell* **50**:809–818.
7. Plaut M, Pierce JH, Watson CJ, Hanley-Hyde J, Nordon RP and Paul WE (1989) Mast cell lines produce lymphokines in response to cross-linkage of FcεRI or to calcium ionophores. *Nature* **339**:64-67.
8. Tunon de Lara JM, Okayama Y, McEuen AR, Heusser CH, Church MK and Walls AF (1994) Release and inactivation of interleukin-4 by mast cells. *Ann New York Acad Sci* **725**:50–58.

9. Bradding P, Feather IH, Howarth PH *et al* (1992) Interleukin-4 is located to and released by human mast cells. *J Exp Med* **176**:1381–1386.

10. Thompson CB (1995) Distinct roles for costimulatory ligands B7-1 and B7-2 in T helper cell differentiation. *Cell* **81**:979–982.

11. Bluestone J (1995) New perspectives of CD28-B7 mediated T cell costimulation. *Immunity* **2**:555–559.

12. Paul WE (1991) Interleukin-4 production by FcεR+ cells. *Skin Pharmacol* **4**:8–14.

13. MacGlashan DW, White JM, Huang SK, Ono SJ, Schroeder J and Lichtenstein LM (1994) Secretion of IL-4 from basophils: the relationship between IL-4 mRNA and protein in resting and stimulated basophils. *J Immunol* **152**:3006–3016.

14. Fuleihan R, Ahern D and Geha RS (1995) Expression of the CD40 ligand in T lymphocytes and induction of IgE isotype switching. *Int Arch Allergy Immunol* **107**:43–44.

15. Klaus S, Berberich I, Shu G and Clark EA (1994) CD40 and its ligand in the regulation of humoral immunity. *Semin Immunol* **6**:279–286.

16. Stockinger B, Zal T, Zal A and Gray D (1996) B cells solicit their own help from T cells. *J Exp Med* **183**:891–899.

17. Gauchat J-F, Henchoz S, Mazzei G *et al* (1993) Induction of human IgE synthesis in B cells by mast cells and basophils. *Nature* **365**:340–343.

18. Scharenberg AM and Kinet JP (1995) Early events in mast cell signaling. *Chem Immunol* **61**:72–87.

19. Weiss A (1994) Signal transduction by lymphocyte antigen receptors. *Cell* **76**:263–274.

20. Rao A (1994) NF-ATp: a transcription factor required for the coordinate induction of several cytokine genes. *Immunol Today* **15**:274–281.

21. Schreiber SL and Crabtree GR (1992) The mechanism of action of cyclosporin A and FK506. *Immunol Today* **13**:136–142.

22. Kubo M, Kincaid RL and Ransom JT (1994) Activation of the interleukin-4 gene is controlled by the unique calcineurin-dependent transcriptional factor NF(P). *J Biol Chem* **269**:19441–19446.

23. Kubo M, Kincaid RL, Webb DR and Ransom JT (1994) The Ca^{2+}/calmodulin activated phosphoprotein phosphatase calcineurin is sufficient for positive transcriptional regulation of the mouse IL-4 gene. *Int Immunol* **6**:179–188.

24. Mitchell PJ and Tijan R (1989) Transcriptional regulation in mammalian cells by sequence-specific DNA binding proteins. *Science* **245**:371–378.

25. Ernst P and Smale ST (1995) Combinatorial regulation of transcription. I: General aspects of transcriptional control. *Immunity* **2**:311–319.

26. Levine M and Manley JL (1989) Transcriptional repression of eukaryotic promoters. *Cell* **59**:405–408.

27. Renkawitz R (1990) Transcriptional repression in eukaryotes. *Trends Genet* **6**:192–197.

28. Rooney JW, Hodge MR, McCaffrey PG, Rao A and Glimcher LH (1994) A common factor regulates both Th1 and Th2-specific cytokine gene expression. *EMBO J* **13**:625–633.

29. Tara D, Weiss DL and Brown MA (1995) Characterization of the constitutive and inducible components of a T cell activation responsive element. *J Immunol* **154**:4592–4602.

30. Szabo SJ, Gold JS, Murphy TL and Murphy KM (1993) Identification of cis-acting regulatory elements controlling interleukin-4 gene expression in T cells: roles for NF-Y and NF-ATc. *Mol Cell Biol* **13**:4793–4805.

31. Bruhn KW, Nelms K, Boulay J-L, Paul WE and Lenardo MJ (1993) Molecular dissection of the mouse interleukin-4 promoter. *Proc Natl Acad Sci USA* **90**:9707–9711.

32. Abe E, Malefyt R, Matsuda I, Arai K and Arai N (1992) An 11-base-pair DNA sequence motif apparently unique to the human interleukin 4 gene confers responsiveness to T cell activation signals. *Proc Natl Acad Sci USA* **89**:2864–2868.

33. Hodge MR, Rooney JW and Glimcher LH (1995) The proximal promoter of the IL-4 gene is composed of multiple essential regulatory sites that bind at least two distinct factors. *J Immunol* **154**:6397–6405.

34. Li-Weber M, Davydov IV, Krafft H and Krammer PH (1994) Role of NF-Y and IRF-2 in the regulation of human IL-4 gene expression. *J Immunol* **153**:4122–4133.

35. Rooney JW, Hoey T and Glimcher LH (1995) Coordinate and cooperative roles for NF-AT and AP-1 in the regulation of the murine IL-4 gene. *Immunity* **2**:473–483.

36. Li-Weber M, Eder A, Krafft-Czepa H and Krammer PH (1992) T cell specific negative regulation of transcription of the human cytokine IL-4. *J Immunol* **148**:1913–1918.

37. Li-Weber M, Krafft H and Krammer PH (1993) A novel enhancer element in the human IL-4 promoter is suppressed by a position-independent silencer. *J Immunol* **151**:1371–1382.

38. Todd MD, Grusby MJ, Lederer JA, Lacy E, Lichtman AH and Glimcher LH (1993) Transcription of the interleukin 4 gene is regulated by multiple promoter elements. *J Exp Med* **177**:1663–1674.

39. Shaw J-P, Utz PJ, Durand DB, Toole JJ, Emmel EA and Crabtree GR (1988) Identification of a putative regulator of early T cell activation genes. *Science* **241**:202–205.

40. McCaffrey PG, Perrino BA, Soderling TR and Rao A (1993) NF-ATp, a T lymphocyte DNA binding protein that is a target for calcineurin and immunosuppressive drugs. *J Biol Chem* **268**:3747–3752.

41. Northrop JP, Ho SN, Timmerman LA, Nolan GP, Admon A and Crabtree GR (1994) NF-AT components define a family of transcription factors targeted in T cell activation. *Nature* **369**:497–502.

42. McCaffrey PG, Luo C, Kerppola TK *et al* (1993) Isolation of the cyclosporin-sensitive T cell transcription factor NFATp. *Science* **262**:750–754.

43. Ho SN, Thomas DJ, Timmerman LA, Li X, Francke U and Crabtree GR (1995) NFATc3, a lymphoid-specific NFATc family member that is calcium-regulated and exhibits distinct DNA binding specificity. *J Biol Chem* **270**:19898–19907.

44. Hoey T, Sun Y-L, Williamson K and Xu X (1995) Isolation of two new members of the NF-AT gene family and functional characterization of the NF-AT proteins. *Immunity* **2**:461–472.

45. Masuda ES, Naito Y, Tokumitsu H *et al* (1995) NFATx, a novel member of the nuclear factor of activated T cells family that is expressed predominantly in the thymus. *Mol Cell Biol* **15**:2697–2706.

46. Park J, Yaseen NR, Hogan P, Rao A and Sharma S (1995) Phosphorylation of the transcription factor NFATp inhibits its DNA binding activity in cyclosporin A-treated human B and T cells. *J Biol Chem* **270**:20653–20659.

47. Xanthoudakis S, Viola JPB, Shaw KTY *et al* (1996) An enhanced immune response in mice lacking the transcription factor NFAT1. *Science* **272**:892–895.

48. Hodge M, Ranger AM, Hoey T, Grusby MJ and Glimcher LH (1996) Hyperproliferation and dysregulation of IL-4 expression in NF-ATp-deficient mice. *Immunity* **4**:397–405.

49. Swain SL, Weinberg AD, English M and Huston G (1990) IL-4 directs the development of Th2-like helper effectors. *J Immunol* **145**:3796–3806.

50. Le Gros G, Ben-Sasson SZ, Seder R, Finkelman FD and Paul WE (1990) Generation of interleukin 4 (IL-4)-producing cells *in vivo* and *in vitro*: IL-2 and IL-4 are required for *in vitro* generation of IL-4-producing cells. *J Exp Med* **172**:921–929.

51. Rothman P, Kreider B, Azam M *et al* (1994) Cytokines and growth factors signal through tyrosine phosphorylation of a family of related transcription factors. *Immunity* **1**:457–468.

52. Schindler C, Kashleva H, Pernis A, Pine R and Rothman P (1994) STF-IL-4: a novel IL-4 induced signal transducing factor. *EMBO J* **13:**1350–1356.
53. Hou J, Schindler U, Henzel WJ, Ho TC, Brasseur M and McKnight SL (1994) An interleukin-4-induced transcription factor: IL-4 STAT. *Science* **265:**1701–1707.
54. Kotanides H, Moczygemba M, White MF and Reich NC (1995) Characterization of the interleukin-4 nuclear activated factor/STAT and its activation independent of the insulin receptor substrate proteins. *J Biol Chem* **270:**19481–19486.
55. Lederer JA, Perez VL, DesRoches L, Kim SM, Abbas AK and Lichtman AH (1996) Cytokine transcriptional events during helper T cell subset differentiation. *J Exp Med* **184:**397–406.
56. Ho I-C, Hodge M, Rooney JW and Glimcher LH (1996) The proto-oncogene c-maf is responsible for tissue-specific expression of interleukin-4. *Cell* **85:**973–983.
57. Czarnetzki BM (1987) Mechanisms and mediators in urticaria. *Semin Dermatol* **6:**272–282.
58. Gordon JR, Burd PR and Galli SJ (1991) Mast cells as a source of multifunctional cytokines. *Immunol Today* **11:**458–464.
59. Smith TJ, Ducharme LA and Weis JH (1994) Preferential expression of interleukin-12 or interleukin-4 by bone marrow mast cells derived in mast cell growth factor or interleukin 3. *Eur J Immunol* **24:**822–826.
60. Weiss DL, Hural J, Tara D, Timmerman LA, Henkel G and Brown MA (1996) Nuclear factor of activated T cells is associated with a mast cell interleukin 4 transcription complex. *Mol Cell Biol* **16:**228–235.
61. Gross DS and Garrard WT (1988) Nuclease hypersensitive sites in chromatin. *Annu Rev Biochem* **57:**159–197.
62. Henkel G and Brown MA (1994) PU.1 and GATA: components of a mast cell-specific interleukin 4 intronic enhancer. *Proc Natl Acad Sci USA* **91:**7737–7741.
63. Siden E (1993) Regulated expression of germline antigen receptor genes in mast cell lines from the murine embryo. *J Immunol* **150:**4427–4437.
64. Smale S and Baltimore D (1989) The 'initiator' as a transcriptional control element. *Cell* **57:**103–113.
65. Weis L and Reinberg D (1992) Transcription by RNA polymerase II: initiator-directed formation of transcription-competent complexes. *FASEB J* **6:**3300–3309.
66. Riley LK, Morrow JK, Danton MJ and Coleman MS (1988) Human terminal deoxyribonucleotidyltransferase: Molecular cloning and structural analysis of the gene and 5′ flanking region. *Proc Natl Acad Sci USA* **85:**2489–2493.

7 Cytokine Signal Transduction and its Role in Isotype Class Switching

SYLVIA K. CHAI and PAUL ROTHMAN
Columbia University, New York, USA

7.1 INTRODUCTION

Immunoglobulins (Ig) can be classified according to their heavy chain constant (C_H) regions, into eight serological isotypes or classes, each of which is encoded by an individual C_H region gene. The early immune response to antigenic challenge is dominated by the expression of IgM and later switches to the expression of other Ig isotypes such as IgG, IgA, or IgE. Individual B cells have the ability to change from μ to γ, α or ε chain production in a process termed class switching. Normally class switching is mediated by a nonhomologous recombination event which involves the looping-out and deletion of intervening C_H genes, which thereby juxtaposes a downstream C_H gene 3' to the expressed V_H–D–J_H gene (1–4). The intervening C_H genes, deleted during the recombinatorial process, can be found as circular forms that are eventually lost from the cell.

The recombinatorial event of class switching commonly involves genomic regions which are composed of tandemly repeated sequences, the switch (S) regions, located 5' of each C_H region gene with the exception of C_δ. These repeated elements are comprised of various short motifs which have been suggested to serve as recognition sites for S region-specific recombinases. However, unlike the site-specific recombination of V_H–D–J_H joining, which is mediated by well-conserved heptamer/nonamer sequences, switch recombination does not appear to be site specific, and may occur between disparate nucleotides of tandemly repeated donor and acceptor elements (3, 5, 6).

In the mouse, S region repeats vary in length from 10–80 nucleotides and encompass regions which span from 2.5 kb (Sε) to 10 kb (Sγ1). Each S region has its own characteristic short and long repeats, most of which share homology with one another. For example, the GAGCT motif found in the Sμ region is also the predominant motif found in the Sε region (7). Although the Sμ and Sε regions share a high degree of homology with one another, switch recombination involving Sε is infrequent, as reflected by the scarcity of IgE in serum as compared to Ig of other isotypes. It is likely that the low level of switching to IgE is secondary to the regulation of this event by cytokines (see below). It is also possible that physical

IgE Regulation: Molecular Mechanisms. Edited by D. Vercelli. © 1997 John Wiley & Sons Ltd.

features of the Sε region, such as its relatively short length, nucleotide composition, and/or its distal location within the C_H locus, contribute to the low frequency of class switching to IgE (see also Chapter 8).

Immunoglobulin class switching, with the exception of switching to IgD, is preceded by the generation of truncated RNA molecules called sterile germline transcripts. These sterile transcripts initiate 5′ of the S regions from multiple sites within the I region (a promoter region) (8–13), and typically include the S region and C_H gene. A stable form of these nascent RNAs, which consists of an I exon spliced to the exons of the C_H genes, can be readily identified in cells prior to switching. Germline transcripts cannot be formed from a heavy chain allele after switching since the I region is deleted during the recombination event.

The data indicate that there may be an exact correlation between class switching and the appearance of germline transcripts. Also, the cytokines which regulate class switching may do so by regulating the appearance of these transcripts (14). This highly correlative association is suggestive of a causal relationship, but this has yet to be unequivocally demonstrated. The well-conserved structure of the sterile transcripts suggests that they themselves perform a functional role, either as RNA molecules with a stabilizing function, or as encoders of short, essential polypeptides. Alternatively, germline transcripts themselves may not be essential, but rather, transcription *per se* may be essential for targeting switch recombination. Changes in chromatin structure, or in topoisomerase activity might also be influenced by transcriptional activity, as demonstrated by the interleukin (IL)-4 induced changes in methylation, and in DNAse I hypersensitivity patterns at the $\gamma 1$ locus. Germline transcription may also be an associated epiphenomenon of other cytokine-induced events (e.g. S region-specific recombinases) which are essential for switching (see also Chapters 8–10).

To define the importance of germline transcription in class switch recombination, gene targeting techniques have been employed to mutate the heavy chain locus. For example, the Ig heavy chain ε locus was mutated in an Abelson murine leukemia virus-transformed pre-B cell line (18.81A20) by homologous recombination to ascertain whether constitutive transcription through the Sε region was sufficient to target this locus for class switching. Culture of wild-type 18.81A20 cells with lipopolysaccharide (LPS) and IL-4 normally induces germline ε transcripts prior to class switching to the ε locus (15). The heavy chain locus of the mutant cell line, EPKO-EμV$_H$, contains the Ig heavy chain Eμ enhancer plus the V$_H$ gene promoter instead of the Iε region (which includes the LPS/IL-4 responsive promoter and the Iε exon). The mutant cell line is able to transcribe the ε locus independently of IL-4. Significantly, the mutant cell line is also able to switch to ε in the absence of IL-4. Therefore, in the 18.81A20 cell line, the alteration in switching to ε, which results from altered transcriptional activity at this locus, indicates that transcription through the ε locus is sufficient to permit some level of class switching to ε. However, the level of switching to ε in EPKO-EμV$_H$ cells cultured with LPS alone or with LPS/IL-4 is more than 10-fold lower than that of parent cells cultured with LPS/IL-4 (11). The mechanism for this decreased ability to switch remains unclear. Mice with a similar replacement mutation in their B cells have also been generated. Their phenotype is similar to that reported for the EPKO-EμV$_H$ mutant cell line; IL-4-independent switching occurs at a much lower frequency than expected (16).

The importance of germline transcription in class switching is also supported by other gene targeting experiments involving alterations of the I region promoters and exons. Analysis of murine B cells which lack either the Iγ1 or Iγ2b regions (including the I promoters and exons) have shown that sequences within these regions are necessary for switching to γ1 and γ2b, respectively (9, 12). The promoter activity associated with these I regions may be necessary for targeting Sγ1 or Sγ2b switch recombination. However, the deletion of these I regions eliminates all transcriptional activity through the corresponding S regions, and abolishes the production of the corresponding germline transcripts. Therefore, it is possible that the switching defect associated with these mutant murine B cells results from the absence of germline transcripts. Alternatively, I region sequences may contain elements, such as binding sites for a switch recombinase, which are required for switch recombination. Recently, gene targeting experiments in mice, utilizing the human metallothionine II$_A$ promoter to replace the Iγ1 promoter, have demonstrated that switch recombination to IgG1 can be directed by this heterologous promoter only with complementation by the 3', 114 bp Iγ1 exon (which includes the splice donor site of the exon) (9). Mutant B cells lacking this 114 bp portion transcribe through the γ1 locus 10–20 fold less frequently. Therefore, it is not clear whether the dependence on this 114 bp sequence stems from the presence of the splice donor sequences or from the increased level of γ1 transcription in these B cells. Although the requirement for spliced germline transcripts for class switching appears controversial, the above data clearly demonstrates a requirement for germline transcription prior to switching. The regulation of these transcripts therefore appears to represent the key process in controlling specific class switching events, such as switching to IgE (see also Chapters 8–10).

7.2 CYTOKINES AND CLASS SWITCHING

There are several CD4$^+$ Th-cell derived cytokines which have a profound effect on immunoglobulin isotype switching, demonstrating a very elaborate, fine-tuned immunoregulatory mechanism. These cytokines can exert their effects in a positive or negative fashion and can even play reciprocal roles in switch regulation as exemplified by the activities of IL-4, IL-10, IL-13, and interferon (IFN)-γ. The ability of IL-4 to regulate the production of specific isotypes was initially observed when T-cell supernatants enhanced the production of IgG1 and IgE, and inhibited the production of IgG2b and IgG3 in mitogen-activated (LPS-activated) murine B cells (17–19). The subsequent purification and cloning of the active component in these murine T-cell supernatants identified the pertinent factor as IL-4 (14). The role played by IL-4 in the induction of IgE in the murine model was further confirmed when IgE responses during helminth infection were shown to be inhibited by the injection of antibodies directed against IL-4 (20). Also, IL-4-deficient mice lacked detectable IgE production during helminth infection (21). IL-4 does not seem to be an absolutely necessary component for the induction of IgG1; the addition of antibodies directed against IL-4 only partially inhibits the IgG1 response *in vivo* and *in vitro* (14). Furthermore, in IL-4-deficient mice, the magnitude of IgG1 response is only partially reduced, not obliterated, unlike the situation for the IgE response. There are, therefore, other alternate signals responsible for the production of IgG1. This example of functional dichotomy is not unusal among the reported activities of other cytokines, and indicates a fine tuning of cytokine selectivity and responsiveness.

Cytokines can also play reciprocal roles in the regulation of switching as exemplified by the antagonistic effects of IL-4 and IFN-γ, as IFN-γ inhibits the IL-4 induction of both IgG1 and IgE. Correspondingly, IFN-γ also represses IL-4-induced ε and γ1 germline transcription (22, 23). Interestingly, IFN-γ and IL-4 are produced by different CD4$^+$ Th cells (Th1 and Th2, respectively). IL-4-producing Th2 clones (which also produce IL-5, IL-6, and IL-10) are able to stimulate an IgE response and in contrast, IFN-producing Th1 clones (which also produce TNF-α/β and IL-2) inhibit IgE induction (24). Thus, these two subsets of T cells appear to have opposite actions on switching to IgE through the production of these cytokines. Although the mechanism underlying the antagonist activities of IL-4 and IFN-γ remains undefined, the identification of the signaling pathways activated by these cytokines has led to some new models of cross-regulation (see below and see also Chapter 5).

The cytokine regulation of similar Ig class switching responses in humans has been demonstrated for IL-4 and IL-13, which direct human B cells to produce IgG4 and IgE (25–28). IL-13, while having some properties different from those of IL-4, nevertheless has growth promoting effects on human B cells, and induces B-cell switching to IgG4 and IgE, independently of IL-4. These two cytokines do not exert an additive, synergistic effect, which is compatible with recent data indicating that the α subunits of their receptors are shared (29). Murine IL-13 does not share the isotype switching properties of its human counterpart (30), as murine B cells have not been shown to respond to IL-13, presumably because they lack the IL-13 receptor. This is compatible with the observation that IL-4-deficient mice fail to produce IgE in response to parasitic infection (21), and so IL-13 cannot supplant IL-4 function in this case. An example of negative regulatory control of human B cell IgE responses is found with IFN-α/γ and IL-10 activity. For example, IL-4-induced IgE secretion by human B cells was also found to be blocked by co-culture with IFN-γ and IFN-α (28). Also, IL-10 prevents IL-4-induced IgE synthesis by inhibiting the accessory cell function of monocytes (31) (see also Chapters 1 and 5).

7.3 REGULATION OF THE GERMLINE ε PROMOTER

As discussed above, different cytokines are known to stimulate the production of particular germline transcripts. Since germline transcription appears to be an essential component of the switching process, the elements that regulate these transcripts are the key link between cytokines and Ig isotype-specific immune responses. This model would predict that there would be cytokine-inducible *cis*-acting elements in and around the promoter region of these germline transcripts. In recent years, several cytokine-inducible activities, localized to the regions 5′ of the S regions have been characterized. In general, these cytokine responsive elements can be isolated to small, discrete regions located within 300 bp upstream of the germline transcription initiation start site. In addition to the identification of these cytokine responsive promoter regions, cytokine-inducible protein–DNA interactions within these regions have been demonstrated using EMSA (electrophoretic mobility shift assays). These activities involve various DNA binding proteins, and their binding to specific sites in several different I regions. Here, we will describe the response elements and the DNA binding proteins that have been implicated in the regulation of switching to IgE by cytokines.

7.4 IL-4 RESPONSIVE ELEMENTS

The first evidence of an IL-4 responsive element in B cells arose from studies examining IL-4-inducible activity at the murine major histocompatibility complex (MHC) Aα locus. Nuclear extracts, as assayed by EMSA, using DNA fragments representing a 1.3 kb region upstream of this MHC gene, contained IL-4-inducible DNA binding activity. This activity correlated with the MHC class II gene expression of B lineage cells (32). The core of this identity region corresponded to the sequence ATGT/GCTAGG (termed BRE) as determined through footprinting assays and sequencing. This sequence was the first element to be shown to bind an IL-4-inducible DNA binding factor.

A similar IL-4-inducible DNA binding activity was later identified in association with IL-4-inducible immunoglobulin switching to IgE (33, 34). A 1.1 kb region of DNA surrounding the germline ε (Iε) promoter was found to confer LPS/IL-4-inducible germline transcription activity to a heterologous reporter gene stably transfected into a pre-B cell line. Analyses of constructs transiently transfected into a lymphoma B cell line demonstrated that LPS/IL-4-inducibility could be conferred by a 179 bp segment of DNA overlapping the Iε transcription initiation site. With the use of EMSA, and with the Iε region as a probe, three DNA–protein complexes (complexes 1, 2, and 3) were detected in extracts derived from B lymphoid cells. One of these complexes, complex 3, was present constitutively in these cells. In later studies, the nuclear protein responsible for complex 3 formation was found to bind a specific sequence within the well conserved 179 bp region. This sequence is distinct from those associated with complexes 1 and 2, and was found to bind the early B-cell specific transcription factor, BSAP (B-cell specific activator protein) (35). BSAP, also known as NF-HB, is a mammalian homolog of the sea urchin transcription factor, TSAP (36). The formation of complex 3 could be competed with the NF-HB site from the 5′ Sγ2a region, or with a BSAP binding site from the histone

H2A-2.2 promoter. The deletion or mutation of the complex 3 binding site eliminated transcription imparted by the Iε promoter, as determined by assays using substituted Iε:CAT (cloramphenicol acetyltransferase) reporter constructs. Reintroduction of the BSAP binding site restored the IL-4/LPS inducibility of CAT. Two other complexes (termed complex 1 and 2) detected with the Iε probe in EMSA were induced by IL-4. Cold competition assays showed that these IL-4 complexes were competed by the BRE element from the MHC Aα locus. These competition experiments suggested that the same IL-4-inducible factors bound to elements at these two IL-4-inducible enhancer elements.

Another IL-4-inducible element was subsequently identified upstream of the CD23 gene. Köhler and Rieber (37) identified an IL-4-inducible factor (termed NF-IL-4) which is post-translationally activated by IL-4 in lymphoid and monocytic cells. By using deletional mutants, derived from the 360 base pair region (between exon II and exon Ib) spanning a region 5′ of the CD23 gene, fused to a luciferase reporter construct, they were able to demonstrate that binding of NF-IL-4 to their IL-4 response element is essential for the initiation of gene transcription in response to IL-4. Homologous binding sequences for NF-IL-4 were identified in the promoter regions of the IL-4-inducible CD23b and IgHε genes (5′ TYCYRRGAA-3′).

Similarly, Kotanides and Reich (38) described an IL-4-inducible factor similar to NF-IL-4, which they termed IL-4 NAF (IL-4 nuclear activated factor). Using nuclear extracts derived from human monocytic cells, they were able to demonstrate that an IL-4- and an IFN-γ-inducible factor bound to the IFN-γ response region derived from the FcγRI gene. This sequence has a homologous counterpart within the 129 bp region of the germline ε promoter initially described by Rothman and co-workers (33, 34).

Further dissection of the 129 bp IL-4 response region situated in the germline ε promoter confirmed the above findings. The minimal 179 bp promoter was found to contain binding sites for CCAAT box/enhancer binding protein (C/EBP) and NF-κB, in addition to the previously characterized NF-IL-4/IL-4 NAF site (37, 38). By analysis of a series of 5′ deletion constructs and linker-scanning mutations, a 46 bp fragment (-129 to -79) was identified to confer IL-4 inducibility to a minimal c-fos promoter (39). The sequence comprising this region is highly conserved between human and mouse and can also be found in the promoter region for murine γ1 germline transcripts. This region is sufficient to transfer IL-4 inducibility to another promoter as long as the binding sites for C/EBP and NF-IL-4/NAF are left intact.

IL-4 response elements, which behave similarly to those identified in murine systems, have been identified in the human germline promoter (40, 41). Deletional and mutational analyses of this region (around 100 bp upstream of the germline transcription start site) have correlated with the abrogation of IL-4-mediated transcriptional activity in reporter constructs. In EMSA, a single, as yet unidentified, IL-4-inducible complex binds a ^{32}P-labeled IL-4 response element. This human element has also been reported to contain repressor activity (40). This region lacks significant homology with its murine counterpart and is situated markedly upstream of that reported in the murine system.

7.5 THE CD40 RESPONSE ELEMENT

Costimulation of B cells with IL-4 and CD40 induces an increase in IgE and IgG4 production (26, 42–44). CD40/CD40 ligand (CD40L) interaction is also known to induce germline transcription of many heavy chain genes in the absence of cytokine costimulation (45). Thus, the CD40–CD40L interaction synergizes with IL-4, but its effects may ensue independent of cytokine stimulation. Deletion mutants of the human Iε promoter region have defined a CD40L-responsive element, situated between -27 to $+78$ (relative to the germline transcription initiation site) (46). A consensus sequence for BSAP resides within the CD40 response element. This putative BSAP binding site is highly homologous to the murine BSAP binding site (35). Notably, CD40L-expressing L cells upregulate BSAP expression in murine B cells (47).

7.6 THE HMG-I(Y) BINDING SITE

Recent work studying the murine Iε promoter has identified a binding site for the HMG-I(Y) protein. HMG-I(Y), an abundant non-histone chromosomal protein, can bind at the transcription initiation sites of the germline ε promoter (Figure 7.1). This site is one of the few sites involved in the negative regulation of germline ε transcripts. Co-transfection of an expression construct directing the synthesis of antisense HMG-I(Y) RNA increases ε promoter activity. Footprinting studies indicate that HMG-I(Y) shares a binding site at the ε promoter with NF-BRE (an IL-4-inducible nuclear protein) (48). The mechanism of this negative regulation by HMG-I(Y), and the involvement of NF-BRE, has not been clearly defined to date. This work also reports that the immunosuppressive agent, rapamycin, preferentially suppresses IL-4-induced IgE production, and acts by inhibiting the activation of the human germline ε promoter and by inhibiting the IL-4-induced phosphorylation of HMG-I(Y).

7.7 IL-4-INDUCED CYTOKINE SIGNAL TRANSDUCTION INCORPORATES THE JAK/STAT PATHWAY

The IL-4 receptor is comprised of two polypeptide chains, one necessary for ligand binding (IL-4R α chain), and the other operating in signal transduction (γ chain) (49–52). In addition to IL-4, it appears that IL-13 also uses the IL-4R α chain for activating cells. However, the IL-13 receptor complex also contains a ligand-specific binding chain. The IL-4R α chain is a widely expressed 140 kDa transmembrane protein composed of 825 amino acids, with a large (569 amino acid) cytosolic tail containing several well-defined motifs. In the extracellular domain, the IL-4R α chain bears the paired extracellular cysteine residues and the conserved WSXWS motif characteristic of the cytokine receptor superfamily (53). The cytoplasmic

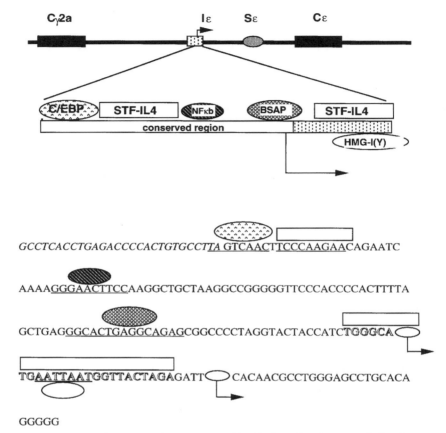

Figure 7.1. The murine Iε germline promoter. The binding sites for transcription factors are boxed, and indicated on the schematic diagram (top), as well as on the sequence (bottom). The arrows mark the major transcription initiation sites

region of the receptor contains several regions required for IL-4 signaling. In the membrane proximal region of the cytoplasmic domain is a 'box 1 motif' which is a binding site for receptor-associated Janus-activated kinases (JAK) (see below). In addition, there are two acidic 'insulin-like' domains (54, 55), one of which is essential for the activation of the IRS1/IRS2 molecules. Scattered in the cytoplasmic domain are five tyrosine residues that are conserved in human and murine receptor molecules. When tyrosine is phosphorylated, four of these residues can act as docking sites for the Stat6 signaling molecule (see below). Like other members of the cytokine receptor superfamily, the IL-4R α chain has neither endogenous kinase activity nor recognizable kinase domains (56, 57).

The second chain of the IL-4 receptor complex is the common γ chain. This chain, which is also used by other cytokines such as IL-2, IL-7, and IL-15 for signaling, is absent in patients with X-linked SCID (severe combined immunodeficiency). Although it appears that the γ chain is normally activated in response to IL-4, it is unclear whether the γ chain is an absolute requirement for signal transduction or for signal transduction in all cells (58, 59). For example, neither IL-4 nor IL-13 receptor function is completely abrogated by the absence of a γ chain (29, 60–62). There are also data to indicate that the IL-4R α chain alone is able to function without its γ chain partner (63). This is consistent with findings that some IL-4 responsive cell lines do not express the γ chain (60, 62). Interestingly, the homodimerization of the IL-4R α chain can induce germline ε transcripts in B-cell lines (63). Whether signaling from the homodimerization of the IL-4R α chain is able to induce class switching to IgE has not yet been determined.

Because neither the IL-4R α or γ chain encode any enzymatic activity, it appears that downstream targeting events require the activation of proteins that associate with these receptor chains. One of the earlier signaling events occurring after cytokine (i.e. IL-4) receptor engagement is the activation of JAKs. The JAKs represent a unique family of tyrosine kinases involved in the signal transduction of many different cytokines (64–73). The four members, Jak1, Jak2, Jak3, and Tyk2, have molecular weights ranging from 125 to 135 kDa, and share an overall sequence identity of 35–45% (64, 67, 74). All members, with the exception of Jak3, are expressed in many different tissues, consistent with the wide distribution of cytokine activity. In contrast, Jak3 is only expressed in hematopoietic cells.

In terms of IL-4 signaling, Jak1 has been shown to associate with the IL-4R α chain, while Jak3 associates with the γ chain. Both these JAKs are activated in response to IL-4. Interestingly, the IL-13 receptor associates with the Tyk2 kinase. Correspondingly, IL-13 activates the Jak1 and Tyk2 kinases. The present model for IL-4 signaling suggests that the dimerization of the receptor chains by ligand allows the JAKs to activate the receptor complex, possibly by cross-phosphorylation/activation. The activation of the JAKs then leads to the tyrosine phosphorylation of the IL-4R α chain. This tyrosine phosphorylation is essential for the signaling cascade as it allows the IL-4R α chain to act as a docking site for other signaling proteins. Among these proteins is a member of the STAT (signal transducers and activators of transcription) family of transcription factors, Stat6 (Figure 7.2).

Signal transducers and activators of transcription

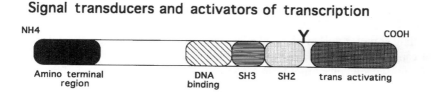

Figure 7.2. Schematic structure of STAT proteins, with the different domains so far identified

The JAK kinases are required for the tyrosine phosphorylation and activation of STATs, although it is not clear yet whether JAKs phosphorylate STATs directly. Following their activation through tyrosine phosphorylation, the STAT factors homo- or heterodimerize to form the major portions of unique DNA binding factors (38, 75), and translocate to the nucleus, where they activate transcription. This transcriptional activation results from the interaction of transcription factors with specific DNA sequences (consensus sequences) found in the promoter (e.g. Iε) of the relevant gene, thereby initiating events leading to transcription. Tyrosine phosphorylation and activation of STATs leads to the transcriptional activation of unique, but overlapping, patterns of target genes, which characterize specific cellular responses to cytokines and extracellular stimuli.

The STATs were recognized for their dual functions of signal transduction in the cytoplasm and of activation of transcription in the nucleus, hence the name STAT. To date, six members of the STAT family, STATs 1–6, have been identified and characterized (60, 76–83). STATs are widely expressed in different cell types and tissues, with the exception of Stat4 which is expressed predominantly in testis and in cells of hematopoietic origin. The STAT proteins share sequence similarities in blocks of amino acids spanning the length of the 700 amino acid protein (64). Several of these regions have been shown to encode functionally important domains. Two of these regions have been shown to be essential for the activation of the STATs. A Src homology region (SH2) domain is present in all STAT proteins. Comparison of this 100–120 amino acid motif in different STATs reveals that the NH$_2$-terminal portion of this region is conserved, while the COOH-terminus of this SH2 region is more divergent. Specific interactions between STATs and other proteins occur through the interaction of the SH2 domain with specific motifs containing phosphotyrosine residues. The first of these interactions that has been shown to be important is the interaction between the SH2 of STATs and specific docking sites present within the cytoplasmic domains of cytokine receptors. The tyrosine phosphorylation of these sites allows the STAT molecules to be drawn into the receptor complex. Experimental proof of this model was shown using short peptides, containing a 'docking site' from the IL-6 receptor, which were able to confer Stat3 recruitment ability to a heterologous receptor (84). Conversely, swapping STAT SH2 domains can change the receptors to which the chimeric STATs are recruited and activated (85).

A second motif essential for STAT activation is a conserved tyrosine residue adjacent to the SH2 domain. Once the STAT molecules are drawn into the receptor complex, this residue is phosphorylated. This phosphorylation is thought to be performed by the activated JAK kinases that are present in the dimerized receptor complex. Once the STATs are phosphorylated, they dimerize to form the active signaling complex we have termed STF (signal transducing factor). It is this complex that can translocate to the nucleus and bind DNA.

There are four other motifs in STATs that are important in their function. The carboxy-terminal regions of STATs contain sequences important in their ability to activate transcription once they are bound to promoter elements. Although somewhat divergent in composition, such transactivating domains have been identified in Stat1,

Stat2, and recently in Stat6 (86, 87). A region that determines the DNA binding specificity of the different STAT molecules is present downstream to the SH2 region (88, 89). Although all STAT molecules can bind to certain conserved elements, there are also elements that preferentially bind certain STATs. For example, Stat6 can bind elements that other STATs cannot bind (see below). Another conserved region present in all STATs is found in the amino terminus of these molecules. Although the exact function of this region is unknown, it appears to be essential for STAT function. Similarly, adjacent to the SH2 domain, lies a region spanning approximately 50 amino acids, with distant but meaningful homology to the Src homology region 3 domains (SH3). Again, the function of this region remains unknown. Thus the STAT molecules contain six regions that appear to be important in their function.

7.8 REGULATION OF GERMLINE ε TRANSCRIPTS BY STATS

The factors NF-IL-4, IL-NAF, IL-4 STAT (described above) in all likelihood correspond to the recently defined transcription factor Stat6. Schindler *et al* (75) also defined an IL-4-inducible DNA binding factor (STF-IL-4), with a strong affinity for a GAS (gamma activating site: see below) probe, confirming previous studies (Figure 7.3). Additionally, they demonstrated that this IL-4-inducible factor binds to a GAS-like element in the IL-4-inducible promoter of IgHε. The IL-4-dependent activation of STF-IL-4 is rapid, does not require *de novo* protein synthesis, and results in the sequential appearance of binding activity first in the cytoplasm, then in the nucleus. Activation of STF-IL-4 is sensitive to tyrosine kinase inhibitors and the active factor is tyrosine phosphorylated. STF-IL-4 is different from STF-IFN-γ (Stat1 homodimers), in that the STF-IL-4 complex, when bound to a GAS probe, migrates more slowly than the bound STF-IFN-γ complex. In addition, an oligonucleotide, derived from the IgHε germline promoter which binds an IL-4-inducible complex (34) competes for binding of STF-IL-4 but not for binding of STF-IFN-γ. Thus, these data together indicated that a probable component of this STF-IL-4 is a STAT.

The importance of Stat6 as a major component of STF-IL-4 was realized with the subsequent purification and cloning of STF-IL-4 (78). As indicated by its functional characteristics, the factor was found to be a new member of the STAT family, and was initially named IL-4 STAT. Following this, the components of this Stat6 recognition code were defined, and as suspected, the code comprised a GAS consensus-like element, 5'-TTCNNNNGAA-3'. Further validation of Stat6 function in IL-4-induced switching was confirmed by characterization of several different Stat6-deficient mice (90–92). The three types of Stat6-deficient mice were generated in a slightly different fashion, but generally yielded similar results at the protein level, with minor exceptions. In all three cases there were obvious disruptions of IL-4-mediated responses.

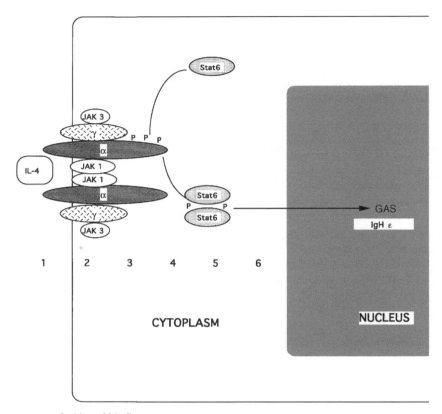

1 Ligand binding

2 Receptor dimerization

3 Transphosphorylation of JAKs

4 JAKs phosphorylate tyrosines on the IL-4 receptor

5 STAT proteins are drawn into the receptor complex.
   Phosphorylation of tyrosine on STATs. STAT dimerization.

6 STAT translocation to nucleus, and GAS binding by STAT
   containing complexes.

Figure 7.3. Signal transduction through the IL-4 receptor. The different steps in the process are numbered and identified at the bottom

(1) In lymph node cells derived from mutant mice, the IL-4-inducible expression of CD23 and MHC class II antigens was abrogated (90–92);

(2) IgG1 and IgE responses in antigen-stimulated lymph node B cells derived from mutant mice were significantly impaired (92);

(3) Spleen-derived, resting B cells of Stat6-deficient mice could not respond to IL-4 and anti-IgM antibody stimulation *in vitro* (92);

(4) Serum IgE levels were not detectable after *Nippostrongylus brasiliensis* infection in Stat6-deficient mice, while IgG1 levels post-infection were 10 times lower than that of infected wild-type mice;

(5) the examination of lymph node B cells revealed an absence of IgE-producing B cells (91).

In general, lymphocytes derived from Stat6-deficient mice were unable to respond to IL-4 *in vivo* or *in vitro*, and these findings agreed with those obtained in IL-4-deficient mice studies (21), in anti-IL-4 antibody studies (93), and in anti-IL-4 receptor antibody studies (20). Thus, overwhelming evidence indicates that Stat6 is an absolute requirement for the generation of an IgE response. In some of these Stat6-deficient mice, an increase of IgM, IgG1, IgG2a, IgG2b, and IgG3 serum levels was reported, leading to the speculation that Stat6 may somehow be involved in the negative regulation of switching to those isotypes (90, 91).

Although the role of Stat6 in switching to IgE is clear, the role of other STATs in switching to IgE and other isotypes remains undefined. IFN-γ induces the activation of Stat1. Stat1-deficient mice are deficient in IFN-γ signaling, but otherwise appear to be able to respond to all other cytokines. Analysis of these mice reveals low serum IgG2a levels, with or without LPS and IFN-γ stimulation *in vitro* (D. Levy and D. Kuehner, unpublished data). Additionally, analysis of these B cells demonstrates that IFN-γ does not suppress the IL-4 induction of switching to IgG1. Therefore it is likely that Stat1 plays an important role in regulating switching. Whether the Stat1 molecule itself is involved, or exerts this activity through the induction of the other mediators, is not yet defined.

Similarly, it is likely that STATs play a role in the regulation of switching induced by IL-10. IL-10 has been shown to activate both Stat1 and Stat3. These activated STATs form both homodimers and heterodimers (e.g. Stat1:Stat1, Stat1:Stat3, and Stat3:Stat3). It remains to be seen which of these different factors are important in the induction of switching by IL-10. Another cytokine which has been described to play a major role in switch induction is TGF-β. TGF-β can induce switching to IgA in both mice and humans. However, the TGF-β receptor is quite distinct from that of other cytokines and has not been shown to induce the activation of the JAK:STAT pathway.

The identification of the JAK:STAT pathway has helped answer many questions about how the specificity of cytokine biologic responses is maintained. Extensive studies have indicated that different STAT proteins are elicited in response to different cytokine-receptor interactions. For example, although Jak1 is activated by both IL-4 and IFN-γ, Stat1 is activated in response to IFN-γ, while only Stat6 is activated in response to IL-4 (78, 89). This specificity is based on the specificity of STAT-receptor peptide interactions. The Stat1 and Stat6 proteins bind directly and selectively to phosphopeptides derived from their activating receptors (IFN-γ and IL-4, respectively). An additional level of biological specificity relies on the ability to bind different target DNA sequences. Activated Stat1 is partial to binding a site with the consensus sequence 5′-TTCNNNGAA-3′ while Stat6 is partial to binding the consensus sequence 5′-TTC<u>NNNN</u>GAA-3′. These elements were initially termed GAS (gamma activating sites), as they were first shown to be important elements in several IFN-α/γ-inducible genes (94, 95). Recently, similar, if not identical, GAS elements have been described in the promoter of genes induced by other cytokines (95–98). Interestingly, Stat6 binding sites, which do not bind other STAT proteins, are present in IL-4-inducible genes.

The finding that both IL-4 and IFN-γ induce the activation of STAT proteins (Stat6 and Stat1, respectively) has raised the question of how these cytokines antagonize each other's activities. At least some of this antagonism relies on their opposing effects on transcriptional activation. For example, IL-4 inhibits the induction of germline γ3 and γ2a transcripts and correspondingly reduces switching to IgG3 and IgG2a. Similarly, IFN-γ inhibits the IL-4-dependent induction of germline γ1 and ε transcripts and switching to IgG1 and IgE. Although both Stat1 and Stat6 dimers can bind to IFN-γ response (GAS) elements, IFN-γ but not IL-4 can activate transcription from these elements. Although it is tempting to suggest that the binding of Stat6 dimers to these elements could repress transcriptional activation by IFN-γ, this has not been demonstrated.

The mechanism by which IFN-γ inhibits IL-4 function is even more difficult to understand. Again, the data suggests that IFN-γ antagonizes the IL-4-dependent induction of Ig class switching by repressing the induction of germline transcripts. It appears that this inhibition occurs through elements present in the Iε promoter. For example, studies of the minimal 179 bp germline ε promoter (23) indicate that IFN-γ represses IL-4 induction of this *cis*-responsive element. To date, no Stat1 binding elements (i.e. GAS) have been identified within this region. Although there are two Stat6 binding sites within this region, EMSA have shown that, *in vitro*, neither of these sites can bind Stat1 dimers. An IFN-γ responsive element within the germline ε promoter has not been identified. Thus, it remains a mystery as to how IFN-γ and IL-4 are able to play such opposite roles over the same promoter regions. IFN-γ does not appear to alter the IL-4 induction of Stat6 dimers that can bind DNA. It is entirely possible that there are other unidentified regulatory elements within this region that are able to bind either Stat1 or other IFN-γ-inducible transcription factors. Alternatively, Stat1 may somehow regulate the ability of Stat6 to activate transcription, either by directly altering Stat6 function, or by regulating the function of other factors that bind to the Iε promoter.

7.9 OTHER POSSIBLE ROLES FOR STAT6 IN IGE PRODUCTION

Many of the pleiotropic effects of IL-4 rely on signaling events mediated by Stat6. However, this Stat6-mediated signaling requirement is not the exclusive domain of B cells. IL-4 not only affects B-cell function, but it also mediates the differentiation of naive CD4$^+$into Th2 cells (the producers of IL-4, IL-5, IL-10, and IL-13). In Stat6-

deficient mice (90–92), IL-4-mediated Th2 cell differentiation and corresponding cytokine production are severely impaired. This phenomenon is consistent with the notion that Stat6 is essential for mediating various signals induced by IL-4. Thus, Stat6 influences switching at the ε locus in at least two ways: (i) by mediating IL-4 signals on the B cell surface; and (ii) by affecting the function of Th2 cells, the producers of IL-4. Similarly, other STATs that affect Th cell differentiation are important regulators of IgE production. For example, IL-12 can induce naive Th cells to differentiate to Th1 cells. IL-12 signals through the Stat4 molecule. Recently, Stat4-deficient mice have been shown to lack the ability to generate a strong Th1 response. Since Th1 cells produce IFN-γ, their induction during an immune response antagonizes Th2 cells and IL-4-mediated responses, such as switching to IgE. Thus, through their regulation of Th1 and Th2 differentiation, STATs can also affect switching.

7.10 THE MECHANISM OF SYNERGY BETWEEN IL-4 AND CD40

In addition to signals initiated by cytokines, isotype switching also requires a second signal provided by direct cell contact with activated Th cells (26). This phenomenon reflects the requirement for the interaction between CD40 and CD40L, molecules found on the surface of B and T cells, respectively (99–102). This interaction has been observed to synergize with IL-4-initiated switch events at the γ1 and ε locus, as demonstrated by a corresponding increase in both germline transcription and class switching. The mechanism by which IL-4 and the CD40–CD40L interaction synergize to induce switching is not yet defined. Clearly, some component of this synergy uses different elements within the region controlling germline transcripts. This region includes both the proximal germline promoters and, in mice, the 3′ Cα enhancer region. Thus, using a CD40L-expressing baculovirus system, resting B cells can be stimulated to generate γ1 and ε germline transcripts in the absence of cytokines, and this transcriptional activation is unaffected by mutating the DNA binding site for an IL-4-inducible factor (NF-IL-4γ1) (45, 103). CD40–CD40L interaction has been shown to activate other pathways, such as NF-κB and perhaps BSAP (see above). The effect of CD40–CD40L interactions on germline ε transcripts and switching might merely reflect the activation of these factors, which are clearly important in the production of germline ε transcripts.

It is also possible that the CD40–CD40L interaction may play an activating role for STATs. For example, serine as well as tyrosine phosphorylation of STATs has been shown to be important in transcriptional activation of genes (104). There is some evidence for this as Stat1 can be phosphorylated at serine 727, a potential MAPK (mitogen-activated protein kinase) site, with a corresponding increase in transcriptional activation (104, 105). Stat3 can also be phosphorylated at an analogous serine residue with a corresponding increase in DNA binding activity (106).

Thus the CD40–CD40L induced signal, supposedly not affecting changes in STAT DNA binding activity, may influence germline transcription at the ε locus by providing a second, synergizing signal via other signal transduction pathways. However, there is presently no evidence that any post-translational modification, other than tyrosine phosphorylation, is important in the activation of Stat6.

The importance of the STATs in cytokine signaling has been most dramatically demonstrated in the phenotype of Stat1-deficient and Stat6-deficient mice. As described above, there are obvious and profound defects in specific immunoglobulin responses in these mutant mice. Although it has not been unequivocally demonstrated, the impairment of these immunoglobulin responses may support the contention that STATs are important in the regulation of germline transcription and thus, class switching. Interestingly, IL-4 and IL-13 seem to approach the induction of IgE through different mechanistic paths; however, these paths seem to merge at the point of activation of Stat6. Therefore, the regulation of STAT activity may ultimately prove to be an important mode for the regulation of switching to IgE.

ACKNOWLEDGMENTS

This work was supported by NIH Grants AI 33450-04 (P.R.), the Pew Scholars Program (P.R.), the Pfizer Corporation (P.R.), Asthma and Allergy Foundation of America (P.R.), the Leukemia Society of America (P.R.) and Arthritis Foundation (S.K.C.).

REFERENCES

1. Honjo T and Kataoka T (1978) Organization of immunoglobulin heavy chain genes and allelic deletion model. *Proc Natl Acad Sci USA* **75**:2140–2144.
2. Iwasato T, Shimizu A, Honjo T and Yamagishi H (1990) Circular DNA is excised by immunoglobulin class switch recombination. *Cell* **62**:143–149.
3. Von Schwedler U, Jack HM and Wabl M (1990) Circular DNA is a product of the immunoglobulin class switch rearrangement. *Nature* **345**:452–456.
4. Matsuoka M, Yoshida K, Maeda T, Usuda S and Sakano H (1990) Switch circular DNA formed in cytokine-treated mouse splenocytes. *Cell* **62**:135–142.
5. Szurek P, Petrini J and Dunnick W (1985) Complete nucleotide sequence of the murine γ3 switch region and analysis of switch recombination sites in two γ3-expressing hybridomas. *J Immunol* **135**:620–626.
6. Winter E, Krawinkel U and Radbruch A (1987) Directed Ig class switch recombination in activated murine B cells. *EMBO J* **6**:1663–1671.
7. Nikaido T, Yamawaki KY and Honjo T (1982) Nucleotide sequences of switch regions of immunoglobulin Cε and Cγ genes and their comparison. *J Biol Chem* **257**:7322–7329.
8. Gauchat JF, Lebman DA, Coffman RL, Gascan H and De Vries J (1990) Structure and expression of germline epsilon transcripts in human B cells induced by interleukin 4 to switch to IgE production. *J Exp Med* **172**:463–473.
9. Jung S, Rajewsky K and Radbruch A (1993) Shutdown of class switch recombination by deletion of a switch region control element. *Science* **259**:984–987.

10. Lutzker S and Alt FW (1988a) Structure and expression of germ line immunoglobulin γ2b transcripts. *Mol Cell Biol* **8**:1849–1852.

11. Xu L, Gorham B, Bottaro A, Alt FW and Rothman P (1993) Replacement of germ-line ε promoter by gene targeting alters control of immunoglobulin heavy chain class switching. *Proc Natl Acad Sci USA* **90**:3705–3709.

12. Zhang J, Bottaro A, Li S, Stewart V and Alt FW (1993) A selective defect in IgG2b switching as a result of targeted mutation of the Iγ2b promoter and exon. *EMBO J* **12**:3529–3537.

13. Yancopoulos GD, DePinho RA, Zimmerman KA, Lutzker SG and Rosenberg N (1986) Secondary genomic rearrangement events in pre-B cells: VHDJH replacement by a LINE-1 sequence and directed class switching. *EMBO J* **5**:3259–3266.

14. Coffman RL, Lebman DA and Rothman P (1993) The mechanism and regulation of immunoglobulin isotype switching. *Adv Immunol* **54**:229–270.

15. Rothman P, Lutzker S, Cook W, Coffman R and Alt FW (1988) Mitogen plus interleukin 4 induction of Cε transcripts in B lymphoid cells. *J Exp Med* **168**:2385–2389.

16. Bottaro A, Lansford R, Xu L, Zhang J, Rothman P and Alt FW (1994) S region transcription *per se* promotes basal IgE class switch recombination but additional factors regulate the efficiency of the process. *EMBO J* **13**:665–674.

17. Coffman RL and Carty J (1986) A T cell activity that enhances polyclonal IgE production and its inhibition by interferon-γ. *J Immunol* **136**:949–954.

18. Bergstedt LS, Sideras P, MacDonald HR and Severinson E (1984) Regulation of Ig class secretion by soluble products of certain T-cell lines. *Immunol Rev* **78**:25–50.

19. Isakson PC, Puré E, Vitetta ES and Krammer PH (1982) T cell-derived B cell differentiation factor(s). Effect on the isotype switch of murine B cells. *J Exp Med* **155**:734–748.

20. Finkelman FD, Holmes J, Katona IM *et al* (1990) Lymphokine control of *in vivo* immunoglobulin isotype selection. *Annu Rev Immunol* **8**:303–333.

21. Kuhn R, Rajewsky K and Müller W (1991) Generation and analysis of interleukin-4 deficient mice. *Science* **254**:707–710.

22. Berton MT, Uhr JW and Vitetta ES (1989) Synthesis of germ-line γ1 immunoglobulin heavy-chain transcripts in resting B cells: induction by interleukin 4 and inhibition by interferon-γ. *Proc Natl Acad Sci USA* **86**:2829–2833.

23. Xu L and Rothman P (1994) IFN-γ represses ε germline transcription and subsequently down-regulates switch recombination to ε. *Int Immunol* **6**:515–521.

24. Gajewski TF and Fitch FW (1988) Anti-proliferative effect of IFN-γ in immune regulation. I. IFN-γ inhibits the proliferation of Th2 but not Th1 murine helper T lymphocyte clones. *J Immunol* **140**:4245–4252.

25. Gascan H, Gauchat JF, Roncarolo MG, Yssel H, Spits H and De Vries J (1991) Human B cell clones can be induced to proliferate and to switch to IgE and IgG4 synthesis by interleukin 4 and a signal provided by activated CD4+ T cell clones. *J Exp Med* **173**:747–750.

26. Gascan H, Gauchat JF, Aversa G, Van Vlasselaer P and De Vries J (1991) Anti-CD40 monoclonal antibodies or CD4+ T cell clones and IL-4 induce IgG4 and IgE switching in purified human B cells via different signaling pathways. *J Immunol* **147**:8–13.

27. Punnonen J, Aversa G, Cocks BG *et al* (1993) Interleukin-13 induces interleukin-4-independent IgG4 and IgE synthesis and CD23 expression by human B cells. *Proc Natl Acad Sci USA* **90**:3730–3734.

28. Pene J, Rousset F, Briere F *et al* (1988) IgE production by normal human lymphocytes is induced by interleukin 4 and suppressed by interferons γ and α and prostaglandin E2. *Proc Natl Acad Sci USA* **85**:6880–6884.

29. Hilton DJ, Zhang JG, Metcalf D, Alexander WS, Nicola NA and Willson TA (1996) Cloning and characterization of a binding subunit of the interleukin 13 receptor that is also a component of the interleukin 4 receptor. *Proc Natl Acad Sci USA* **93**:497–501.
30. De Waal Malefyt R, Figdor CG and De Vries J (1993) Effects of interleukin 4 on monocyte functions: comparison to interleukin 13. *Res Immunol* **144**:629–633.
31. Punnonen J, De Waal Malefyt R, Van Vlasselaer P, Gauchat JF and De Vries J (1993) IL-10 and viral IL-10 prevent IL-4-induced IgE synthesis by inhibiting the accessory cell function of monocytes. *J Immunol* **151**:1280–1289.
32. Boothby M, Gravallese E, Liou HC and Glimcher LH (1988) A DNA binding protein regulated by IL-4 and by differentiation in B cells. *Science* **242**:1559–1562.
33. Rothman P, Chen YY, Lutzker S *et al* (1990) Structure and expression of germ line immunoglobulin heavy-chain ε transcripts: interleukin-4 plus lipopolysaccharide-directed switching to Cε. *Mol Cell Biol* **10**:1672–1669.
34. Rothman P, Li SC, Gorham B, Glimcher L, Alt F and Boothby M (1991) Identification of a conserved lipopolysaccharide-plus-interleukin-4-responsive element located at the promoter of germ line ε transcripts. *Mol Cell Biol* **11**:5551–5561.
35. Liao F, Birshtein BK, Busslinger M and Rothman P (1994) The transcription factor BSAP (NF-HB) is essential for immunoglobulin germ-line ε transcription. *J Immunol* **152**:2904–2911.
36. Barberis A, Widenhorn K, Vitelli L and Busslinger M (1990) A novel B-cell lineage-specific transcription factor present at early but not late stages of differentiation. *Genes Dev* **4**:849–859.
37. Köhler I and Rieber E (1993) Allergy-associated Iε and Fcε receptor II (CD23b) genes activated via binding of an interleukin-4-induced transcription factor to a novel responsive element. *Eur J Immunol* **23**:3066–3071.
38. Kotanides H and Reich NC (1993) Requirement of tyrosine phosphorylation for rapid activation of a DNA binding factor by IL-4. *Science* **262**:1265–1267.
39. Delphin S and Stavnezer J (1995) Characterization of an interleukin 4 (IL-4) responsive region in the immunoglobulin heavy chain germline ε promoter: regulation by NF-IL-4, a C/EBP family member and NF-κB/p50. *J Exp Med* **181**:181–192.
40. Albrecht B, Peiritsch S and Woisetschlager M (1994) A bifunctional control element in the human IgE germline promoter involved in repression and IL-4 activation. *Int Immunol* **6**:1143–1151.
41. Ichiki T, Takahashi W and Watanabe T (1993) Regulation of the expression of human Cε germline transcript—identification of a novel IL-4 responsive element. *J Immunol* **150**:5408–5417.
42. Rousset F, Garcia E and Banchereau J (1991) Cytokine-induced proliferation and immunoglobulin production of human B lymphocytes triggered through their CD40 antigen. *J Exp Med* **173**:705–710.
43. Zhang K, Clark EA and Saxon A (1991) CD40 stimulation provides an IFN-γ-independent and IL-4-dependent differentiation signal directly to human B cells for IgE production. *J Immunol* **146**:1836–1842.
44. Jabara HH, Fu SM, Geha RS and Vercelli D (1990) CD40 and IgE: synergism between anti-CD40 monoclonal antibody and interleukin-4 in the induction of IgE synthesis by highly purified human B-cells. *J Exp Med* **172**:1861–1864.
45. Jumper MD, Splawski JB, Lipsky PE and Meek K (1994) Ligation of CD40 induces sterile transcripts of multiple Ig H chain isotypes in human B cells. *J Immunol* **152**:438–445.
46. Fujita K, Jumper MD, Meek K and Lipsky PE (1995) Evidence for a CD40 response element, distinct from the IL-4 response element, in the germline ε promoter. *Int Immunol* **7**:1529–1533.
47. Wakatsuki Y, Neurath MF, Max EE and Strober W (1994) The B cell-specific transcription factor BSAP regulates B cell proliferation. *J Exp Med* **179**:1099–1108.

48. Kim J, Reeves R, Rothman P and Boothby M (1995) The non-histone chromosomal protein HMG-I(Y) contributes to repression of the immunoglobulin heavy chain germline ε RNA promoter. *Eur J Immunol* **25**:798–808.

49. Schreiber RD and Aguet M (1994) The interferon-γ receptor. In: Nicola NA (Ed.) *Guidebook to Cyokines and their Receptors*, pp. 120–123. Oxford University Press, New York.

50. Ohara J and Paul WE (1987) Receptors for B-cell stimulatory factor-1 expressed on cells of haematopoietic lineage. *Nature* **325**:537–540.

51. Izuhara K, Yang G, Miyajima A, Howard M and Harada N (1993) Structure of IL-4 and its receptor. *Res Immunol* **144**:584–590.

52. Russell S, Johnston J, Noguchi M *et al* (1994) Interaction of IL-2Rβ and γ chains with Jak1 and Jak3: implications for XSCID and XCID. *Science* **266**:1042–1045.

53. Miyajima A, Kitamura T, Harada N, Yokota T and Arai K (1992) Cytokine receptors and signal transduction. *Annu Rev Immunol* **10**:295–331.

54. Keegan AD, Nelms K, White M, Wang L-M, Pierce JH and Paul WE (1994) An IL-4 receptor region containing an insulin receptor motif is important for IL-4-mediated IRS-1 phosphorylation and cell growth. *Cell* **76**:811–820.

55. Idzerda RL, March CJ, Mosley B *et al* (1990) Human interleukin 4 receptor confers biological responsiveness and defines a novel receptor superfamily. *J Exp Med* **171**:861–876.

56. Cosman D (1993) The hematopoietin receptor superfamily. *Cytokine* **5**:95–106.

57. Kishimoto T, Taga T and Akira S (1994) Cytokine signal transduction. *Cell* **76**:253–262.

58. Obiri NI, Debinski W, Leonard WJ and Puri RK (1995) Receptor for interleukin 13. Interaction with interleukin 4 by a mechanism that does not involve the common γ chain shared by receptors for interleukins 2, 4, 7, 9, and 15. *J Biol Chem* **270**:8797–8804.

59. He YW, Adkins B, Furse RK and Malek TR (1995) Expression and function of the γ subunit of the IL-2, IL-4, and IL-7 receptors. Distinct interaction of γ chain in the IL-4 receptor. *J Immunol* **154**:1596–1605.

60. Lin JX, Migone TS, Friedmann M *et al* (1995) The role of shared receptor motifs and common STAT proteins in the generation of cytokine pleiotropy and redundancy by IL-2, IL-4, IL-7, IL-13, and IL-15. *Immunity* **2**:331–339.

61. Zurawski SM, Vega FJ, Huyghe B and Zurawski G (1993) Receptors for interleukin-13 and interleukin-4 are complex and share a novel component that functions in signal transduction. *EMBO J* **12**:2663–2670.

62. Zurawski SM, Chomarat P, Djossou O *et al* (1995) The primary binding subunit of the human interleukin-4 receptor is also a component of the interleukin-13 receptor. *J Biol Chem* **270**:13869–13878.

63. Reichel M, Nelson BH, Greenberg PD and Rothman PB (1997) The IL-4 receptor α-chain cytoplasmic domain is sufficient for activation of JAK-1 and STAT6 and the induction of IL-4-specific gene expression. *J. Immunol.* **158**:5860–5867.

64. Darnell JE, Kerr I and Stark G (1994) Jak-STAT pathways and transcriptional activation in response to IFNs and other extracellular signaling proteins. *Science* **264**:1415–1420.

65. Wilks AF, Harpur AG, Kurban RR, Ralph SJ, Zurcher G and Ziemiecki A (1991) Two novel protein-tyrosine kinases, each with a second phosphotransferase-related catalytic domain, define a new class of protein kinase. *Mol Cell Biol* **11**:2057–2065.

66. Firmbach-Kraft I, Byers M, Shows T, Dalla-Favera R and Krolewski JJ (1990) Tyk2, prototype of a novel class of non-receptor tyrosine kinase genes. *Oncogene* **5**:1329–1336.

67. Ihle J, Wittuhn B, Quelle F *et al* (1994) Signaling by the cytokine receptor superfamily: JAKs and STATs. *Trends Biol Sci* **19**:222–227.

68. Velazquez L, Fellous M, Stark GR and Pellegrini S (1992) A protein tyrosine kinase in the interferon α/β signaling pathway. *Cell* **70**:313–322.

69. Watling D, Guschin D, Müller M et al (1993) Complementation by tyrosine kinase JAK2 of a mutant cell line defective in the interferon-γ signal transduction pathway. *Nature* **366:**166–170.
70. Witthuhn BA, Silvennoinen O, Miura O et al (1994) Involvement of the Jak-3 Janus kinase in signalling by interleukins 2 and 4 in lymphoid and myeloid cells. *Nature* **370:**153–157.
71. Barbieri G, Velazquez L, Scrobogna M, Fellous M and Pellegrini S (1994) Activation of the protein tyrosine kinase tyk2 by interferon α/β. *Eur J Biochem* **223:**427–435.
72. Johnston J, Kawamura M, Kirken R et al (1994) Phosphorylation and activation of the Jak-3 Janus kinase in response to interleukin-2. *Nature* **370:**151–153.
73. Mueller M, Laxton C, Briscoe B et al (1993) Complementation of a mutant cell line: central role of the 91-kDa polypeptide of ISGF-3 in the interferon-α and -γ signal transduction pathways. *EMBO J* **12:**4221–4228.
74. Schindler C, Shuai K, Prezioso VR and Darnell JE (1992) Interferon-dependent tyrosine phosphorylation of a latent cytoplasmic transcription factor. *Science* **257:**809–813.
75. Schindler C, Kashleva H, Pernis A, Pine R and Rothman P (1994) STF-IL-4: A novel IL-4 induced signal transducing factor. *EMBO J* **13:**1350–1356.
76. Shuai K, Schindler C, Prezioso VR and Darnell JE (1992) Activation of transcription by IFN-γ: tyrosine phosphorylation of a 91-kD DNA binding protein. *Science* **258:**1808–1812.
77. Larner AC, David M, Feldman GM et al (1993) Tyrosine phosphorylation of DNA binding proteins by multiple cytokines. *Science* **261:**1730–1733.
78. Hou J, Schindler U, Henzel W, Ho TC, Brasseur M and McKnight SL (1994) An interleukin-4 induced transcription factor: IL-4 Stat. *Science* **265:**1701–1705.
79. Rothman P, Kreider B, Levy D et al (1994) Cytokines signal through tyrosine phosphorylation of a family of related transcription factors. *Immunity* **1:**457–468.
80. Szabo SJ, Jacobson NG, Dighe AS, Gubler U and Murphy KM (1995) Developmental commitment to the Th2 lineage by extinction of IL-12 signaling. *Immunity* **2:**665–675.
81. Greenlund AC, Morales MO, Viviano BL, Yan H, Krolewski J and Schreiber RD (1995) Stat recruitment by tyrosine-phosphorylated cytokine receptors: an ordered reversible affinity-driven process. *Immunity* **2:**677–687.
82. Ihle JN and Kerr IM (1995) Jaks and Stats in signaling by the cytokine receptor superfamily. *Trends Genet* **11:**69–74.
83. Briscoe J, Guschin D and Müller M (1994) Signal transduction. Just another signaling pathway. *Curr Biol* **4:**1033–1035.
84. Stahl N, Farruggella T, Boulton T, Zhong Z, Darnell JE and Yancopoulos G (1995) Choice of STATs and other substrates specified by modular tyrosine-based motifs in cytokine receptors. *Science* **267:**1349–1353.
85. Heim MH, Kerr IM, Stark GR and Darnell JE (1995) Contribution of STAT SH2 groups to specific interferon signaling by the JAK–STAT pathway. *Science* **267:**1347–1353.
86. Qureshi SA, Leung S, Kerr IM, Stark GR and Darnell JE (1996) Function of Stat2 protein in transcriptional activation by α interferon. *Mol Cell Biol* **16:**288–293.
87. Lu B, Reichel M and Rothman P (1996) Carboxy terminus of Stat6 is a transcriptional activator. (submitted for publication).
88. Horvath CM, Wen Z and Darnell JE (1995) A STAT protein domain that determines DNA sequence recognition suggests a novel DNA-binding domain. *Genes Dev* **9:**984–994.
89. Schindler U, Wu P, Rothe M, Brasseur M and McKnight SL (1995) Components of a Stat recognition code: evidence for two layers of molecular selectivity. *Immunity* **2:**689–697.
90. Kaplan MH, Schindler U, Smiley S and Grusby MJ (1996) Stat6 is required for mediating responses to IL-4 and for the development of Th2 cells. *Immunity* **4:**313–319.

91. Shimoda K, Van Deursen J, Sangster MY *et al* (1996) Lack of IL-4-induced Th2 response and IgE class switching in mice with disrupted Stat6 gene. *Nature* **380**:630–633.

92. Takeda K, Tanaka T, Shi W *et al* (1996) Essential role of Stat6 in IL-4 signalling. *Nature* **380**:627–630.

93. Finkelman FD, Katona IM, Urban JJ, Snapper CM, Ohara J and Paul WE (1986) Suppression of *in vivo* polyclonal IgE responses by monoclonal antibody to the lymphokine B-cell stimulatory factor 1. *Proc Natl Acad Sci USA* **83**:9675–9678.

94. Decker T, Lew DJ, Cheng YS, Levy DE and Darnell JE (1989) Interactions of α- and γ-interferon in the transcriptional regulation of the gene encoding a guanylate-binding protein. *EMBO J* **8**:2009–2014.

95. Lew DJ, Decker T and Darnell JE (1989) α interferon and γ interferon stimulate transcription of a single gene through different signal transduction pathways. *Mol Cell Biol* **9**:5404–5411.

96. Pearse RN, Feinman R, Shuai K, Darnell JE and Ravetch JV (1993) Interferon γ-induced transcription of the high-affinity Fc receptor for IgG requires assembly of a complex that includes the 91-kDa subunit of transcription factor ISGF3. *Proc Natl Acad Sci USA* **90**:4314–4318.

97. Kanno Y, Kozak CA, Schindler C *et al* (1993) The genomic structure of the murine ICSBP gene reveals the presence of a gamma interferon-responsive element, to which an ISGF3 α subunit (or similar) molecule binds. *Mol Cell Biol* **13**:3951–3963.

98. Strehlow I, Seegert D, Frick C *et al* (1993) The gene encoding IFP53/tryptophanyl-tRNA synthetase is regulated by γ-interferon activation factor (GAF). *J Biol Chem* **268**:16590–16595.

99. Armitage R, Fanslow W, Strockbine L *et al* (1992) Molecular and biological characterization of a murine ligand for CD40. *Nature* **357**:80–82.

100. Lederman S, Yellin MJ, Krichevsky A, Belko J, Lee JJ and Chess L (1992) Identification of a novel surface protein on activated CD4$^+$ T cells that induces contact-dependent B cell differentiation. *J Exp Med* **175**:1091–1101.

101. Hollenbaugh D, Grosmaire LS, Kullas CD *et al* (1992) The human T cell antigen gp39, a member of the TNF gene family, is a ligand for the CD40 receptor: expression of a soluble form of gp39 with B cell co-stimulatory activity. *EMBO J* **11**:4313–4321.

102. Spriggs MK, Armitage RJ, Strockbine L *et al* (1992) Recombinant human CD40 ligand stimulates B cell proliferation and immunoglobulin E secretion. *J Exp Med* **176**:1543–1550.

103. Warren WD and Berton MT (1995) Induction of germ-line $\gamma 1$ and ε Ig gene expression in murine B cells. *J Immunol* **155**:5637–5646.

104. Wen Z, Zhong Z and Darnell JE (1995) Maximal activation of transcription by STAT 1 and STAT 3 requires both tyrosine and serine phosphorylation. *Cell* **82**:241–250.

105. Ihle JN (1996) STATs: Signal transducers and activators of transcription. *Cell* **84**:331–334.

106. Zhang X, Blenis J, Li HC, Schindler C and Chen-Kiang S (1995) Requirement of serine phosphorylation for formation of STAT-promoter complexes. *Science* **267**:1990–1994.

8 Switch Transcripts and Cytokine Regulation of Class Switching

GREGOR SIEBENKOTTEN and ANDREAS RADBRUCH*
*Miltenyi Biotec GmbH, Bergisch Gladbach and *Deutsches
Rheumaforschungszentrum Berlin, Germany*

Apart from V(D)J rearrangement, immunoglobulin class switching is the only known case of cell differentiation in vertebrates for which recombination is required. Because this is an irreversible process, and because recombination-induced DNA strand breaks are a risk for the integrity of the genome, this differentiation step has to be especially tightly regulated. Thus induction of class switch recombination requires at least two kinds of signals: one signal which activates the recombination enzymes as such and a second signal, which directs these enzymes towards certain C_H genes.

8.1 ACTIVATION OF THE SWITCH RECOMBINATION MACHINERY

Class switch recombination can be induced at high frequency upon activation in resting B cells and is obviously actively shut off in terminally differentiated plasma blasts (1, 2). The recombination machinery can be induced by stimulation with T cell-independent antigens, by polyclonal activation with anti-immunoglobulin (Ig)-dextran (3) or, in mice, with bacterial lipopolysaccharides (LPS) (4). The central physiological signal, however, is cross-linking of CD40 on the B cells by its ligand (CD40L), expressed on activated T cells, basophils, mast cells, and eosinophils (5, 6).

In the course of T-cell dependent immune responses, triggering of CD40 during cognate interaction of primed T cells with B cells—which have taken up and are presenting antigen—rescues B cells from undergoing apoptosis and switches on the recombination machinery. Class switch is induced in the T-cell zone of secondary lymphoid organs very early, at the beginning of the formation of germinal centers (7). Induction of class switching occurs after the onset of somatic mutation (8) and before differentiation of the cells into plasma or memory cells (9). Patients suffering from X-linked hyper-IgM syndrome, caused by a defect of the CD40L gene, show drastically decreased serum levels of Ig classes other than IgM and IgD (10–13).

IgE Regulation: Molecular Mechanisms. Edited by D. Vercelli. © 1997 John Wiley & Sons Ltd.

Mice rendered deficient in CD40 or CD40L by targeted mutation show IgM but no IgG, IgE, or IgA responses to T-cell dependent antigens, while the serum levels of the different isotypes are normal in response to T-cell independent antigens (14–17). A soluble form of CD40L has been identified (18) to which no specific function could be attributed so far (19). Some of the effects of CD40 cross-linking might be indirect and result from signals transmitted after homotypic adhesion of the B cells, appearing after CD40 signal-induced upregulation of the adhesion molecules intercellular adhesion molecule-1 (ICAM-1) and leukocyte function-associated antigen-1 (LFA-1) (20, 21).

After class switch recombination the inactive IgH allele, which is not under selective pressure, is in most cases recombined to the same C_H gene as the active one (22–25). This indicates that the class switch recombination machinery is precisely directed towards specific C_H genes. To this end, a second set of signals is required. These signals are mostly, if not always, delivered by cytokines, expressed by T cells and antigen-presenting or accessory cells. The kind of antigen and the route of invasion can, therefore, indirectly determine the major Ig isotypes and thus the function of the specific antibodies in a given immune response.

Cytokine signals direct class switching by activating certain switch regions for recombination. This activation is indicated by changes in the methylation pattern within and $5'$ of the switch (S) region (26, 27) and the appearance of DNaseI hypersensitive sites (28, 29). Most strikingly, it strictly correlates with the appearance of specific transcripts, which initiate heterogeneously at a promoter region $5'$ of the S region and terminate at the normal poly A sites of the corresponding C_H gene segment. These transcripts are called germline or switch transcripts. The possible functional relevance of these transcripts is discussed below.

One cytokine can specifically direct class switching to more than one isotype. In addition, cytokines can selectively suppress a class switch, paralleled by the suppression of specific switch transcripts. The major antipodes in the functional diversification of immune responses into humoral and cell-mediated reactions, interleukin (IL)-4 and interferon (IFN)-γ, are also antagonists in the regulation of class switching.

IL-4 activates B cells, and by inducing the generation of T helper 2 (Th2) cells, it suppresses inflammatory and cell-mediated responses. In mice, IL-4 directs class switching to IgG1, which dominates in most responses to protein antigens, and to IgE. IL-4 regulates switching to IgG1 and IgE (30) in a dose-dependent manner, with low doses required for IgG1 and high doses for IgE switching (31, 32). In humans it directs class switching to IgG4 and IgE (33) and perhaps also to IgG1 and IgG3, although the evidence for this is not that clear (34). In mice IL-4 suppresses class switching to IgG3, which prevails in reactions to carbohydrates, like those on bacterial cell walls, and class switching to IgG2b (35, 36). IL-13 elicits the same effect as IL-4 in humans, probably by signal transduction through a shared component of the IL-4 and IL-13 receptors (37–39).

IFN-γ activates macrophages, elicits inflammatory responses, cell-mediated immune responses, and antibody-dependent cell-mediated cytotoxicity (ADCC). It directs class switching to IgG2a, the major antibody secreted in virus-induced immune reactions, and to IgG3 in the mouse (31, 40–42). It suppresses class switching to IgG1 and IgE in mice (31, 43, 44) and to IgG4 and IgE in man (45, 46).

Finally, transforming growth factor (TGF)-β targets class switching to IgG2b and IgA in mice (47, 48), directs the switch to IgA1 and IgA2 in man (49, 50) and may specifically inhibit class switching to IgE in man (45, 51).

All the effects of the various cytokines described above on class switch recombination could be correlated to specific appearance or disappearance, respectively, of switch transcripts of the corresponding C_H genes. The described cytokines are, however, not the only regulators of switching to particular classes. Mice rendered deficient for IFN-γ receptor can still produce IgG3 and IgG2b (42) and IL-4-deficient mice can still produce IgG1 and IgE (52, 53), although in much lower quantities. This is most likely not due to leakiness in regulation, but to redundant signaling by other inductive factors, such as IL-13 instead of IL-4 in man.

8.2 SEQUENTIAL SWITCHING

Upon stimulation with more than one cytokine, or with one cytokine which activates more than one C_H gene, a B cell can switch Ig isotype more than once. Stimulation with IL-4, for example, often although not obligatorily, leads to a sequential switch from IgM via IgG1 to IgE in mice (54–56) and, at least in B-cell cultures, the time between the two recombinations is long enough to allow substantial expression of IgG1 (32, 55, 57). Sequential recombination might simply be due to a simultaneous strong activation of the long Sγ1 region (10 kb) and a weak activation of the short Sε region (2 kb), since low IgE switch frequency is an intrinsic feature of Sε (56). In human B cells frequent sequential switching to IgE via IgG4 has been reported (58, 59). The low frequency of class switching to IgE leads to a limitation within the repertoire of IgE molecules. This oligoclonality could be of importance for the main function of IgE, i.e. activation of mast cells and basophils by cross-linking of IgE bound to their high-affinity Fcε receptors. Cross-linking could be hampered by IgE molecules of too many different specificities on the cell surface. An excess of IgG1 (or IgG4) antibodies of the same repertoire could on the other hand increase the threshold of undesirable IgE-mediated immune responses by masking the antigen (60, 61). Since other cytokines activate more than one S region at a time, other preferentially sequential switch programs may exist, but have not been described in much detail.

8.3 CONTROL OF SWITCH TRANSCRIPTION

The nature of the B-cell activation signal influences the control of class switching by cytokines. When murine B cells are activated by anti-Ig-dextran instead of LPS or CD40L, IL-4 directs switching only to IgE and cannot induce switching to IgG1, and

TGF-β leads to switching to IgA and not to IgG2b (62). Thus, more than one factor is required for the induction of a switch transcript, yet only one has to be induced specifically by a cytokine.

The elements, which act as transcriptional promoters or enhancers and are essential for recombination, are located 5' of each S region and 3' of the Cα gene. They have been shown to bind several transcription factors, which are activated upon stimulation of resting B cells.

NF-κB binding sites have been identified within murine Sγ1, Sγ3 and Sγ2b (63), 5' of Sγ3 (64), Sε (65), Sγ1 and human Sα2 (66). Several binding sites have been found in the regulatory region 3' of Cα (67). Interestingly, mice with a targeted disruption of the p50 subunit of NF-κB (68) have defects in class switching which resemble those observed in mice with a deletion in the 3' control region (69).

The B cell lineage-specific activator protein (BSAP) has several binding sites in the IgH locus, i.e. in Sμ (70) and Sα (71), 5' of Sγ2a (72) and Sε (73) and at multiple sites in the regulatory elements 3' of Cα (67) in mice. It seems to have activating as well as repressing functions at distinct stages of B-cell development. BSAP knock-out mice show a block at the very early CD43$^+$ stage of B-cell development (74) and could therefore not elucidate the function of this protein in class switching (see also Chapters 7 and 10 in this book).

The prime candidates for specific effects of cytokines on class switching and the most important signal transduction pathways of many cytokine receptors seem to be the JAK (Janus kinase)/STAT (signal transducer and activator of transcription) pathways. By analyses of mice with targeted mutations, Stat1 has been shown to be absolutely required for signal transduction in response to IFN-α and IFN-γ, but not for signaling triggered by the many other factors for which Stat1 has been reported to be involved (75, 76). Stat6 has been shown to be indispensable for most of the effects of IL-4 and has been described as a unique signal transducer of the IL-4 receptor so far. Stat6 binding sites have been identified in the Iγ1 and the Iε promoter (65, 77). Consequently, comparable to the situation in IL-4-deficient mice, serum IgG1 in Stat6-deficient mice is reduced and IgE is apparently absent (78–80). Thus, at least for IL-4 and IFN-γ, STATs appear to be the major factors conferring high specificity to the cytokine induction of specific switch transcripts.

8.4 SWITCH TRANSCRIPTS AND THE MECHANISM OF RECOMBINATION

The recombination machinery seems to be extremely active. A switch obviously starts with intra-S region deletions, followed by primary and often secondary switch recombinations and finishes with deletions within the resulting hybrid switch regions (23, 81, 82).

Switch recombination occurs by a looping-out process, by which the deleted part is closed to a circle. These circles can be easily isolated from switching cells (83–

85). The existence of the reciprocal products of recombination suggests that the donor and the acceptor S regions are cut in a concerted action. The sequences of the recombination breakpoints on the circles and on the chromosomes show no structural difference (86); thus, both products seem to be generated similarly. Sometimes, instead of being excised as a circle, the DNA between two S regions is inverted (87, 32). Therefore, it seems likely that S regions are aligned before they are cut completely. Inversions are rare, indicating that during cutting and rejoining the recombination machinery preserves the information at the $5'$ and at the $3'$ part of an S region (see also Chapter 11).

Small regions of homology at many breakpoints of switch recombination suggest a mechanism comparable to that described in a model for non-homologous recombination in double strand break repair. Proteins of this system may be part of the switch recombination machinery (86). Double strand breaks have been shown to appear in S regions upon stimulation of B cells with LPS (88). According to the double strand break repair model, exonuclease(s) may generate $3'$ overhangs in both partners of recombination after the strand break. These single strands are then aligned by specialized protein(s) (89). In case some complementary bases exist at the ends, the strands will pair, which leads to the observed small homologies. Using the $3'$ ends as a primer (even if the ends are connected solely by protein) the remaining gaps are filled by DNA repair polymerase. This synthesis might occur without proofreading and run through some hundred base pairs, as suggested by Dunnick *et al* (86) and Li *et al* (90). Proofreading might be affected during somatic hypermutation. This would lead to products that, after segregation of the chromatides during the next cell division, show mutations only at one side of the recombination breakpoint (86). It has been shown that DNA synthesis is required for switch recombination (91–93).

Switch transcripts play a central although not fully understood role in class switch recombination. All such transcripts of mouse and man analyzed so far have the same structure. They start $5'$ of the S region with a small exon, called I exon, run through the S region and the complete C_H gene segment until its polyadenylation site. They are processed in such a way that the I exon is spliced to the first C_H exon and the transcribed S region is an intron (36, 94). Although $S\mu$ is anyway transcribed from the V_H promoter after VDJ recombination, an additional transcript with the structure of a switch transcript is initiated within the Ig_H intron enhancer. After recombination, hybrid switch transcripts are synthesised, consisting of $I\mu$ and the juxtaposed C_H sequence (95). Due to stop codons in the I exon, switch transcripts are generally not translated. However, open reading frames or cryptic translation products have been described for the murine α and μ switch transcript, respectively (96, 97), but no function has been attributed to them so far.

The role of transcription and the transcripts in switch recombination has been analyzed extensively by targeted mutation experiments in mice. If transcription is specifically inhibited by deletion of the promoters $5'$ of $I\gamma1$ or $I\gamma2b$ or by deletion of the J_H locus, together with the $I\mu$ promoter, the corresponding S region cannot participate in switch recombination any more (81, 98, 99). However, it is not transcription as such, which is sufficient to activate an S region for recombination. When the Iε promoter, together with the Iε exon, is replaced by a V$_H$ promoter plus the Ig$_H$ intron enhancer, the S region is transcribed, but rarely recombined (100). Similarly, if the Iγ1 promoter and Iγ1 exon are replaced by the human metallothionein IIa promoter, considerable transcription, but no recombination is observed (101). When, however, a tiny sequence of 114 bp containing the Iγ1 splice donor site in its middle is retained in the transcription unit, switching to IgG1 occurs at normal levels (101). This strongly suggests that processing of the transcripts is essential for switch recombination. In another experiment, in which the Iα promoter and exon have been replaced by a complete hypoxanthine guanine phosphoribosyltransferase (HPRT) mini-gene, switch recombination appears to be unaffected or only slightly reduced (102). Transcription extends through the S region and the Cα sequence but no splicing from a splice donor site in the HPRT gene to Cα has been observed so far (66). The primary transcript, however, is cut at the poly-A site 3' of the HPRT gene and thus 5' of the S region sequence. Cutting the switch transcript 5' of the S region, as the key feature of the initiation of switch recombination, would fit all of the described experiments (66). The RNA cleavage could help to stabilize a DNA/RNA hybrid of the S region, displace one DNA strand, as described by Reaban and Griffin (103) and Daniels and Lieber (104), and thus could make it sensitive to endonuclease attack or to transcription-coupled nucleotide excision repair (90) initiating recombination. Because splicing can occur at the nascent transcript (105, 106), the process of splicing itself might have an effect on recombination. For yeast mitochondria, an endonuclease has been described, which includes an excised intron RNA as a catalytic component, and catalyzes cleavage of a DNA strand by partial reverse splicing (107, 108) (see also Chapters 7 and 9).

Alternatively, the switch transcript as such might be the component conferring specificity to the recombination machinery. Processed switch transcripts differ from productive Ig transcripts in that they carry an I$_H$ exon instead of a VDJ exon. I$_H$ exons have no obvious consensus sequence. Thus, it seems unlikely that they take part in the recombination by means of their sequence, except along the lines described above. However, the spliced-out intronic S region might attract the switch recombination machinery to an S region in the DNA and, thus, confer S region specificity to the recombinase.

The results reported for gene-targeting experiments, replacing or deleting control regions of class switching, differ essentially from those obtained by using extrachromosomal switch substrates. For such substrates to be recombined, transcription but not splicing seems to be required (104, 109). This difference could be due to relaxed substrate requirements, e.g. cuts in the S region could be generated by different mechanisms in substrates replicating extrachromosomally. For V(D)J rearrangement, it has been shown that the cleavage activity of the recombinase on extrachromosomal substrates is fundamentally different from that on recombination signal sequences within chromatin or genomic DNA (110). It could also be that the much shorter transcripts from switch substrates do not have to be spliced, to let the transcribed S region fragments fit the recombination enzyme(s). It remains to be elucidated how the switch transcripts and/or their processing are coupled to recombination in this unique process of cell differentiation.

REFERENCES

1. Esser C and Radbruch A (1990) Immunoglobulin class switching: molecular and cellular analysis. *Annu Rev Immunol* **8:**717–735.
2. Klein S and Radbruch A (1994) Inhibition of class switch recombination in plasma cells. *Cell Immunol* **157:**106–117
3. Snapper CM and Mond JJ (1993) Towards a comprehensive view of immunoglobulin class switching. *Immunol Today* **14:**15–17.
4. Kearney JF, Cooper MD and Lawton AR (1976) B cell differentiation induced by lipopolysaccharide. IV. Development of immunoglobulin class restriction in precursors of IgG synthesizing cells. *J Immunol* **117:**1567–1572
5. Banchereau J, Bazan F, Blanchard D *et al* (1994) The CD40 antigen and its ligand. *Annu Rev Immunol* **12:**881–922.
6. Gauchat J-F, Henchoz S, Fattah D *et al* (1995) CD40 ligand is functionally expressed on human eosinophils. *Eur J Immunol* **25:**863–865.
7. Toellner KM, Gulbranson-Judge A, Taylor DR, Sze DM and MacLennan IC (1996) Immunoglobulin switch transcript production in vivo related to the site and time of antigen-specific B cell activation. *J Exp Med* **183:**2303-2312.
8. Liu YJ, Malisan F, Debouteiller O *et al* (1996) Within germinal centers, isotype switching of immunoglobulin genes occurs after the onset of somatic mutation. *Immunity* **4:**241–250.
9. Feuillard J, Taylor D, Casamayor-Palleja M, Johnson GD and MacLennan IC (1995) Isolation and characteristics of tonsil centroblasts with reference to Ig class switching. *Int Immunol* **7:**121–130
10. Aruffo A, Farrington M, Hollenbaugh D *et al* (1993) The CD40 ligand, gp39, is defective in activated T cells from patients with X-linked hyper-IgM syndrome. *Cell* **72:**291–300.
11. Allen RC, Armitage RJ, Conley ME *et al* (1993) CD40 ligand gene defects responsible for X-linked hyper-IgM syndrome. *Science* **259:**990–993.
12. Korthauer U, Graf D, Mages HW *et al* (1993) Defective expression of T-cell CD40 ligand causes X-linked immunodeficiency with hyper-IgM. *Nature* **361:**539–541.
13. DiSanto JP, Bonnefoy JY, Gauchat JF, Fischer A and de Saint Basile G (1993) CD40 ligand mutations in X-linked immunodeficiency with hyper-IgM. *Nature* **361:**541–543.
14. Kawabe T, Naka T, Yoshida K *et al* (1994) The immune response in CD40-deficient mice: impaired immunoglobulin class switching and germinal center formation. *Immunity* **1:**167–178.
15. Xu J, Foy TM, Laman JD *et al* (1994) Mice deficient for the CD40 ligand. *Immunity* **1:**423–431.
16. Renshaw BR, Fanslow WC, Armitage RJ *et al* (1994) Humoral immune responses in CD40 ligand-deficient mice. *J Exp Med* **180:**1889–1900.
17. Castigli E, Alt FW, Davidson L *et al* (1994) CD40-deficient mice generated by recombination-activating gene-2-deficient blastocyst complementation. *Proc Natl Acad Sci USA* **91:**12135–12139.
18. Graf D, Muller S, Korthauer U, van Kooten C, Weise C and Kroczek RA (1995) A soluble form of TRAP (CD40 ligand) is rapidly released after T cell activation. *Eur J Immunol* **25:**1749–1754.

19. Pietravalle F, Lecoanet Henchoz S, Aubry JP, Elson G, Bonnefoy JY and Gauchat JF (1996) Cleavage of membrane-bound CD40 ligand is not required for inducing B cell proliferation and differentiation. *Eur J Immunol* **26**:725–728.

20. Katada Y, Tanaka T, Ochi H *et al* (1996) B cell–B cell interaction through intercellular adhesion molecule-1 and lymphocyte functional antigen-1 regulates immunoglobulin E synthesis by B cells stimulated with interleukin-4 and anti-CD40 antibody. *Eur J Immunol* **26**:192–200.

21. Kehry MR (1996) CD40-mediated signaling in B cells. Balancing cell survival, growth, and death. *J Immunol* **156**:2345–2348.

22. Radbruch A, Müller W and Rajewsky K (1986) Class switch recombination is IgG1 specific on active and inactive IgH loci of IgG1-secreting B-cell blasts. *Proc Natl Acad Sci USA* **83**:3954–3957

23. Winter E, Krawinkel U and Radbruch A (1987) Directed Ig class switch recombination in activated murine B cells. *EMBO J* **6**:1663–1671.

24. Schultz C, Petrini J, Collins J *et al* (1990) Patterns and extent of isotype-specificity in the murine H chain switch DNA rearrangement. *J Immunol* **144**:363–370.

25. Irsch J, Irlenbusch S, Radl J, Burrows PD, Cooper MD and Radbruch AH (1994) Switch recombination in normal IgA1⁺ B lymphocytes. *Proc Natl Acad Sci USA* **91**:1323–1327.

26. Stavnezer-Nordgren J and Sirlin S (1986) Specificity of immunoglobulin heavy chain switch correlates with activity of germline heavy chain genes prior to switching. *EMBO J* **5**:95–102.

27. Burger C and Radbruch A (1990) Protective methylation of immunoglobulin and T cell receptor (TcR) gene loci prior to induction of class switch and TcR recombination. *Eur J Immunol* **20**:2285–2291.

28. Schmitz J and Radbruch A (1989) An interleukin 4-induced DNase I hypersensitive site indicates opening of the γ1 switch region prior to switch recombination. *Int Immunol* **1**:570–575.

29. Berton MT and Vitetta ES (1990) Interleukin 4 induces changes in the chromatin structure of the γ1 switch region in resting B cells before switch recombination. *J Exp Med* **172**:375–378.

30. Bergstedt-Lindqvist S, Moon HB, Persson U, Moller G, Heusser C and Severinson E (1988) Interleukin 4 instructs uncommitted B lymphocytes to switch to IgG1 and IgE. *Eur J Immunol* **18**:1073–1077.

31. Severinson E, Fernandez C and Stavnezer J (1990) Induction of germ-line immunoglobulin heavy chain transcripts by mitogens and interleukins prior to switch recombination. *Eur J Immunol* **20**:1079–1084.

32. Siebenkotten G, Esser C, Wabl M and Radbruch A (1992) The murine IgG1/IgE class switch program. *Eur J Immunol* **22**:1827–1834.

33. Lundgren M, Persson U, Larsson P *et al* (1989) Interleukin 4 induces synthesis of IgE and IgG4 in human B cells. *Eur J Immunol* **19**:1311–1315.

34. Fujieda S, Zhang K and Saxon A (1995) IL-4 plus CD40 monoclonal antibody induces human B cells γ subclass-specific isotype switch: switching to γ1, γ3, and γ4, but not γ2. *J Immunol* **155**:2318–2328.

35. Rothman P, Lutzker S, Gorham B, Stewart V, Coffman R and Alt FW (1990) Structure and expression of germline immunoglobulin γ3 heavy chain gene transcripts: implications for mitogen and lymphokine directed class-switching. *Int Immunol* **2**:621–627.

36. Lutzker S and Alt FW (1988) Structure and expression of germ line immunoglobulin γ2b transcripts. *Mol Cell Biol* **8**:1849–1852.

37. Punnonen J, Aversa G, Cocks BG *et al* (1993) Interleukin 13 induces interleukin 4-independent IgG4 and IgE synthesis and CD23 expression by human B cells. *Proc Natl Acad Sci USA* **90**:3730–3734.

38. de Vries JE, Punnonen J, Cocks BG, de Waal Malefyt R and Aversa G (1993) Regulation of the human IgE response by IL-4 and IL-13. *Res Immunol* **144**:597–601.

39. Keegan AD, Johnston JA, Tortolani PJ *et al* (1995) Similarities and differences in signal transduction by interleukin 4 and interleukin 13: analysis of Janus kinase activation. *Proc Natl Acad Sci USA* **92**:7681–7685.

40. Snapper CM, McIntyre TM, Mandler R *et al* (1992) Induction of IgG3 secretion by interferon γ: a model for T cell-independent class switching in response to T cell-independent type 2 antigens. *J Exp Med* **175**:1367–1371.

41. Collins JT and Dunnick WA (1993) Germline transcripts of the murine immunoglobulin γ2a gene: structure and induction by IFN-γ. *Int Immunol* **5**:885–891.

42. Huang S, Hendriks W, Althage A *et al* (1993) Immune response in mice that lack the interferon-γ receptor. *Science* **259**:1742–1745.

43. Snapper CM and Paul WE (1987) Interferon-γ and B cell stimulatory factor-1 reciprocally regulate Ig isotype production. *Science* **236**:944–947.

44. Berton MT, Uhr JW and Vitetta ES (1989) Synthesis of germ-line γ1 immunoglobulin heavy-chain transcripts in resting B cells: induction by interleukin 4 and inhibition by interferon γ. *Proc Natl Acad Sci USA* **86**:2829–2833.

45. Gauchat JF, Gascan H, de Waal Malefyt R and de Vries JE (1992) Regulation of germ-line ε transcription and induction of ε switching in cloned EBV-transformed and malignant human B cell lines by cytokines and CD4⁺ T cells. *J Immunol* **148**:2291–2299.

46. Kitani A and Strober W (1993) Regulation of Cγ subclass germ-line transcripts in human peripheral blood B cells. *J Immunol* **151**:3478–3488.

47. McIntyre TM, Klinman DR, Rothman P *et al* (1993) Transforming growth factor β 1 selectively stimulates immunoglobulin G2b secretion by lipopolysaccharide-activated murine B cells. *J Exp Med* **177**:1031–1037.

48. Lebman DA, Park MJ, Hansen-Bundy S and Pandya A (1994) Mechanism for transforming growth factor β regulation of α mRNA in lipopolysaccharide-stimulated B cells. *Int Immunol* **6**:113–119.

49. Islam KB, Nilsson L, Sideras P, Hammarstrom L and Smith CI (1991) TGF-β1 induces germ-line transcripts of both IgA subclasses in human B lymphocytes. *Int Immunol* **3**:1099–1106.

50. Nilsson L, Islam KB, Olafsson O *et al* (1991) Structure of TGF-β1-induced human immunoglobulin Cα1 and Cα2 germ-line transcripts. *Int Immunol* **3**:1107–1115.

51. Ichiki T, Takahashi W and Watanabe T (1992) The effect of cytokines and mitogens on the induction of Cε germline transcripts in a human Burkitt lymphoma B cell line. *Int Immunol* **4**:747–754.

52. Kühn R, Rajewsky K and Müller W (1991) Generation and analysis of interleukin-4 deficient mice. *Science* **254**:707–710.

53. von der Weid T, Kopf M, Köhler G and Langhorne J (1994) The immune response to *Plasmodium chabaudi* malaria in interleukin-4-deficient mice. *Eur J Immunol* **24**:2285–2293.

54. Yoshida K, Matsuoka M, Usuda S, Mori A, Ishizaka K and Sakano H (1990) Immunoglobulin switch circular DNA in the mouse infected with *Nippostrongylus brasiliensis*: evidence for successive class switching from μ to ε via γ1. *Proc Natl Acad Sci USA* **87**:7829–7833.

55. Mandler R, Finkelman FD, Levine AD and Snapper CM (1993) IL-4 induction of IgE class switching by lipopolysaccharide-activated murine B cells occurs predominantly through sequential switching. *J Immunol* **150**:407–418.

56. Jung S, Siebenkotten G and Radbruch A (1994) Frequency of immunoglobulin E class switching is autonomously determined and independent of prior switching to other classes. *J Exp Med* **179**:2023–2026.

57. Hodgkin PD, Castle BE and Kehry MR (1994) B cell differentiation induced by helper T cell membranes: evidence for sequential isotype switching and a requirement for lymphokines during proliferation. *Eur J Immunol* **24**:239–246.

58. Jabara HH, Loh R, Ramesh N, Vercelli D and Geha RS (1993) Sequential switching from μ to ε via γ4 in human B cells stimulated with IL-4 and hydrocortisone. *J Immunol* **151**:4528–4533.

59. Zhang K, Mills FC and Saxon A (1994) Switch circles from IL-4-directed ε class switching from human B lymphocytes. Evidence for direct, sequential, and multiple step sequential switch from μ to ε Ig heavy chain gene. *J Immunol* **152**:3427–3435.

60. Rihet P, Demeure CE, Dessein AJ and Bourgois A (1992) Strong serum inhibition of specific IgE correlated to competing IgG4, revealed by a new methodology in subjects from a *S. mansoni* endemic area. *Eur J Immunol* **22**:2063–2070.

61. Hussain R, Poindexter RW and Ottesen EA (1992) Control of allergic reactivity in human filariasis. Predominant localization of blocking antibody to the IgG4 subclass. *J Immunol* **148**:2731–2737.

62. Mond JJ, Vos Q, Lees A and Snapper CM (1995) T cell independent antigens. *Curr Opin Immunol* **7**:349–354.

63. Wuerffel R, Jamieson CE, Morgan L, Merkulov V, Sen R and Kenter AL (1992) Switch recombination breakpoints are strictly correlated with DNA recognition motifs for immunoglobulin Sγ3 DNA-binding proteins. *J Exp Med* **176**:339–349.

64. Gerondakis S, Gaff C, Goodman DJ and Grumont RJ (1991) Structure and expression of mouse germline immunoglobulin γ3 heavy chain transcripts induced by the mitogen lipopolysaccharide. *Immunogenetics* **34**:392–400.

65. Delphin S and Stavnezer J (1995) Regulation of antibody class switching to IgE: characterization of an IL-4-responsive region in the immunoglobulin heavy-chain germline ε promoter. *Ann NY Acad Sci* **764**:123–135.

66. Stavnezer J (1996) Antibody class switching. *Adv Immunol* **61**:79–146.

67. Michaelson JS, Singh M, Snapper CM, Sha WC, Baltimore D and Birshtein BK (1996) Regulation of 3' IgH enhancers by a common set of factors, including κB-binding proteins. *J Immunol* **156**:2828–2839.

68. Snapper CM, Zelazowski P, Rosas FR *et al* (1996) B cells from p50/NF-κB knockout mice have selective defects in proliferation, differentiation, germ-line C_H transcription, and Ig class switching. *J Immunol* **156**:183–191.

69. Cogne M, Lansford R, Bottaro A *et al* (1994) A class switch control region at the 3' end of the immunoglobulin heavy chain locus. *Cell* **77**:737–747.

70. Xu L, Kim MG and Marcu KB (1992) Properties of B cell stage specific and ubiquitous nuclear factors binding to immunoglobulin heavy chain gene switch regions. *Int Immunol* **4**:875–887.

71. Waters SH, Saikh KU and Stavnezer J (1989) A B-cell-specific nuclear protein that binds to DNA sites 5' to immunoglobulin Sα tandem repeats is regulated during differentiation. *Mol Cell Biol* **9**:5594–5601.

72. Liao F, Giannini SL and Birshtein BK (1992) A nuclear DNA-binding protein expressed during early stages of B cell differentiation interacts with diverse segments within and 3' of the Ig$_H$ chain gene cluster. *J Immunol* **148**:2909–2917.

73. Liao F, Birshtein BK, Busslinger M and Rothman P (1994) The transcription factor BSAP (NF-HB) is essential for immunoglobulin germ-line ε transcription. *J Immunol* **152**:2904–2911.

74. Urbánek P, Wang ZQ, Fetka I, Wagner EF and Busslinger M (1994) Complete block of early B cell differentiation and altered patterning of the posterior midbrain in mice lacking Pax5/BSAP. *Cell* **79**:901–912.

75. Meraz MA, White JM, Sheehan KC *et al* (1996) Targeted disruption of the Stat1 gene in mice reveals unexpected physiologic specificity in the JAK–STAT signaling pathway. *Cell* **84:**431–442.

76. Durbin JE, Hackenmiller R, Simon MC and Levy DE (1996) Targeted disruption of the mouse Stat1 gene results in compromised innate immunity to viral disease. *Cell* **84:**443–450.

77. Lundgren M, Larsson C, Femino A, Xu M, Stavnezer J and Severinson E (1994) Activation of the Ig germ-line γ1 promoter. Involvement of C/enhancer-binding protein transcription factors and their possible interaction with an NF-IL-4 site. *J Immunol* **153:**2983–2995.

78. Kaplan MH, Schindler U, Smiley ST and Grusby MJ (1996) Stat6 is required for mediating responses to IL-4 and for development of Th2 cells. *Immunity* **4:**313–319.

79. Takeda K, Tanaka T, Shi W *et al* (1996) Essential role of Stat6 in IL-4 signalling. *Nature* **380:**627–630.

80. Shimoda K, van Deursen J, Sangster MY *et al* (1996) Lack of IL-4-induced Th2 response and IgE class switching in mice with disrupted Stat6 gene. *Nature* **380:**630–633.

81. Gu H, Zou Y-R and Rajewsky K (1993) Independent control of immunoglobulin switch recombination at individual switch regions evidenced through cre-lox-P-mediated gene targeting. *Cell* **73:**1155–1164.

82. Zhang K, Cheah HK and Saxon A (1995) Secondary deletional recombination of rearranged switch regions in Ig isotype-switched B cells. A mechanism for isotype stabilization. *J Immunol* **154:**2237–2247.

83. Iwasato T, Shimizu A, Honjo T and Yamagishi H (1990) Circular DNA is excised by immunoglobulin class switch recombination. *Cell* **62:**143–149.

84. Matsuoka M, Yoshida K, Maeda T, Usuda S and Sakano H (1990) Switch circular DNA formed in cytokine-treated mouse splenocytes: evidence for intramolecular DNA deletion in immunoglobulin class switching. *Cell* **62:**135–142.

85. von Schwedler U, Jack HM and Wabl M (1990) Circular DNA is a product of the immunoglobulin class switch rearrangement. *Nature* **345:**452–456.

86. Dunnick W, Hert GZ, Scappino L and Gritzmacher C (1993) DNA sequences at immunoglobulin switch region recombination sites. *Nucleic Acids Res* **21:**365–372.

87. Jäck HM, McDowell M, Steinberg CM and Wabl M (1988) Looping out and deletion mechanism for the immunoglobulin heavy-chain class switch. *Proc Natl Acad Sci USA* **85:**1581–1585

88. Kenter AL and Wuerffel RA (1995) Detection of double strand breaks in immunoglobulin Sγ3 DNA from normal activated B cells—implications for switch recombination. In: EMBO workshop *Lymphocyte neoplasia and DNA rearrangements in the immune system.* Abstract Book, p. 78.

89. Roth D and Wilson J (1988) Illegitimate recombination in mammalian cells. In: Kucherlapati R and Smith GR (Eds) *Genetic Recombination*, pp 621–653. American Society for Microbiology, Washington DC.

90. Li J, Daniels GA and Lieber MR (1996) Asymmetric mutation around the recombination break point of immunoglobulin class switch sequences on extrachromosomal substrates. *Nucleic Acids Res* **24:**2104–2111.

91. Severinson Gronowicz E, Doss C and Schröder J (1979) Activation to IgG secretion by lipopolysaccharide requires several proliferation cycles. *J Immmunol* **123:**2057–2062.

92. Chu CC, Paul WE and Max EE (1992) Analysis of DNA synthesis requirements for deletional switching in normal B cells. In: *Proceedings of the 8th International Congress of Immunology*, pp. 34.

93. Lundgren M, Strom, L, Bergquist LO *et al* (1995) Cell cycle regulation of immunoglobulin class switch recombination and germ-line transcription: potential role of Ets family members. *Eur J Immunol* **25**:2042–2051.

94. Lennon GG and Perry RP (1985) Cμ-containing transcripts initiate heterogeneously within the IgH enhancer region and contain a novel 5′-nontranslatable exon. *Nature* **318**:475–478.

95. Li SC, Rothman PB, Zhang J, Chan C, Hirsh D and Alt FW (1994) Expression of Iμ-Cγ hybrid germline transcripts subsequent to immunoglobulin heavy chain class switching. *Int Immunol* **6**:491–497.

96. Radcliffe G, Lin YC, Julius M, Marcu KB and Stavnezer J (1990) Structure of germ line immunoglobulin α heavy-chain RNA and its location on polysomes. *Mol Cell Biol* **10**:382–386.

97. Bachl J, Turck CW and Wabl M (1996) Translatable immunoglobulin germ-line transcript. *Eur J Immunol* **26**:870–874.

98. Jung S, Rajewsky K and Radbruch A (1993) Shutdown of class switch recombination by deletion of a switch region control element. *Science* **259**:984–987.

99. Zhang J, Bottaro A, Li S, Stewart V and Alt FW (1993) A selective defect in IgG2b switching as a result of targeted mutation of the Iγ2b promoter and exon. *EMBO J* **12**:3529–3537.

100. Bottaro A, Lansford R, Xu L, Zhang J, Rothman P and Alt FW (1994) S region transcription *per se* promotes basal IgE class switch recombination but additional factors regulate the efficiency of the process. *EMBO J* **13**:665–674.

101. Lorenz M, Jung S, Radbruch A (1995) Switch transcripts in immunoglobulin class switching. *Science* **267**:1825–1828.

102. Harriman GR, Bradley A, Das S, Rogers Fani P and Davis AC (1996) IgA class switch in Iα exon-deficient mice. Role of germline transcription in class switch recombination. *J Clin Invest* **97**:477–485.

103. Reaban ME and Griffin JA (1990) Induction of RNA-stabilized DNA conformers by transcription of an immunoglobulin switch region. *Nature* **348**:342–344.

104. Daniels GA and Lieber MR (1995) Strand specificity in the transcriptional targeting of recombination at immunoglobulin switch sequences. *Proc Natl Acad Sci USA* **92**:5625–5629.

105. Spector DL (1993) Macromolecular domains within the cell nucleus. *Annu Rev Cell Biol* **9**:265–315.

106. Wuarin J and Schibler U (1994) Physical isolation of nascent RNA chains transcribed by RNA polymerase II: evidence for cotranscriptional splicing. *Mol Cell Biol* **14**:7219–7225.

107. Zimmerly S, Guo H, Eskes R, Yang J, Perlman PS and Lambowitz AM (1995) A group II intron RNA is a catalytic component of a DNA endonuclease involved in intron mobility. *Cell* **83**:529–538.

108. Yang J, Zimmerly S, Perlman PS and Lambowitz AM (1996) Efficient integration of an intron RNA into double-stranded DNA by reverse splicing. *Nature* **381**:332–335.

109. Leung H and Maizels N (1992) Transcriptional regulatory elements stimulate recombination in extrachromosomal substrates carrying immunoglobulin switch-region sequences. *Proc Natl Acad Sci USA* **89**:4154–4158.

110. Stanhope-Baker P, Hudson KM, Shaffer AL, Constantinescu A and Schlissel MS (1996) Cell type-specific chromatin structure determines the targeting of V(D)J recombinase activity *in vitro*. *Cell* **85**:887–897.

9 Local and General Control Elements of Immunoglobulin Class Switch Recombination

ANDREA BOTTARO and FREDERICK W. ALT
Howard Hughes Medical Institute, The Children's Hospital, and the Center for Blood Research and Department of Genetics, Harvard Medical School, Boston MA, USA

9.1 CLASS SWITCH RECOMBINATION: MECHANISM AND SPECIFICITY

During a humoral immune response, a naive B lymphocyte differentiates into antibody-secreting plasma cells or long-lived memory B cells. These differentiative events are effected by signals from surface receptors on the B lymphocyte; such receptors include the antigen-specific immunoglobulin (Ig) receptor and additional receptors for signals from other immune system cells. A key event along this activation/differentiation pathway is Ig heavy (H) chain class switching, a process which changes the constant (C) region of the Ig H chain produced by the B cell from IgM/IgD to that of another class of Ig: IgG, IgE or IgA.

In the context of the complete Ig molecule, the different Ig H chain constant regions (referred to as H chain isotypes) provide the multiplicity of effector functions required for the efficient neutralization/elimination of antigen during the humoral immune response. The specific activation of the different isotypes depends on the nature of the antigen (e.g. bacterial wall polysaccharides versus virus envelope proteins versus parasite antigens), the microenvironment at the site of the response (recruitment of different immune system cells) and perhaps phenomena intrinsic to the B cell, such as specific 'commitments' to certain types of responses (see below).

This high degree of complexity of class switching, as well as the need to coordinate this process with the other cellular events taking place during B cell activation, requires strict control. Our laboratory has been involved in elucidating the molecular elements that regulate class switching in mice—both at the level of the single Ig H chain C genes as well as at the level of the entire Ig H locus. Here we will review findings from our laboratory and other studies in this field, and we will discuss them in the context of our present understanding of humoral immunity and of regulation of gene expression.

IgE Regulation: Molecular Mechanisms. Edited by D. Vercelli. © 1997 John Wiley & Sons Ltd.

9.1.1 The Mechanism of Class Switching: S Region Recombination and S Region Binding Proteins

In the murine H chain locus, eight C_H gene segments are clustered in a 150 kb region 3′ of the variable (V), diversity (D) and joining (J) segments that encode the antigen-recognizing portion of the H chain (1). Proof that class switching occurs via a DNA rearrangement process came only a few years after the discovery of VDJ recombination (2–6); however, our understanding of the mechanism of class switch recombination (CSR) has proceeded at a much slower pace.

The targets of CSR are large (several kb long), repetitive sequences called S regions, located upstream of every C_H gene that can undergo switch recombination (i.e. all but $C\delta$) (7–9). During switching, the S region upstream of the first IgH gene, $C\mu$, recombines with one of the downstream S regions with excisional deletion of the intervening sequences (Figure 9.1), generating a new transcription unit composed of

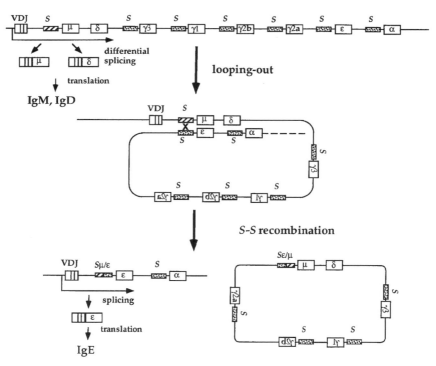

Figure 9.1. The looping-out and deletion mechanism for class switching. Top, a schematic of the murine Ig H locus after VDJ recombination. The individual C_H genes are indicated by a greek letter; S regions are shown (Sμ, striped box; downstream S regions, dotted boxes). Looping out (middle) brings Sμ and one of the downstream S_H regions in close proximity, intrachromosomal recombination removes the intervening sequences as a DNA circle (bottom right), and a new transcription unit is generated (bottom left)

the same VDJ exon together with downstream C_H exons (10–12; reviewed in 13, 14).

S regions can be classified according to sequence similarity into $S\mu$-like ($S\mu$, $S\varepsilon$, $S\alpha$) and $S\gamma$-like. Even within a single group the similarities can be quite limited, although all share some motifs, such as the pentanucleotides GAGCT, GGGGT (reviewed in 15). Their structure is reminiscent of other repetitive elements, such as hypervariable minisatellites, which also have been correlated with enhanced recombinational activity (16). Unlike VDJ recombination, which occurs precisely at the edge of the signal sequences, CSR can fall anywhere within or even in proximity of the S regions (reviewed in 15). The analysis of rearranged S regions has nevertheless lead to potential insights into the switch mechanism (15, 17, 18), suggesting for instance a functional correlation between DNA replication and CSR (19). Preferential recombination sites within the S regions have also been observed, the location of which has been correlated with the binding of specific factors (20–22).

Many activities in nuclear extracts from resting and/or activated B cells have been found to bind to S regions, and several of the actual factors have been identified (20, 23–26). Some (BSAP/Pax5, NF-κB, Oct) are well known DNA-binding factors involved in transcriptional regulation; another, $S\mu$BP-2, shares homology with DNA helicases, but has limited specificity (27, 28). Finally, a number of factors have been characterized only in terms of their binding activities. Despite the wealth of data concerning some of these S region binding factors, any evidence of their actual involvment in CSR is still missing.

9.1.2 Directed, Committed, or Random Class Switching

It has long been known that *in vivo* humoral immune responses towards certain antigens tend to be dominated reproducibly by one or a few Ig isotypes and that, in the mouse, this specificity can be strain dependent—suggesting a significant genetic influence (reviewed in 29). In principle, three models can be formulated to fit this observation. The random switch model postulates a completely random class switch process, in which each activated B cell undergoes switching to one isotype in a stochastic fashion, and during the immune response only the cells that express the 'correct' isotype are selected and expanded. The directed switch model hypothesizes that a B cell is selectively induced to switch to one or few isotypes by external signals at the time of activation, according to the nature of the antigen and the microenvironment at the site of the response. The committed switch model suggests that a developing B cell receives signals that 'preset' its switching ability, so that only a subset of isotypes will be activated when the same B cell encounters antigen. The 'directed' and 'committed' models are not mutually exclusive, as one can imagine that external factors at the time of B-cell activation induce and/or select only the cells that are 'committed' to switch to a certain isotype.

Several observations support the directed or the committed models versus the random switch model. Thus, there is a strict correlation between the signals that can be delivered to resting B cells *in vitro*, in terms of combination of activators and cytokines, and the pattern of class switching of the cultured cells (30–34; reviewed in 35, 36). In addition, the correlation between inducing factor(s) and switching isotype(s) is paralleled by the specific transcriptional activation of the target C_H gene(s) in its germline configuration before the actual recombination event takes place (reviewed in 13, 36). Finally, in murine switched B lineage cells (hybridomas, myelomas, plasmacytomas) there is a significant correlation of the switch pattern on the expressed Ig H allele with that of the non-expressed allele, which is by definition not subject to selection (37–40).

9.1.3 The Specificity of Switching: Class Switch Induction by Cytokines and Activators

There is a vast and continuously expanding literature concerning the ability of specific reagents to induce selective patterns of class switching (30, 32–34, 41; reviewed in 35, 36, 42). Most of these studies were performed *in vitro*, with a few well-characterized B-cell lines or with primary B-cell populations. *In vivo* studies on germline transcription and switching and on the role of cytokines in the induction of specific isotypes show a significant degree of correlation with the *in vitro* observations (43–47). From the *in vitro* studies a model has emerged which views class switch induction as the combined result of two different types of signals delivered to the B cell, which in concert determine the outcome of the differentiation process (reviewed in 48).

The first type of signal, the activator, is thought to initiate the cascade of B-cell activation events including induction of proliferation and determination of competency to switch. At least three classes of activators have been defined: those which induce antigen receptor signaling, those which trigger other specific surface receptors (such as CD40) which are critical for B-cell activation, and those which trigger non-specific polyclonal activation (such as bacterial lipopolysaccharide, LPS). The mechanism of CD40 and surface Ig signaling and the role of these pathways during the initiation of an *in vivo* immune response are now relatively well characterized (reviewed in 49, 50). In this context, the use of these pathways for *in vitro* B-cell activation is considered a representative, although simplified, model for the study of the physiology of B-cell activation. On the other hand, the mode of action of bacterial lipopolysaccharides in B cells is not well understood, starting with the nature of their receptor. It remains debatable whether LPS-activated B cells correspond to any actual counterpart *in vivo*. Nevertheless, LPS culture of mouse B cells has been the most powerful, and until relatively recently, the only, tool for class switch induction *in vitro*.

The study of switching in LPS cultures led to the observation that addition of certain cytokines could dramatically modify the isotype(s) of Ig produced, leading to the definition of the second class of signals necessary for class switching. Cytokines may play multiple roles in influencing class switching. They can directly effect the induction of switching to a certain isotype, they can increase the frequency of cells expressing a particular isotype within a population by selectively expanding these cells, or they can modify secretion levels of all or some isotypes. Only cytokines which mediate the first class of effects can be considered bona fide switch factors. In the murine system, the best characterized so far are interleukin (IL)-4, which induces switching to IgG1 and IgE (32, 41), interferon (IFN)-γ, which induces switching to IgG2a (34, 51) and IgG3 (52), TGF-β which induces switching to IgG2b (53) and IgA (33, 54). IL-5, on the other hand, probably increases Ig secretion in general (55–57), but in some culture systems may directly enhance the rate of switch recombination (58, 59).

9.1.4 Class Switch Induction and Germline Transcription of C_H Genes

Transcripts of C_H genes in their germline configuration were first noticed to precede switch recombination in LPS-treated cell lines (60, 61). C_H gene germline transcripts have now been defined for all murine and most human constant genes that undergo class switching (reviewed in 36, 62). All share a number of basic characteristics. All originate from TATA-less promoters upstream of the S region and have multiple initiation sites. All germline C_H transcripts also contain one or more exons (called I exons) spliced onto the first C_H exon; it is generally believed that the I exons render these transcripts sterile (i.e. unable to encode any significant peptide) due to the presence of multiple stop codons in all reading frames. Finally, the expression of germline C_H transcripts is controlled by factors known to induce class switching to the respective genes, the only exception being the Iμ transcripts, which are constitutively expressed in B cells (63).

9.1.5 The Structure and Function of I Region Promoters

Many studies have focused on the nature of I region promoters as a means to gain insight into the molecular aspects of CSR regulation. The most extensively characterized promoters in the mouse are Iγ1, Iε and Iα promoters.

The Iε region contains at least two major sites for DNA binding proteins: one is IL-4-inducible and overlaps with the 5′-most transcription initiation sites, and the other is constitutive and maps further upstream (64). The IL-4 inducible factor, nuclear factor-B cell responsive element (NF-BRE), is also responsible for IL-4-dependent activation of the major histocompatibility complex (MHC) II-Aα gene (64), and competes for its site with the non-histone chromosomal protein high mobility group (HMG)-I(Y), which thus acts as a repressor of Iε transcription (65). The constitutively expressed binding protein, initially called NF-Iε3 (64), has been identified as the pre-B- and B-cell specific transcription factor BSAP/Pax5, and shown to probably be required for Iε transcription (66). Another relevant protein binding to the Iε IL-4-inducible site is STF–IL-4 (67), a putative member of the growing family of signal transduction and activation of transcription (STAT) factors, which are responsible for the early transcriptional response to a number of cytokines (reviewed in 68). STF–IL-4 (and another IL-4 inducible activity binding in the γ1 promoter, NF–IL-4-γ1, see below) also bind to the so-called GAS sites (68, 69), which are responsible for IFN-γ-activation of several genes (reviewed in 70). Thus, competition of IL-4- and IFN-γ-induced factors for their respective binding sites may represent a mechanism for the mutually repressive action of these two cytokines in a number of gene systems, including regulation of germline C_H transcripts. The human counterpart to STAT–IL-4, called IL-4 nuclear activation factor (NAF), has been shown to be Stat6, a major element of IL-4 receptor signaling (71). Indeed, Stat6 mutant mice have a block in IL-4 signaling and do not switch to IgE (72, 73) (see also Chapters 7 and 10).

The Iγ1 promoter also has several transcription factor binding sites besides the NF–IL-4-γ1 binding site mentioned above (69); other potential regulatory sequences include a CCAAT box/enhancer binding protein (C/EBP) site, a PU box (which binds ets family members), an IFN-α/β responsive site ($\alpha\beta$-IRE), and a TIE (TGF-β inhibitory element) which binds a c-fos containing complex (74). Other DNAse hypersensitive sites correlating with Iγ1 promoter induction are located further upstream (75) and downstream (76, 77; W. Dunnick, personal communication) of the Iγ1 promoter/exon region. Notably, Iγ1 promoter elements are able to confer mitogen and IL-4 inducibility to a heterologous promoter, pointing to the presence of a bona fide enhancer element in this region (74).

Our knowledge of the murine Iα promoter region is not as detailed. Two significant elements have been identified, one activating transcription factor/cAMP responsive element (ATF/CRE) site responsible for the basal activity of the promoter, and a series of TGF-β-responsive sites (at least three copies) necessary for its inducibility (78). In addition, a B-cell specific enhancer element has been identified immediately 3' of the Cα membrane exons (79), and a TGF-β-dependent enhancer is located within the human Iα1 promoter (80).

9.2 IDENTIFICATION AND FUNCTIONAL DISSECTION OF CSR CONTROL ELEMENTS BY GENE TARGETING

Several models can be formulated concerning the role of germline transcripts in CSR. They may be of no functional significance, just a by-product of increased C_H gene accessibility. Alternatively, the I exon sequences and/or their promoter could target the recombinase to the nearby S region, or the germline transcripts could actually be part of a ribonucleoprotein recombinase complex. Finally, the function of germline transcription could be to open up the S region chromatin complexes for the recombinase to act, or to form specific recombination-prone ribonucleic acid structures (such as DNA:RNA triple helices, or supercoiled DNA) (81–83) during S region transcription, with no specific role for the I regions.

Our laboratory has chosen to approach the problem of CSR regulation and mechanism by 'molecular dissection', introducing mutations into candidate regulatory regions (each mutation testing a specific functional hypothesis) and assessing the effects on CSR. This approach, which required the analysis of several mutations was made efficient and cost-effective by the development of the *RAG2*-deficient blastocyst complementation assay (84). This strategy takes advantage of the fact that mice lacking a functional *RAG2* gene do not develop mature T and B cells because of a block in VDJ recombination (85). When totipotent embryonic stem (ES) cells are injected into blastocysts from these mice, the mature B and T cells in the resulting chimeras are entirely derived from the injected cells. Therefore, upon injection of homozygous mutant ES cell lines (obtained in culture from heterozygous knock-out cell lines), it is possible to analyze the effect of the mutation in a pure mutant B-cell population without the need for germline transmission (84).

9.2.1 I Regions/Promoters Locally Control Class Switching

The first mutation we tested was aimed at addressing the basic question of whether integrity of the I region was necessary for normal class switch recombination. We replaced the entire Iγ2b region and its promoter sequences with a G418-resistance (neo$_r$) gene in the opposite transcriptional orientation. The result of this mutation on LPS-induced Cγ2b CSR was clear: homozygous mutant B cells failed to express substantial levels of γ2b transcripts; switching to IgG2b was almost completely abolished; and switching to other Ig C$_H$ genes was unchanged (86). These findings, together with independent mutational studies of the Iγ1 exon (87), provided strong evidence that integrity of the I region sequences is required for normal CSR, and clearly implicated this region as a controlling element for class switching.

9.2.2 The Mode of Action of the Local Control Elements: Germline Transcripts and Germline Transcription

The findings concerning the Iγ1 and Iγ2b mutations just described left open the question of whether transcription through an S region would be sufficient to induce CSR, even in the absence of I exon transcripts. To specifically address this point, we replaced the Iε region and its IL-4-dependent promoter with a general B-cell expression cassette, containing a V$_H$ promoter (V$_H$P) linked to the intronic Ig H enhancer, Eμ. This mutation was independently introduced into an Abelson murine leukemia virus-transformed pre-B-cell line known to switch to IgE upon stimulation with LPS and IL-4 (88), and into ES cells for analysis with the RAG2$^{-/-}$ blastocyst complementation method (89). Whereas IL-4 treatment is absolutely required for germline transcription of and CSR to the Cε gene in normal cells, mutant cells harboring the Iε replacement mutation transcribed the targeted Sε region at substantial levels following LPS stimulation in the absence of IL-4 and also underwent CSR to Cε in the absence of IL-4 treatment. However, the level of CSR to Cε, following treatment of mutant cells with either LPS or LPS/IL-4, was significantly reduced (about five-fold in the pre-B-cell line, and 10–100-fold in the mutant B cells) compared to that of normal cells.

The Iε replacement studies indicated that replacement of the Iε promoter/exon region with a different, constitutive promoter rendered the Sε region competent for CSR, but that optimal efficiency of this process required an intact Iε region (for instance, we cannot rule out the possibility that the inserted neo$_r$ gene somehow inhibited the process). From these findings, it seems possible that class switching may be functionally regulated at two independent levels: transcription to make the S regions specifically 'accessible' (competence), and an unknown process, dependent on the integrity of the I region transcription unit (promoter and/or exon), that may increase the actual rate of CSR (efficiency). The inability of germline transcription through the S region *per se* to induce high levels of CSR is also suggested by results in other systems: anti-IgD/IL-4-activated B cells are able to transcribe high levels of Iγ1, but require IL-5 to initiate class switching (59) and peritoneal B1a (Ly-1 B) cells are able to induce germline γ1 transcripts like 'conventional' B2 cells do, but switch at a much lower frequency (90). In these cases, we would hypothesize that the I region/promoter-dependent, CSR-driving mechanism is absent or less active in anti-IgD/IL-4-stimulated blasts without IL-5 addition, or in B1a cells.

The actual nature of the I-region dependent, CSR-driving mechanism is still an object of speculation. One possibility is that the germline transcripts, after all, play an active role in CSR. This model is supported by the recent observation that CSR in Iγ1-promoter replacement mutants was dependent on the presence of a 114 bp fragment containing the Iγ1 exon donor splice site (91). Although strongly suggestive of a role for I exon splicing in CSR, the fact that the absence of the 114 bp region also reduced the actual level of transcription through the S region by a factor of at least 10 may also indicate that this mutation affects some undefined regulatory element, interference with which may decrease CSR efficiency. Indeed, replacement of the entire Iα exon (splice donor included) with an hypoxanthine phosphoribosyltransferase (hprt) minigene supported non TGF-β-dependent IgA switching at normal levels, despite the lack of Cα-containing spliced transcripts (92). In this case, it has been proposed that polyadenylation of the hprt minigene would generate a truncated S region-containing transcript which could replace the normal spliced-out S region in its switch-promoting function (14, 92) (see also Chapter 8 in this book).

In an alternative model, the relevant elements are the I region promoters. Direct physical interaction—through DNA looping-out—is probably responsible for the synergistic activity of distant pairs of promoters and enhancers, including the intronic Eμ enhancer and V$_H$ promoters (93, 94), and it is mediated by the action of 'tethering' proteins binding at the two sites. Similarly, interaction between transcriptional regulatory elements upstream of Sμ and the target S$_H$ region, perhaps through the action of additional general regulatory elements (see below), could bring the Sμ/S$_H$ regions in close proximity, facilitating their interaction or their common recognition by the putative CSR recombinase complex (Figure 9.2). The results of the Iα replacement mentioned above may be consistent with this hypothesis because this targeted mutation left the Iα promoter intact, and therefore may have allowed the binding of all necessary factors (92). The different impact on CSR efficiency of the different I region targeting experiments could, therefore, depend on the way the mutations (i.e. the deleted regions and the replacing elements) affected the ability of Sμ and the targeted S regions to achieve physical proximity. In both mouse and human the distance between Sμ and the first of the other S regions is about 50–60 kb

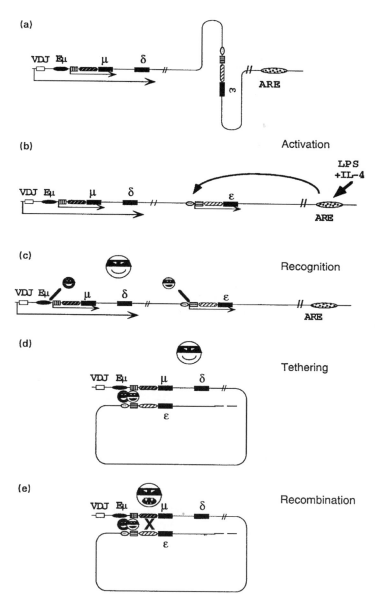

Figure 9.2. The 'tethering' model of class switch recombination. (a) in resting B cells, the 3′ portion of the Ig H locus is inactive. (b) external signals (such as LPS and IL-4) induce B-cell activation. An activation-responsive transcriptional regulatory element (ARE) in the Ig H locus in turn activates transcription from the germline promoters. (c) at this stage, elements upstream of Sμ and of the target S region are recognized by specific 'tethering factors' (small gray smileys), which bring the two S regions in close proximity (d).(e) Switch recombinase (large, white smiley) is activated, and can catalyze the reaction between the two S regions. It is possible that the ARE plays a more direct role in the tethering process, for instance Sμ and S$_H$ could both anchor at different sites of the ARE

(1, 95), suggesting that distance could indeed be a major factor with respect to control of CSR, and that the large intron may have been conserved as part of the switch recombination control system.

9.2.3 The Eμ Intronic Enhancer Region is a Local CSR Control Element

The μ gene, like the other switching C_H genes, is also organized into a germline transcription unit (63), with a 700 bp Iμ exon located immediately downstream of the Eμ intronic enhancer, which serves as its promoter (96). Flanking the Eμ enhancer are two matrix attachment regions (MARs) (97–99), which have also been proposed to contribute to Ig H gene expression. Due to the central role of Sμ in class switching, the characterization of the elements that control CSR at this switch region is of great interest. The first evidence that elements upstream of Sμ may regulate class switching derived from the studies in which a deletion extending from the J_H segments to downstream of the Eμ enhancer was introduced into the murine germline (100). These mutants failed to switch at Sμ, although internal Sγ1 deletions were still observed in activated B cells, indicating that downstream S regions were still CSR competent. Again, absence of transcription in these mutants did not allow the detailed mechanism of the block to be elucidated.

To gain better insight into the relevant *cis*-acting switch control elements at the μ locus, we have recently analyzed the effects of different mutations of the Eμ enhancer region, one (Eμ-del) deleting the Eμ and the flanking MARs (101) and one replacing these sequences with a transcribed neo$_r$ gene (Eμ-repl) (102). Hybridoma analysis shows that Eμ-del mutant alleles have a significant, although not complete, decrease in the ability to perform CSR (A.B., F. Young, J. Chen, M. Serwe, F. Sablitzky and F.W.A., in preparation). Yet, the majority of these homozygous mutant hybridomas show detectable steady-state transcription through the targeted allele. These data suggest that the Eμ complex may play a significant role in determining CSR efficiency independent of its transcriptional enhancing activity. Surprisingly, however, when the Eμ complex was replaced with a neo$_r$ gene driven by the pgk promoter, CSR activity was maintained at normal levels (A.B., F. Young, J. Chen, M. Serwe, F. Sablitzky and F.W.A., in preparation). Therefore, whatever the role played by the Eμ region in facilitating CSR, it does not appear to be sequence-specific, nor does it appear to require the presence of MARs. On the other hand, the pgk-neo$_r$ gene may contain elements inherently able to replace CSR-promoting sequences. In this regard, the pgk promoter was also used to drive the hprt minigene used to replace the Iα region and to maintain switching to IgA (92). Furthermore, replacement of most of the Iγ2b exon with pgk-neo$_r$ leads to LPS- and LPS-IL-4-driven IgG2b switching, while deletion of the pgk-neo$_r$ gene causes a complete block of γ2b CSR (A. Vo, J. Zhang, A.B. and F.W.A., unpublished). Of potential relevance to these findings, it has been hypothesized that the pgk-neo$_r$ gene may be able to compete for the function of the 3′ IgH enhancer complex (103, 104; see below).

9.2.4 The IgH 3′ enhancer region

Because of the central role of Sμ in class switching, mutation of the Eμ enhancer complex affects switching throughout the Ig H locus. However, this should not be taken to mean that Eμ regulates CSR competence of all Ig H genes. Indeed, there is evidence that in Eμ-deleted B cells, downstream genes may still be switch-competent (namely, they undergo internal S region deletions) (100 and A.B., F. Young, J. Chen, M. Serwe, F. Sablitzky and F.W.A., in preparation). Therefore, the Eμ complex likely represents a local CSR regulator similar in function to downstream I region elements; but in this case, such regulation affects the common donor Sμ region and, thus, generally, impacts on the control of the CSR process.

The existence of general control elements able to exert their function over the entire Ig H locus has been suspected for some time, either by analogy with other multigene systems, or because of general regulatory similarities between genes in the two duplication units of the human Ig H locus (105). Moreover, the existence of transcriptional regulatory elements 3′ of the Ig H locus was strongly suggested by the ability of Eμ-deleted B lineage cells to still express high levels of Ig H transcripts (106, 107) and by the activation of myc genes in Ig H translocations in which Eμ and myc were disjoined (108). Following a general search, a transcriptional enhancer element was identified about 25 kb 3′ of the rat Ig H locus (109). This element, termed 3′ E$_H$ or 3′αE, was later identified in the mouse as well (110, 111), where it comprises two DNAse hypersensitive sites (now called HS1 and HS2). The 3′E$_H$ has enhancer activity in activated and terminally differentiated B cells, but appears to be suppressed at earlier stages of development (110, 112, 113). Later, two additional hypersensitive sites (HS3, HS4), corresponding to two independent enhancer elements, were located 13 and 17 kb downstream of HS1/2, respectively (110, 112, 113).

9.2.5 Molecular Aspects of the 3′E$_H$ Function: Binding Factors and Regulation

The multi-element nature of the 3′E$_H$ region suggests complex regulatory mechanisms. Initial studies showed the HS1,2 complex to have the highest activity in terminally differentiated B cells (110). DNA accessibility and methylation studies confirmed this pattern (112). Following the identification of the additional hypersensitive sites, studies have focused on the interplay between the different elements and on the role of DNA binding factors whose specific sites are clustered within the HS elements. Extensive studies were performed on the enhancer activity of the different HS sites, alone and in combination, in B cell lines at different stages of development (114, 115). Complexes of all four HS sites are the most efficient transcriptional activators in terminally differentiated B cells, the single elements having much lower or no activity. At any given developmental stage, in general, there is little correlation between the level of activity of each single site and their combined effect, suggesting a significant level of positive and negative interaction between elements. HS1-4 complexes were also able to induce copy number-dependent and position-independent expression of a reporter gene, features characteristic and defining of locus control regions (LCRs) (114).

A number of transcription factor DNA binding sites have been identified in the different HS sites, most notably sites for ets family members (116, 117), for the AP-1 complex (c-fos and jun-B) (118), for the E47/E12 helix–loop–helix/basic domain proteins (119), for Oct (116, 120), for BSAP/Pax 5 (which can act as an activator or a repressor of different elements at different stages of development) (117, 120–122) and for NF-κB (123). Mice with a null mutation of the NF-κB key component p50 (124) display a defect in germline transcription similar to that of $3'E_H$ neo$_r$ replacement mice, raising the possibility that NF-κB plays a critical role in $3'E_H$-mediated transcriptional activation (125). To add yet another level of complexity, several factors, namely BSAP, NF-κB and Oct, can exert either positive or negative effects on the different elements according to the differentiation stage and to the presence or absence of other binding proteins at neighboring sites (120, 123).

9.2.6 The $3'E_H$ Region is a General Regulator of CSR

Based on the properties described above, the $3'E_H$ was a promising candidate for a general regulatory element of the Ig H locus, and an obvious target for a knock-out experiment. Indeed, replacement of the $3'E_H$ with a pgk-neo$_r$ gene revealed a striking phenotype in mutant B cells: switching to most Ig H genes was essentially abolished in cultures stimulated with LPS, with or without IL-4, with the exception of $\gamma1$ and α, while in the serum of homozygous mutant chimeras a very strong reduction of IgG3 and IgG2a was observed (104). This deficiency was paralleled by the inability to express germline transcripts from the affected genes *in vitro*, suggesting that the $3'E_H$ mutation affects the function of a major regulatory element of Ig H germline transcription, hence blocking CSR. On the other hand, the expression of normal levels of VDJ-μ, VDJ-$\gamma1$ and VDJ-α mRNAs in *in vitro* activated B-cell blasts indicates that the mutation does not affect the function of V_H promoters in high-expressing B cells (104). Others have further shown that myelomas with a deletion of the Eμ intronic enhancer ceased Ig H transcription upon neo$_r$ replacement of the $3'$ enhancer HS1/2 elements (126). Thus, the $3'E_H$ complex and Eμ appear to be able to substitute for each other in enhancing transcription of rearranged Ig H genes in Ig-secreting B cells; moreover, Eμ and $3'E_H$(HS1/2) have been shown to act cooperatively to drive expression from the V_H promoter (127).

The initial experiments in the $3'E_H$ HS1/2 neo$_r$ replacement focused on LPS-induced class switching (104); however, the $3'E_H$ mutation also affects anti-CD40- and anti-IgD-induced CSR (A.B, M. Tian, C. Snapper and F.W.A., unpublished). These data, and direct evidence that different pathways can activate the $3'E_H$ (113, 118), suggest that all switch-activation pathways may utilize the same Ig H control element(s). However, two observations point to the likely existence of other higher-order regulatory elements not affected by the $3'E_H$ mutation: first, IgG1 and IgA switching is essentially normal in the $3'E_H$ mutant mice, indicating that these genes are under separate control (104). Indeed, local enhancer elements are located in proximity to these genes (74, 79, 128), although a formal proof of their function is missing. Second, while IgG2b is absent in LPS cultures from homozygous $3'E_H$ mutant B cells, normal levels of this isotype are present in the serum of chimeras (104), suggesting that particular activation conditions may be able to bypass the requirement for the activity affected by the $3'E_H$ mutation.

9.2.7 The Mode of Action of the General Control Element(s): the Promoter Competition Model

The simplest explanation for the effect of the $3'E_H$ HS1/2 neo$_r$ replacement is that the HS1/2 complex is the main regulatory element of LPS-induced germline transcription, its deletion inhibiting the activity of the I region promoters (Figure 9.3a). Notably, however, the pgk promoter-driven neo$_r$ gene replacing the $3'E_H$ becomes LPS-inducible (103), suggesting that further element(s) exist that can respond to LPS by increasing transcription from the pgk promoter. Indeed, the HS3 and HS4 sites, which have intrinsic enhancer activity in various transcription assays (114, 115) and are not deleted by our mutation, are candidates for such elements.

  Thus, the $3'E_H$ HS1/2 mutation theoretically may not involve the actual LPS-responsive element(s), but may somehow disrupt its ability to induce I region promoter activation. One way this could happen is if the $3'E_H$ control region was comprised of multiple elements, HS1/2 being necessary for germline transcription initiation, and others (e.g. HS3/4) for LPS-responsiveness (Figure 9.3b). Another hypothesis, not mutually exclusive with the previous one, is that the inhibitory effect on germline transcription of the $3'E_H$ replacement could be due to competition of the pgk promoter for the LPS-responsive element, in a way that would not allow expression of the upstream germline promoters (Figure 9.3c). In this model, the differential induction of germline transcripts by cytokines would be dependent on their ability to activate specific transcription factors, which would change the relative 'affinity' of germline promoters for the putative general regulatory element(s). There is increasing evidence that promoter competition is a common regulatory mechanism of gene expression in complex loci. For instance, it may be responsible for imprinting of the Ins-2 and $Igf2$ genes (129, 130), and it was proposed to act at the level of the β-globin LCR to control the temporal expression of the fetal, embryonic and adult globin genes (131–135, 136–138).

  The similarities between the β-globin LCR and the $3'E_H$ enhancer region are certainly intriguing. Like the $3'E_H$ region, the β-globin LCR maps just outside (6–22 kb upstream) of the locus (139, 140), and is comprised of multiple HS sites, each with variable individual transcriptional regulatory activities, but with highly coordinated effects when assayed in combination (comprehensively reviewed in 135, 141, 142). The temporally organized expression of the different β-globin genes is the result of the concerted action of the 5'-LCR and of local regulatory elements in proximity of the individual genes (reviewed in 135, 141, 142), probably through direct physical interaction between the distant elements (131, 132). Moreover, tar-

The IgH 3′enhancer:
an LPS-dependent transcriptional activator?

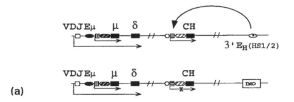

(a)

The IgH 3′enhancer:
element of an
LPS-dependent transcriptional activator?

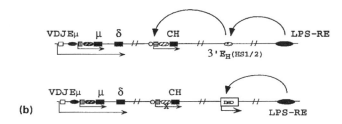

(b)

The IgH 3′enhancer:
simple bystander of an
LPS-dependent transcriptional activator?

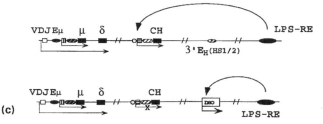

(c)

Figure 9.3. Three models for the effect of the $3'E_H(HS1/2)$ mutation. (a) HS1/2 could constitute a specific enhancer for some I region promoters. HS1/2 replacement with neo_r would thus directly inactivate germline transcription for lack of the enhancer element. (b) HS1/2 could be one of the components of a more complex regulatory element. LPS inducibility would be dependent on a separate LPS-responsive element (LPS-RE), which would activate HS1/2 (perhaps by regulating local accessibility), and HS1/2 would enhance germline transcription. Replacement of HS1/2 with neo_r renders neo_r LPS-inducible, but blocks I region transcription for lack of the enhancer. (c) HS1/2 could have no specific or necessary function in regulating germline transcription. Insertion of neo_r in place of HS1/2, however, would block germline transcription because the pgk promoter would compete for the LPS-responsive enhancer element with the germline promoters. Neo_r would become LPS-inducible, and the out-competed germline promoters would be inactive. Note that the models shown in B and C are not mutually exclusive, since the different $3'E_H$ elements could have partially overlapping functions

geting experiments have shown that insertion of selection markers next to, or replacing, specific HS sites in the β-globin LCR results in disruption of its activity, while the 'clean' deletion of the same elements does not (134, 136, 137).

The competition hypothesis is strongly supported by the observation that a pgk-neo$_r$ gene replacing Cε inhibits switching to the same isotypes as the $3'E_H$ mutation (H. Oettgen, personal communication). This finding is particularly intriguing in light of the fact that other mutations, inserting different hexogenous promoters in the IgH locus (i.e. the polyoma enhancer/HSV tk promoter-driven neo$_r$ genes in the Iγ2b and Iε replacement (86, 89), the latter in conjunction with an Eμ/V$_H$P cassette) do not cause such a defect. These observations, together with the data indicating that pgk promoter-driven selection markers can efficiently replace switch-promoting sequences (e.g. Eμ or Iγ2b, see above), suggest that the pgk promoter may contain some specific element able to locally support CSR by interacting with distant general regulatory elements (thereby out-competing the other I region promoters that depend on the same regulatory elements). We are presently testing this hypothesis directly, using modified versions of the pgk-neo$_r$ gene, with the aim of identifying the specific factors and sites that allow interaction between local and general regulatory elements.

Altogether, therefore, it is becoming increasingly evident that the regulation of the different promoters (V$_H$ promoter, I regions) in the Ig H locus may be more the result of a network of interacting regulatory elements at different hierarchical levels than of linear, specific enhancer–promoter relationships. Besides the obvious functional need to tightly coordinate the expression of several different promoters with different activation requirements, it is possible that this regulatory organization has evolved as a direct system to control CSR by simultaneously modulating the local accessibility and the physical proximity of the rearranging S regions.

9.3 PERSPECTIVES

Our understanding of the molecular regulation of class switching has made a great deal of progress in the past few years, in part due to the advent of gene targeting, and in part because of the influx of knowledge from neighboring fields focusing on gene expression regulation, B-cell activation and signal transduction.

In our opinion, the immediate major goals of research in the field will be to finally clarify the role of germline transcripts/transcription in mediating CSR, to further locate and understand the mode of action of the general regulatory elements such as the $3'E_H$ region, and to continue in the identification of the factors that regulate their activity. Moreover, artificial recombination substrates able to faithfully recapitulate the switch events will need to be developed. Eventually, this knowledge will come together when the actual molecular components of the switch recombination machinery are identified, and a comprehensive model for class switching can be formulated.

Until that time, class switch scientists will keep looking with envy at their colleagues working on VDJ recombination, who in less than 20 years have gone from discovering a rearrangement process to deciphering initial aspects of its biochemistry *in vitro*.

ACKNOWLEDGMENTS

We are grateful to members of the Alt lab, in particular Barry Sleckman, Ming Tian, Rusty Lansford, Ignacio Moreno, John Manis and Faith Young, for useful comments and discussions; to Hans Oettgen (Harvard Medical School) and Wes Dunnick (University of Michigan Medical School) for sharing unpublished results; and to Bortolo Nardini for inspiration. This work was supported by the Howard Hughes Medical Institute and by NIH grant AI31541. A.B. was supported in part by the Italian Telethon Foundation, grant E.122.

REFERENCES

1. Shimizu A, Takahashi N, Yaoita Y and Honjo T (1982) Organization of the constant-region gene family of the mouse immunoglobulin heavy chain. *Cell* **28**:499–506.
2. Honjo T and Kataoka T (1978) Organization of immunoglobulin heavy chain genes and allelic deletion model. *Proc Natl Acad Sci USA* **75**:2140–2144.
3. Yaoita Y and Honjo T (1980) Deletion of immunoglobulin heavy chain genes from expressed allelic chromosome. *Nature* **286**:850–853.
4. Cory S and Adams JM (1980) Deletions are associated with somatic rearrangement of immunoglobulin heavy-chain genes. *Cell* **19**:37–51.
5. Rabbitts TH, Forster A, Dunnick W and Bentley DL (1980) The role of gene deletion in the immunoglobulin heavy chain switch. *Nature* **283**:351–356.
6. Coleclough C, Cooper D and Perry RP (1980) Rearrangement of immunoglobulin heavy chain genes during B lymphocyte development as revealed by studies of mouse plasmacytoma cells. *Proc Natl Acad Sci USA* **77**:1422–1426.
7. Davis MM, Kim SK and Hood LE (1980) DNA sequences mediating class switching in α-immunoglobulins. *Science* **209**:1360–1365.
8. Dunnick W, Rabbitts TH and Milstein C (1980) A mouse immunoglobulin heavy chain deletion mutant: isolation of a cDNA clone and sequence analysis of the mRNA. *Nucleic Acids Res* **8**:1475–1484.
9. Kataoka T, Kawakami T, Takahashi N and Honjo T (1980) Rearrangement of immunoglobulin γ1-chain gene and mechanism for heavy-chain class switch. *Proc Natl Acad Sci USA* **77**:919–923.
10. Jack HM, McDowell M, Steinberg CM and Wabl M (1988) Looping out and deletion mechanism for the immunoglobulin heavy-chain class switch. *Proc Natl Acad Sci USA* **85**:1581–1585.
11. Matsuoka M, Yoshida K, Maeda T, Usuda S and Sakano H (1990) Switch circular DNA formed in cytokine-treated mouse splenocytes: Evidence for intramolecular DNA deletion in immunoglobulin class switching. *Cell* **62**:135–142.
12. von Schwedler U, Jack HM and Wabl M (1990) Circular DNA is a product of the immunoglobulin class switch rearrangement. *Nature* **345**:452–456.

13. Lansford R, Okada A, Chen J *et al* (1996) Mechanism and control of immunoglobulin gene rearrangement. In: Hames BD and Glover DM (eds) *Molecular Immunology*, pp 248–282. Oxford University Press, Oxford.

14. Stavnezer J (1996) Immunoglobulin class switching. *Curr Opin Immunol* **8**:199–205.

15. Dunnick W, Hertz G, Scappino L and Gritzmacher C (1993) DNA sequences at immunoglobulin switch region recombination sites. *Nucleic Acids Res* **21**:365–372.

16. Wahls WP, Wallace LJ and Moore PD (1990) Hypervariable minisatellite DNA is a hotspot for homologous recombination in human cells. *Cell* **60**:95–103.

17. Petrini J and Dunnick WA (1989) Products and implied mechanism of H chain switch recombination. *J Immunol* **142**:2932-2935.

18. Dunnick W and Stavnezer J (1990) Copy choice mechanism of immunoglobulin heavy-chain switch recombination. *Mol Cell Biol* **10**:397–400.

19. Dunnick W, Wilson M and Stavnezer J (1989) Mutations, duplication, and deletion of recombined switch regions suggest a role for DNA replication in the immunoglobulin heavy-chain switch. *Mol Cell Biol* **9**:1850–1856.

20. Wuerffel R, Jamieson C, Morgan L, Merkulov G, Sen R and Kenter A (1992) Switch recombination breakpoints are strictly correlated with DNA recognition motifs for immunoglobulin Sγ3 DNA-binding proteins. *J Exp Med* **176**:339–349.

21. Iwasato T, Arakawa H, Shimizu A, Honjo T and Yamagishi H (1992) Biased distribution of recombination sites within S regions upon immunoglobulin class switch recombination induced by transforming growth factor beta and lipopolysaccharide. *J Exp Med* **175**:1539–1546.

22. Kenter AL, Wuerffel R, Sen R, Jamieson CE and Merkulov GV (1993) Switch recombination breakpoints occur at nonrandom positions in the Sγ tandem repeat. *J Immunol* **151**:4718–4731.

23. Wuerffel RA, Nathan AT and Kenter AL (1990) Detection of an immunoglobulin switch region-specific DNA-binding protein in mitogen-stimulated mouse splenic B cells. *Mol Cell Biol* **10**:1714–1718.

24. Williams M and Maizels N (1991) LR1, a lipopolysaccharide-responsive factor with binding sites in the immunoglobulin switch regions and heavy chain enhancer. *Genes Dev* **5**:2353–2361.

25. Schultz CL, Elenich LA and Dunnick WA (1991) Nuclear protein binding to octamer motifs in the immunoglobulin γ1 switch region. *Int Immunol* **3**:109–116.

26. Xu L, Kim MG and Marcu KB (1992) Properties of B cell stage specific and ubiquitous nuclear factors binding to immunoglobulin heavy chain gene switch regions. *Int Immunol* **4**:875–887.

27. Fukita Y, Mizuta TR, Shirozu M, Ozawa K, Shimizu A and Honjo T (1993) The human Sμbp-2, a DNA-binding protein specific to the single stranded guanine-rich sequence related to the immunoglobulin μ chain switch region. *J Biol Chem* **268**:17463–17470.

28. Mizuta TR, Fukita Y, Miyoshi T, Shimizu A and Honjo T (1993) Isolation of cDNA encoding a binding protein specific to 5'phosphorylated single-stranded DNA with G-rich sequences. *Nucleic Acids Res* **21**:1761–1766.

29. Mosmann TR and Coffman RL (1989) TH1 and TH2 cells: different patterns of lymphokine secretion lead to different functional properties. *Annu Rev Immunol* **7**:145–173.

30. Kearney JF and Lawton AR (1975) B lymphocyte differentiation induced by lipopolysaccharide. I. Generation of cells synthesizing four major immunoglobulin classes. *J Immunol* **115**:671–676.

31. Vitetta ES, Brooks K, Chen YW *et al* (1984) T-cell-derived lymphokines that induce IgM and IgG secretion in activated murine B cells. *Immunol Rev* **78**:137–157.

32. Coffman RL, Ohara J, Bond MW, Carty J, Zlotnik A and Paul WE (1986) B cell stimulatory factor-1 enhances the IgE response of lipopolysaccharide-activated B cells. *J Immunol* **136**:4538–4541.

33. Coffman RL, Lebman DA and Shrader B (1989) Transforming growth factor beta specifically enhances IgA production by lipopolysaccharide-stimulated murine B lymphocytes. *J Exp Med* **170**:1039–1044.
34. Snapper CM and Paul WE (1987) Interferon-γ and B cell stimulatory factor-1 reciprocally regulate Ig isotype production. *Science* **236**:944–947.
35. Finkelman FD, Holmes J, Katona IM *et al* (1990) Lymphokine control of *in vivo* immunoglobulin isotype selection. *Annu Rev Immunol* **8**:303–333.
36. Coffman RL, Lebman DA and Rothman P (1993) The mechanism and regulation of immunoglobulin isotype switching. *Adv Immunol* **54**:229–270.
37. Radbruch A, Müller W and Rajewsky K (1986) Class switch recombination is IgG1 specific on active and inactive IgH loci of IgG1-secreting B-cell blasts. *Proc Natl Acad Sci USA* **83**:3954–3957.
38. Hummel M, Berry JK and Dunnick W (1987) Switch region content of hybridomas: the two spleen cell Igh loci tend to rearrange to the same isotype. *J Immunol* **138**:3539–3548.
39. Winter E, Krawinkel U and Radbruch A (1987) Directed Ig class switch recombination in activated murine B cells. *EMBO J* **6**:1663–1671.
40. Siebenkotten G, Esser C, Wabl M and Radbruch A (1992) The murine IgG1/IgE class switch program. *Eur J Immunol* **22**:1827–1834.
41. Vitetta ES, Ohara J, Myers C, Layton J, Krammer PH and Paul WE (1985) Serological, biochemical, and functional identity of B-cell stimulatory factor 1 and B cell differentiation factor for IgG1. *J Exp Med* **161**:1726–1730.
42. Esser C and Radbruch A (1990) Immunoglobulin class switching: molecular and cellular analysis. *Annu Rev Immunol* **8**:717–735.
43. Kuhn R, Rajewsky K and Müller W (1991) Generation and analysis of interleukin-4-deficient mice. *Science* **254**:707–710.
44. Burstein HJ, Tepper RI, Leder P and Abbas AK (1991) Humoral immune functions in IL-4 transgenic mice. *J Immunol* **147**:2950–2956.
45. Islam KB, Baskin B, Christensson B, Hammarstrom L and Smith CIE (1994) *In vivo* expression of human immunoglobulin germ-line mRNA in normal and in immunodeficient individuals. *Clin Exp Immunol* **95**:3–9.
46. Liu YJ, Malisan F, de Bouteiller O *et al* (1996) Within germinal centers, isotype switching of immunoglobulin genes occurs after the onset of somatic mutation. *Immunity* **4**:241–250.
47. Toellner K-M, Gulbranson-Judge A, Taylor DR, Sze DM-Y and MacLennan ICM (1996) Immunoglobulin switch transcript production *in vivo* related to the site and time of antigen-specific B cell activation. *J Exp Med* **183**:2303–2312.
48. Snapper CM and Mond JJ (1993) Towards a comprehensive view of immunoglobulin class switching. *Immunol Today* **14**:15–17.
49. Parker DC (1993) T cell-dependent B cell activation. *Annu Rev Immunol* **11**:331–360.
50. Klaus GGB (1996) B cell activation. In: Hames BD and Glover DM (eds) *Molecular Immunology*, pp. 248–282. Oxford University Press, Oxford.
51. Snapper CM, Peschel C and Paul WE (1988) IFN-γ stimulates IgG2a secretion by murine B cells stimulated with bacterial polysaccharide. *J Immunol* **140**:2121–2127.
52. Snapper CM, McIntyre TM, Mandler R *et al* (1992) Induction of IgG3 secretion by interferon γ: a model for T cell-independent class switching in response to T cell-independent type 2 antigens. *J Exp Med* **175**:1367–1371.
53. McIntyre TM, Klinman DR, Rothman P *et al* (1993) Transforming growth factor β-1 selectively stimulates immunoglobulin G2b secretion by lipopolysaccharide-activated murine B cells. *J Exp Med* **177**:1031–1037.
54. Sonoda E, Matsumoto R, Hitoshi Y *et al* (1989) Transforming growth factor β induces IgA production and acts additively with interleukin 5 for IgA production. *J Exp Med* **170**:1415–1420.

55. Harriman GR, Kunimoto DY, Elliot JF, Paetkau V and Strober W (1988) The role of IL-5 in IgA B cell differentiation. *J Immunol* **140**:3033–3039.
56. Purkerson JM, Newberg M, Wise G, Lynch KR and Isakson PC (1988) Interleukin 5 and interleukin 2 cooperate with interleukin 4 to induce IgG1 secretion from anti-Ig-treated B cells. *J Exp Med* **168**:1175–1180.
57. Yuan D, Dang T and Sanderson C (1990) Regulation of Ig H chain gene transcription by IL-5. *J Immunol* **145**:3491–3496.
58. Purkerson JM and Isakson PC (1992) Interleukin 5 (IL-5) provides a signal that is required in addition to IL-4 for isotype switching to immunoglobulin (Ig) G1 and IgE. *J Exp Med* **175**:973–982.
59. Mandler R, Chu CC, Paul WE, Max EE and Snapper CM (1993) Interleukin 5 induces Sμ-Sγ1 DNA rearrangement in B cells activated with dextran-anti-IgD antibodies and interleukin 4: a three component model for Ig class switching. *J Exp Med* **178**:1577–1586.
60. Stavnezer-Nordgren J and Sirlin S (1986) Specificity of immunoglobulin heavy chain switch correlates with activity of germline heavy chain genes prior to switching. *EMBO J* **5**:95–102.
61. Yancopoulos GD, DePinho RA, Zimmerman KA, Lutzker SG, Rosenberg N and Alt FW (1986) Secondary genomic rearrangement events in pre-B cells: VHDJH replacement by a LINE-1 sequence and directed class switching. *EMBO J* **5**:3259–3266.
62. Lutzker SG and Alt FW (1988) Immunoglobulin heavy-chain class switching. In: *Mobile DNA*, Berg DE and Howe MM (eds) pp. 691–714. American Society for Microbiology, Washington DC.
63. Lennon GG and Perry RP (1985) Cμ-containing transcripts initiate heterogeneously within the IgH enhancer region and contain a novel 5'-nontranslatable exon. *Nature* **318**:475–478.
64. Rothman P, Li SC, Gorham B, Glimcher L, Alt F and Boothby M (1991) Identification of a conserved lipopolysaccharide-plus-interleukin-4-responsive element located at the promoter of germ line ε transcripts. *Mol Cell Biol* **11**:5551–5561.
65. Kim J, Reeves R, Rothman P and Boothby M (1995) The non-histone chromosomal protein HMG-I(Y) contributes to repression of the immunoglobulin heavy chain germline ε RNA promoter. *Eur J Immunol* **25**:798–808.
66. Liao F, Birshtein BK, Busslinger M and Rothman P (1994) The transcription factor BSAP (NF-HB) is essential for immunoglobulin germ-line ε transcription. *J Immunol* **152**:2904–2911.
67. Schindler C, Kashleva H, Pernis A, Pine R and Rothman P (1994) STF-IL4: a novel IL-4-induced signal transducing factor. *EMBO J* **13**:1350–1356.
68. Ihle JN (1995) The Janus protein tyrosine kinase family and its role in cytokine signaling. *Adv Immunol* **60**:1–35.
69. Berton MT and Linehan LA (1995) IL-4 activates a latent DNA-binding factor that binds a shared IFN-γ and IL-4 responsive element present in the germline γ1 Ig promoter. *J Immunol* **154**:4513–4525.
70. Pellegrini S and Schindler C (1993) Early events in signaling by interferons. *Trends Biochem Sci* **18**:338–342.
71. Fenghao X, Saxon A, Nguyen A, Ke Z, Diaz-Sanchez D and Nel A (1995) Interleukin 4 activates a signal transducer and activator of transcription (Stat) protein which interacts with an interferon-γ activation site-like sequence upstream of the Iε exon in a human B cell line. Evidence for the involvement of Janus kinase 3 and interleukin-4 Stat. *J Clin Invest* **96**:907–914.
72. Shimoda K, van Deursen J, Sangster J *et al* (1996) Lack of IL-4-induced Th2 response and IgE class switching in mice with disrupted Stat6 gene. *Nature* **380**:630–633.
73. Takeda K, Tanaka T, Shi W *et al* (1996) Essential role of Stat6 in IL-4 signaling. *Nature* **380**:627–630.

74. Xu MZ and Stavnezer J (1992) Regulation of transcription of immunoglobulin germ-line γ1 RNA: analysis of the promoter/enhancer. *EMBO J* **11:**145–155.
75. Illges H and Radbruch A (1992) DNA binding sites 5' of the IgG1 switch region comprising IL-4 inducibility and B cell specificity. *Mol Immunol* **29:**1265–1272.
76. Schmitz J and Radbruch A (1989) An interleukin 4-induced DNAse I hypersensitive site indicates opening of the γ1 switch region prior to switch recombination. *Int Immunol* **1:**570–575.
77. Berton MT and Vitetta ES (1990) Interleukin 4 induces changes in the chromatin structure of the γ1 switch region in resting B cells before switch recombination. *J Exp Med* **172:**375–378.
78. Lin YC and Stavnezer J (1992) Regulation of transcription of the germ-line Ig α constant region gene by an ATF element and by novel transforming growth factor-β1-responsive elements. *J Immunol* **149:**2914–2925.
79. Matthias P and Baltimore D (1993) The immunoglobulin heavy chain locus contains another B-cell-specific 3' enhancer close to the α constant region. *Mol Cell Biol* **13:**1547–1553.
80. Nilsson L, Grant P, Larsson I, Pettersson S and Sideras P (1995) The human Iα1 region contains a TGF-β1 responsive enhancer and a putative recombination hotspot. *Int Immunol* **7:**1191–1204.
81. Reaban ME and Griffin JA (1990) Induction of RNA stabilised DNA conformers by transcription of an immunoglobulin switch region. *Nature* **348:**342–344.
82. Dröge P (1993) Transcription-driven site-specific DNA recombination *in vitro*. *Proc Natl Acad Sci USA* **90:**2759–2763.
83. Daniels GA and Lieber MR (1995) RNA:DNA complex formation upon transcription of immunoglobulin switch regions: implications for the mechanism and regulation of class switch recombination. *Nucleic Acids Res* **23:**5006–5011.
84. Chen J, Lansford R, Stewart V, Young F and Alt FW (1993) *RAG-2*-deficient blastocyst complementation: an assay of gene function in lymphocyte development. *Proc Natl Acad Sci USA* **90:**4528–4532.
85. Shinkai Y, Rathbun G, Lam K-P (1992) *RAG-2* deficient mice lack mature lymphocytes owing to inability to initiate V(D)J rearrangement. *Cell* **68:**855–867.
86. Zhang J, Bottaro A, Li S, Stewart V and Alt FW (1993) A selective defect in IgG2b switching as a result of targeted mutation of the Iγ2b promoter and exon. *EMBO J* **12:**3529–3537.
87. Jung S, Rajewsky K and Radbruch A (1993) Shutdown of class switch recombination by deletion of a switch region control element. *Science* **259:**984–987.
88. Xu L, Gorham B, Li SC, Bottaro A, Alt FW and Rothman P (1993) Replacement of germline ε promoter by gene targeting alters control of immunoglobulin heavy chain class switching. *Proc Natl Acad Sci USA* **90:**3705–3709.
89. Bottaro A, Lansford R, Xu L, Zhang J, Rothman P and Alt FW (1994) S region transcription per se promotes basal IgE class switch recombination but additional factors regulate the efficiency of the process. *EMBO J* **13:**665–674.
90. Tarlinton DM, McLean M and Nossal GJV (1995) B1 and B2 cells differ in their potential to switch immunoglobulin isotype. *Eur J Immunol* **25:**3388–3393.
91. Lorenz M, Jung S and Radbruch A (1995) Switch transcripts in immunoglobulin class switching. *Science* **267:**1825–1828.
92. Harriman GR, Bradley A, Das S, Rogers-Fani P and Davis AC (1996) IgA class switch in Iα exon-deficient mice. Role of germline transcription in class switch recombination. *J Clin Invest* **97:**477–485.
93. Cullen KE, Kladde MP and Seyfred MA (1993) Interaction between transcription regulatory regions of prolactin chromatin. *Science* **261:**203–206.

94. Artandi SE, Cooper C, Shrivastava A and Calame K (1994) The basic helix–loop–helix–zipper domain of TFE3 mediates enhancer–promoter interaction. *Mol Cell Biol* **14**:7704–7716.

95. Flanagan JG and Rabbitts TH (1982) Arrangement of human immunoglobulin heavy chain constant region genes implies evolutionary duplication of a segment containing γ, ε and α genes. *Nature* **300**:709–713.

96. Su L-K and Kadesch T (1990) The immunoglobulin heavy-chain enhancer functions as the promoter for Iμ sterile transcription. *Mol Cell Biol* **10**:2619–2624.

97. Cockerill PN (1990) Nuclear matrix attachment occurs in several regions of the IgH locus. *Nucleic Acids Res* **18**:2643–2648.

98. Dickinson LA, Joh T, Kohwi Y and Kowhi-Shigematsu T (1992) A tissue-specific MAR/SAR DNA binding protein with unusual binding site recognition. *Cell* **70**:631–645.

99. Herrscher RF, Kaplan MH, Lelsz DL, Das C, Scheuermann R and Tucker PW (1995) The immunoglobulin heavy chain matrix-associating regions are bound by Bright: a B cell-specific *trans*-activator that describes a new DNA-binding protein family. *Genes Dev* **9**:3067–3082.

100. Gu H, Zou YR and Rajewsky K (1993) Independent control of immunoglobulin switch recombination at individual switch regions evidenced through Cre-loxP-mediated gene targeting. *Cell* **73**:1155–1164.

101. Serwe M and Sablitzky F (1993) V(D)J recombination in B cells is impaired but not blocked by targeted deletion of the immunoglobulin heavy chain intron enhancer. *EMBO J* **12**:2321–2327.

102. Chen J, Young F, Bottaro A, Stewart V, Smith RK and Alt FW (1993) Mutations of the intronic IgH enhancer and its flanking sequences differentially affect accessibility of the JH locus. *EMBO J* **12**:4635–4645.

103. Zhang J (1994) Studies of a germline promoter in the murine IgH constant region and its involvement in class switch recombination. PhD thesis, Harvard University, Cambridge MA.

104. Cogné M, Lansford R, Bottaro A *et al* (1994) A class switch control region at the 3′ end of the IgH locus. *Cell* **77**:737–747.

105. Sideras P, Nilsson L, Islam KB *et al* (1992) Transcription of unrearranged Ig H chain genes in human B cell malignancies. Biased expression of genes encoded within the first duplication unit of the Ig H chain locus. *J Immunol* **149**:244–252.

106. Alt FW, Rosenberg N, Casanova RJ, Thomas E and Baltimore D (1982) Immunoglobulin heavy-chain expression and class switching in a murine leukaemia cell line. *Nature* **296**:325–331.

107. Klein S, Sablitzky F and Radbruch A (1984) Deletion of the IgH enhancer does not reduce immunoglobulin heavy chain production of a hybridoma IgD class switch variant. *EMBO J* **3**:2473–2476.

108. Cory S (1986) Activation of cellular oncogenes in hemopoietic cells by chromosome translocation. *Adv Cancer Res* **47**:189–234.

109. Pettersson S, Cook GP, Bruggemann M, Williams GT, and Neuberger MS (1990) A second B cell-specific enhancer 3′ of the immunoglobulin heavy-chain locus. *Nature* **344**:165–168.

110. Dariavach P, Williams GT, Campbell K, Petterson S and Neuberger MS (1991) The mouse IgH 3′ enhancer. *Eur J Immunol* **21**:1499–1504.

111. Lieberson R, Giannini SL, Birshtein BK and Eckhardt L (1991) An enhancer at the 3′ end of the mouse immunoglobulin heavy chain locus. *Nucleic Acids Res* **19**:933–937.

112. Giannini SL, Singh M, Calvo C-F, Ding G and Birshtein BK (1993) DNA regions flanking the mouse Ig 3′ α enhancer are differentially methylated and DNAse I hypersensitive during B cell differentiation. *J Immunol* **150**:1772–1780.

113. Arulampalam V, Grant PA, Samuelsson A, Lendhal U and Petterson S (1994) Lipopolysaccharide-dependent transactivation of the temporally regulated immunoglobulin heavy chain 3′ enhancer. *Eur J Immunol* **24:**1671–1677.

114. Madisen L and Groudine M (1994) Identification of a locus control region in the immunoglobulin heavy-chain locus that deregulates c-myc expression in plasmacytoma and Burkitt's lymphoma cells. *Genes Dev* **8:**2212–2226.

115. Michaelson JS, Giannini SL and Birshtein BK (1995) Identification of 3′α-hs4, a novel Ig heavy chain enhancer element regulated at multiple stages of B cell differentiation. *Nucleic Acids Res* **23:**975–981.

116. Grant PA, Arulampalam V, Ahrlund-Richter L and Pettersson S (1992) Identification of ets-like lymphoid-specific elements within the immunoglobulin heavy chain 3′ enhancer. *Nucleic Acids Res* **20:**4401–4408.

117. Neurath M, Max EE and Strober W (1995) Pax5 (BSAP) regulates the murine immunoglobulin 3′α enhancer by suppressing binding of NF-αP, a protein that controls heavy chain transcription. *Proc Natl Acad Sci USA* **92:**5336–5340.

118. Grant PA, Thompson CB and Pettersson S (1995) IgM receptor-mediated transactivation of the IgH 3′ enhancer couples a novel Elf-1-AP-1 protein complex to the developmental control of enhancer function. *EMBO J* **14:**4501–4513.

119. Meyer KB, Skogberg M, Margenfeld C, Ireland J and Pettersson S (1995) Repression of the immunoglobulin heavy chain 3′ enhancer by helix–loop–helix protein Id3 via a functionally important E47–E12 binding site: implications for developmental control of enhancer function. *Eur J Immunol* **25:**1770–1777.

120. Singh M and Birshtein BK (1996) Concerted repression of an immunoglobulin heavy-chain enhancer, 3′αE(hs1,2). *Proc Natl Acad Sci USA* **93:**4392–4397.

121. Singh M and Birshtein BK (1993) NF-HB (BSAP) is a repressor of the murine immunoglobulin heavy-chain 3′α enhancer at early stages of B cell differentiation. *Mol Cell Biol* **13:**3611–3622.

122. Neurath MF, Strober W and Wakatsuki Y (1994) The murine Ig 3′ α enhancer is a target site with repressor function for the B cell lineage-specific transcription factor BSAP (NF-HB, Sα-BP). *J Immunol* **153:**730–742.

123. Michaelson JS, Singh M, Snapper CM, Sha WC, Baltimore D and Birshtein BK (1996) Regulation of 3′IgH enhancers by a common set of factors, including κB-binding proteins. *J Immunol* **156:**2828–2839.

124. Sha WC, Liou HC, Tuomanen EI and Baltimore D (1995) Targeted disruption of the p50 subunit of NF-κB leads to multifocal defects in immune responses. *Cell* **80:**321–330.

125. Snapper CM, Zelazowski P, Rosas FR *et al* (1996) B cells from p50/NF-κB knockout mice have selective defects in proliferation, differentiation, germline C_H transcription and Ig class switching. *J Immunol* **156:**183–191.

126. Lieberson R, Ong J, Shi X and Eckhardt LA (1995) Immunoglobulin gene transcription ceases upon deletion of a distant enhancer. *EMBO J* **14:**6229–6238.

127. Mocikat R, Kardinal C and Klobeck HG (1995) Differential interactions between the immunoglobulin heavy chain μ intron and 3′ enhancer. *Eur J Immunol* **25:**3195–3198.

128. Elenich LA, Ford CS and Dunnick WA (1996) The γ1 heavy chain gene includes all of the *cis*-acting elements necessary for expression and properly regulated germline transcripts. *J Immunol* **157:**176–182.

129. Leighton PA, Ingram RS, Eggenschwiler J, Efstradiatis A and Tilghman SM (1995) Disruption of imprinting caused by deletion of the mouse H19 gene region in mice. *Nature* **375:**34–39.

130. Leighton PA, Saam JR, Ingram RS, Stewart CL and Tilgham SM (1995) An enhancer deletion affects both H19 and Igf2 expression. *Genes Dev* **9:**2079–2089.

131. Choi O-RB and Engel JD (1988) Developmental regulation of β-globin switching. *Cell* **55:**17–26.

132. Gallarda JL, Foley KP, Yang Z and Engel JD (1989) The β-globin stage selector element factor is erythroid-specific promoter/enhancer binding protein NF-E4. *Genes Dev* **3:**1845–1859.

133. Foley KP and Engel JD (1992) Individual stage selector element mutations lead to reciprocal changes in β- vs. ε-globin gene transcription: genetic confirmation of promoter competition during globin gene switching. *Genes Dev* **6:**730–744.

134. Kim CG, Epner EM, Forrester WC and Groudine M (1992) Inactivation of the β-globin gene by targeted insertion into the β-globin locus control region. *Genes Dev* **6:**928–938.

135. Engel JD (1993) Developmental regulation of human β-globin gene transcription: a switch of loyalties? *Trends Genet* **9:**304–309.

136. Fiering S, Kim CG, Epner EM and Groudine M (1993) An 'in-out' strategy using gene targeting and FLP recombinase for the functional dissection of complex DNA regulatory elements: analysis of the β-globin locus control region. *Proc Natl Acad Sci USA* **90:**8469–8473.

137. Fiering S, Epner E, Robinson K *et al* (1995) Targeted deletion of 5′HS2 of the murine β-globin LCR reveals that it is not essential for proper regulation of the β-globin locus. *Genes Dev* **9:**2203–2213.

138. Bungert J, Davé U, Lim K-C *et al* (1995) Synergistic regulation of human β-globin gene switching by locus control region elements HS3 and HS4. *Genes Dev* **9:**3083–3096.

139. Grosveld F, Blom van Assendelft G, Greaves D and Kollias G (1987) Position-independent, high-level expression of the human β-globin gene in transgenic mice. *Cell* **51:**975–985.

140. Forrester WC, Takegawa S, Papayannopoulou T, Stamatoyannopoulos G and Groudine M (1987) Evidence for a locus activation region: the formation of developmentally stable hypersensitive sites in globin-expressing hybrids. *Nucleic Acids Res* **15:**10159–10177.

141. Epner E, Kim CG and Groudine M (1992) What does a locus control region control? *Curr Biol* **2:**262–264.

142. Crossley M and Orkin SH (1993) Regulation of the β-globin locus. *Curr Opin Gen Dev* **3:**232–237.

10 Regulation of ε Germline Transcription: Q & A

ALESSANDRA AGRESTI and DONATA VERCELLI
Molecular Immunoregulation Unit, DIBIT, San Raffaele Scientific Institute, Milan, Italy

Isotype switching results from a DNA recombination event that juxtaposes different downstream C_H genes to the expressed VDJ gene, thus changing the effector function but not the specificity of the antibody molecule. Isotype switching is not a random event, but is directed by cytokines in conjunction with the regulation of B-cell proliferation and differentiation (Reviewed in (1, 2)). Molecular analysis has shown that cytokine-dependent induction of isotype switching to a particular C_H gene almost invariably correlates with the transcriptional activation of the same gene in germline configuration. Several murine and human germline transcripts have been cloned, and share structural similarities. The germline transcripts initiate from TATAA-less promoters a few kilobases upstream of the switch region, and proceed through short exons (I_H exons), the switch regions and C_H exons. The I_H exon is then spliced to the first exon of the C_H gene. During recombination, the region containing the germline promoter and the I_H exon is deleted as part of a switch circle (3, 4). Induction of correctly spliced transcripts is thought to be necessary to target the appropriate switch region for recombination and switching (5–7).

The role of germline transcripts in the process of switching is extensively discussed in other sections of this book (Chapters 7–9). Here we shall mainly focus on the patterns of expression of germline transcripts and on the transcription factors that regulate the activity of the human ε germline promoter.

10.1 WHEN AND WHERE ARE GERMLINE TRANSCRIPTS EXPRESSED?

Germline transcripts (γ, α and ε) were selectively detected in human tonsil centrocytes (IgD$^-$, CD38$^+$, CD77$^-$, c-myc$^-$, Fas$^+$) from the germinal center light zone, whereas somatic hypermutation occurred within centroblasts from the germinal center dark zone. These results indicated that within germinal centers, isotype switching is most likely initiated after B cells have undergone affinity maturation by somatic mutation, and positive selection. This would allow the acquisition of distinct

IgE Regulation: Molecular Mechanisms. Edited by D. Vercelli. © 1997 John Wiley & Sons Ltd.

immunoglobulin isotypes (which confer specific effector functions) while keeping the high affinity for the selecting antigen (8). Notably, somatic mutation and isotype switching are two independent processes (i.e. somatic mutation can occur within germinal centers without triggering isotype switching, and isotype switching can occur in B-cell clones that have not undergone somatic mutation).

The apical light zone and outer zone of germinal centers is the region where most germinal center T cells are localized. The apical light zone contains strong CD23-expressing follicular dendritic cells networks. Here the selected centrocytes encounter and present antigen to antigen-specific germinal center T cells (8). These T cells are induced to express CD40 ligand (CD40L) and secrete cytokines (including interleukin (IL)-4), thus providing B cells with both signals required for expansion and isotype switching. Finally, the high affinity switched centrocytes differentiate into memory B cells in the presence of prolonged CD40L signaling, and into plasma cells when CD40L signaling is removed (9). Consistent results have been obtained following the appearance of $\gamma 1$ switch transcripts in mouse spleen sections during primary and secondary antigen-specific antibody responses (10).

In another study, the expression of ε germline transcript following cytokine (IL-4 or IL-13) stimulation has been taken as a litmus test to reveal the presence of functional receptors for the relevant cytokine. IL-4 induced ε germline transcripts in human fetal B cells, as well as in pre-B cells (sIgM$^-$, CD10$^+$, CD19$^+$, cytoplasmic IgM$^+$), but not in pro-B cells (sIgM$^-$, CD10$^+$, CD19$^+$, cytoplasmic IgM$^-$). In contrast, IL-13 was unable to trigger ε germline transcription in either pre- or pro-B cells (11). These data indicate that functional receptors for IL-4 and IL-13 are not expressed synchronously in B-cell ontogeny. Thus IL-4, rather than IL-13, is likely to be responsible for the early commitment of B cells to IgE synthesis.

Isotype switching has been linked to cell division by a number of reports. Recently, it has been shown that switching to IgG1, with expression of IgG1 on the membrane, seems to correlate with the number of cell divisions. B cells were uniformly negative for IgG1 until the third division cycle, when a small proportion of cells became positive, this number increasing with further division rounds to a plateau after six cell divisions. These data have been taken to indicate that switching may require prolonged recruitment of T cell help (12).

10.2 IS IL-4 REALLY NECESSARY FOR ε GERMLINE TRANSCRIPTION?

Some puzzling findings recently obtained in IL-4$^{-/-}$ mice may prompt a reassessment of the role of IL-4 in the induction of ε germline transcription and IgE synthesis and/or of the experimental models used to assess it. IL-4$^{-/-}$ mice with a (129/Ola × C57BL/6)F$_2$ (13) or a (129Sv × C57BL/6)F$_2$ (14) hybrid background were shown to be unable to produce IgE upon infection with *Nippostrongylus brasiliensis* (13). Although expression of ε germline transcripts was not explored at the time, these results were taken to show that switching to IgE is strictly dependent on IL-4. More recently, however, it has been reported that 129/Ola IL-4$^{-/-}$ mice backcrossed to C57BL/6J for 12 generations could produce IgE when treated with anti-IgD antibody (15), although 300-fold less efficiently than control littermates. Interestingly, anti-IgD antibody induced ε germline transcripts with comparable efficiency in IL-4$^{-/-}$ mice and controls, but the levels of productive IgE transcripts were lower by a factor of 200, and serum IgE levels were lower by a factor of 300 in the IL-4$^{-/-}$ mice (15). Consistent with the results obtained in the mice originally generated, no serum IgE was detected after infection with *Nippostrongylus brasiliensis*. However germline – although not productive – IgE transcripts were detected in these mice. Thus, IL-4 does not seem to be necessary for the induction of ε germline transcripts, whereas induction and translation of productive IgE transcripts is more IL-4-dependent. Thus, activation of a germline C_H locus does not necessarily lead to switch recombination.

The report by Morawetz *et al* (15) does not represent an isolated observation. IgE production was also observed in genetically pure BALB/c IL-4$^{-/-}$ mice infected with *Leishmania major* (16), and in IL-4$^{-/-}$ (129/Ola × C57BL/6)F$_2$ repeatedly backcrossed to the SWR strain and immunized with bovine serum albumin (BSA)–2,4,6-trinitrophenol (TNP) in the presence of anti-TNP IgE (17, 18). Morawetz's data are important because the analysis of distinct steps in isotype switching allows the dissection of the role of IL-4 at discrete stages of the switching process.

These data seem to indicate that the requirement for IL-4 in the induction of ε germline transcripts *in vivo* can be overcome by certain modes of B-cell activation. Previous *in vivo* studies, showing that CD40–CD40L interactions lead to IL-4-independent induction of ε germline transcripts in resting murine spleen B cells (19) make this contact-mediated signal a potential candidate for the stimulus to ε germline transcription in the absence of IL-4 *in vivo*. On the other hand, it remains to be explained why a contact-mediated signal efficient enough to circumvent the IL-4 requirement would not be able to trigger the recombination machinery. Indeed, the dramatic reduction in the expression of mature ε transcripts in the presence of vigorous transcription through the switch region points to a more complex, qualitative problem that may affect more than one step in isotype switching.

It is also possible that the signal for induction of germline transcription in the IL-4$^{-/-}$ mice is delivered by a potentially novel cytokine. Like IL-13 in humans, this cytokine would normally be redundant with IL-4. Unlike IL-13, however, it would not be expected to signal through the IL-4R α chain, since antibodies to this molecule had no effect on the levels of productive ε transcripts and IgE production (15) (see also Chapters 5 and 7 in this book).

In closing, a caveat is in order. *In vivo* stimulation with anti-IgD was performed in the original 129Sv × C57BL/6 IL-4$^{-/-}$ mice, and was found to have no effect on IgE levels (14). These same mice showed a major impairment of T helper 2 (Th2) responses, whereas the latter were unaffected in the genetically pure BALB/c IL-4$^{-/-}$ mice generated more recently (16). It may be important to understand how differences in the genetic background of the knock-out mice, and/or in the targeting strategy may contribute to the discrepancies in the results reported by the different groups.

10.3 WHO DOES WHAT TO WHOM: TRANSCRIPTION FACTORS INVOLVED IN THE REGULATION OF THE ε GERMLINE PROMOTER

The general paradigm for promoters is that all slots for nuclear transcription factors need to be filled in order for a gene to fire. This implies a level of tight combinatorial control. Like all weak promoters, the I_H promoters are likely to be limited at multiple steps of the transcription reaction. Thus, the activation function of different transcription factors can operate at different limiting steps in the initiation reaction.

Because transcription through the I_H exon and the S region seems to be required to target the appropriate S region for recombination and switching, the induction of germline transcripts is a key step in determining the isotype specificity of the switching event (see also Chapters 5 and 7 in this book). Different cytokines specifically induce different nuclear factors that activate transcription at the appropriate germline promoter. The specificity in the induction of transcription factors is essential for the specificity of cytokine-induced germline transcript expression and isotype switching (2).

Expression of ε germline transcripts is regulated at the transcriptional level by nuclear factors that bind to the Iε promoter and adjacent regions. In interpreting the results reported in the literature, it is important to bear in mind that the requirements for the induction of ε germline transcription seem to be somewhat different in mice and humans. Two signals, IL-4 and lipopolysaccharide (LPS), are required for murine ε germline transcript expression in most murine B cell lines, whereas IL-4 alone is sufficient in humans. We shall briefly discuss the main features of the transcription factors that have been found to bind and regulate the human ε germline promoter (Figure 10.1).

10.3.1 Stat6

Stat6 (20, 21) belongs to the newly identified family of signal transducers and activators of transcription (STAT) (22, 23). Binding of IL-4 to its receptor leads to transphosphorylation and activation of two receptor-associated cytoplasmic tyrosine kinases, Janus kinase (JAK)-3 and to a lesser extent, JAK-1. These kinases are believed to rapidly (within minutes) induce tyrosine phosphorylation of the IL-4R. At this time Stat6, a latent cytoplasmic factor, is recruited to the receptor complex and is tyrosine phosphorylated. The phosphorylated Stat6 homodimerizes, translocates to the nucleus, and binds to the promoter of a number of genes, contributing to the activation of transcription (20). Stat6 preferentially binds dyad symmetric half-sites separated by four base pairs (TTCNNNNGAA). DNA binding specificity is localized to a region of 180 amino acids at the N terminal side of the putative SH3

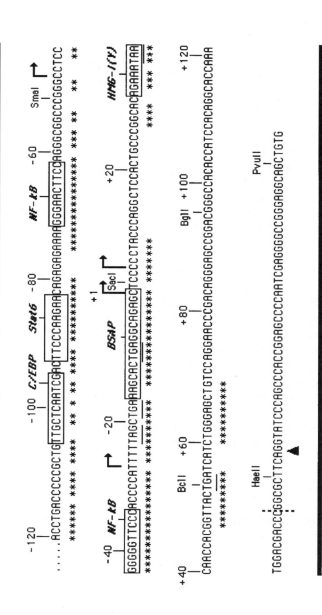

Figure 10.1. Map of the human ε germline promoter. The major transcription start sites in EBV-negative lymphoblastoid B-cell lines (BL-2 and BJAB) were determined by primer extension, and are indicated by arrows. Position +1 corresponds to the major ε RNA start site in BL-2 cells. The splice site for Cε 1 is indicated by an arrowhead. The binding sites for transcription factors identified in the murine and human ε germline promoter are boxed. The asterisks mark a segment highly (>80%) homologous between human and murine sequences. Stop codons are underlined

domain (24). The discovery of JAKs and Stats has finally provided an explanation for the apparent paradox that the IL-4R, as well as the receptors for a number of other cytokines, lacks kinase domains, and yet couples ligand binding to tyrosine phosphorylation (22). Stat6 is not B-cell specific and is induced by IL-4 in monocytes, where it participates in the transcriptional regulation of the IL-4-inducible CD23b promoter, and possibly of the FcγR1 promoter (25). Stat6 binding sites have been identified in the promoters of a number of other IL-4-responsive genes, such as Cε (26–29), Cγ1 and major histocompatibility complex (MHC) class II (25, 28). The presence of homologous responsive elements (RE) in the promoter of different genes underlies the concerted regulation of these genes by a single cytokine. The critical role played by Stat6 in delivering the IL-4-mediated signal has been conclusively proven in Stat6$^{-/-}$ mice, which show profound impairments in IgE and IgG1 class switching, Th2 differentiation and expression of CD23 and MHC class II (30–32) (see also Chapter 7 in this book).

The minimal set of elements in the human ε germline promoter that are required to confer full IL-4 inducibility to a heterologous promoter has not been determined. In the mouse, a region containing the binding sites for Stat6 and a member of the CCAAT box/enhancer binding protein (C/EBP) family is sufficient to transfer IL-4 inducibility to a minimal c-fos promoter (27). Interestingly, the Stat6 binding site in the murine (29) and human ε germline promoter (26) shares a peculiar functional property with the site that binds the non-histone chromosomal protein high mobility group (HMG)-I(Y) (33). Indeed, deletion or mutation of either site results in the loss of IL-4 inducibility, but in a marked increase in basal promoter activity (26, 29). Thus, these elements have a bifunctional activity, i.e., they are required for IL-4-induced promoter activation, but they repress the activity of the promoter in the absence of IL-4. According to these findings, expression of ε germline transcripts and IgE in resting B cells may be low because the germline promoter is kept in a state of repression that requires de-repression through specific pathways. An additional but not necessarily alternative possibility is that the paucity of IgE reflects the intrinsically low accessibility of the ε switch region to the recombination machinery (34) (see also Chapters 8 and 9 in this book).

10.3.2 NF-κB

An IL-4 responsive element located upstream of the major transcription initiation sites in the murine ε germline promoter has been shown to bind three different transcription factors: a member of the C/EBP family, the IL-4-inducible factor Stat6 (NF-IL-4), and NF-κB/p50 (27). Mutation of the NF-κB binding site strongly reduced the IL-4 inducibility of the murine ε promoter (27). The selective importance of NF-κB/p50 for the induction of murine germline transcription has been confirmed by the finding that expression of germline transcripts for several isotypes, including IgE, and switching to the same isotypes, was severely impaired in NF-κB/p50$^{-/-}$ mice (35, 36), but not in mice deficient in RelB (37).

In human B cells, CD40 engagement has been shown to rapidly activate NF-κB, and to support NF-κB-dependent gene expression (37). The human ε germline promoter contains two putative κB binding sites (Figure 10.1), one corresponding to the site identified in the IL-4 responsive element of the murine ε promoter (27), the other located few bases upstream of the B cell lineage-specific activator protein (BSAP) binding site (De Monte, Monticelli and Vercelli, in preparation). Preliminary data obtained in our laboratory clearly indicate that mutation of the downstream κB binding site results in a significant impairment of CD40-induced upregulation of ε germline promoter activity, whereas IL-4 responsiveness is unaffected. The upstream κB binding site is currently under analysis. These results suggest that NF-κB may be specifically involved in mediating the CD40-dependent upregulation of ε germline transcription. It will be interesting to investigate whether BSAP acts in concert with NF-κB and possibly with other factor(s) capable of binding the promoter (see below) (Figure 10.2).

10.3.3 B Cell Lineage-specific Activator Protein (BSAP)

BSAP is encoded by Pax5, a member of the Pax gene family of homeodomain transcription factors, and is the mammalian homologue of the sea urchin tissue-specific transcription activator protein (TSAP), a regulator of late histone genes (38). BSAP is expressed in pro-B, pre-B and mature B lymphocytes, but not in terminally differentiated plasma cells (39). BSAP knock-out mice show a complete block of early B cell differentiation at the pro-preBI stage (40). Binding sites for BSAP have been identified in the promoter of several B-cell related genes, such as CD19 (41),

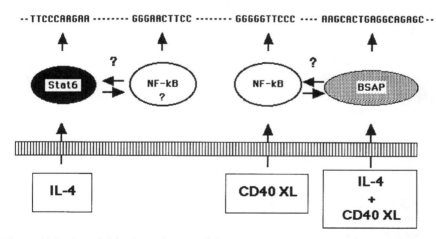

Figure 10.2. A model for the activation of the ε germline promoter based on the cooperation between transcription factors. Stat6 and NF-κB are activated by IL-4 and CD40 engagement, respectively. BSAP is constitutively expressed, and mediates the effects of both IL-4 and CD40 engagement. The sequences indicated correspond to the binding sites for the three transcription factors identified in the germline promoter

the surrogate light chains $\lambda 5$ and V_{preB1} (42), X-box binding protein 1 (43), the tyrosine kinase blk (44), as well as upstream of several immunoglobulin switch regions (μ, $\gamma 1$, $\gamma 2$, ε, α) and in the control region located 3′ of Cα (45, 46). Interestingly, BSAP contributes to the activity of the CD19 promoter (41), but has a negative effect on the 3′ immunoglobulin enhancer (45, 46) and on the promoter of X-box binding protein 1 (43). A deregulation of Pax5 transcription, due to translocation of the Eμ enhancer of the IgH locus next to the Pax5 promoter, has been recently proposed to contribute to the pathogenesis of small lymphocytic lymphomas with plasmacytoid differentiation (47).

Conflicting reports exist about the role of BSAP in the regulation of ε germline transcription in murine B cells. Deletion of the BSAP binding site abrogated induction of ε germline promoter activity in B cells stimulated with IL-4 + LPS. Activity was restored by the introduction of a BSAP binding site from the sea urchin histone gene H2A-2.2 (38). In contrast, deletions in the BSAP binding region were unable to affect the inducibility of the promoter in cells stimulated with IL-4 but not LPS (27). We have shown that BSAP plays an important role in the transcriptional regulation of the human ε germline promoter. Indeed, BSAP is essential both for IL-4-dependent induction and CD40-mediated upregulation of human ε germline transcription (48). Thus BSAP has unique features among the transcription factors that regulate ε germline expression: it is B-cell specific, is constitutively expressed rather than inducible, is involved in activation but not in repression of the promoter, and most importantly, is at the intersection of two signaling pathways (the IL-4- and the CD40-dependent pathways) which are distinct but are both critical for the induction of switching to IgE.

Interestingly, two groups have failed to show an involvement of BSAP in the activation of the ε germline promoter in murine (27) and human (49) B cells. In both cases, however, no extensive deletion of the BSAP binding site was introduced in the reporter vectors, and most importantly, the mutations chosen by the investigators spared a cytosine residue that is highly conserved in all known BSAP binding sites (50). A point mutation (C → A) at this site has been shown to be sufficient to strongly impair BSAP/DNA interactions in human B cells, and to abrogate or strongly impair the activity of the ε germline promoter in murine (38) and human B cells (48) stimulated with IL-4 + LPS or anti-CD40 monoclonal antibody.

10.4 WHY ONLY B CELLS?

Except for BSAP, none of the nuclear factors so far reported to be critical for ε germline transcription in mice or humans (i.e. Stat6, C/EBP, NF-κB, HMG-I(Y)) is expressed exclusively in B cells, and yet, germline transcription is exquisitely B-cell specific. It is tempting to speculate that BSAP, the only B-cell specific transcription factor so far found to bind the ε germline promoter, may somehow contribute to ensuring the B-cell specificity of germline transcription. Our current working hypothesis is that BSAP, in addition to binding DNA at its own site, may regulate

DNA/protein interactions involving other transcription factors (Figure 10.2). The threshold for an efficient activation of the germline promoter would be reached only upon formation of a high-affinity, multi-component complex coordinated by BSAP. Such a model would explain why ε is the only promoter apparently regulated by BSAP, even though binding sites for BSAP have been identified in the vicinity of several germline promoters, such as murine $\gamma 1$, $\gamma 2a$ and α (51, 52). If regulation of the ε germline promoter by BSAP really requires interaction(s) with other transcription factors, it is possible that binding sites for the appropriate BSAP partners are absent in promoters other than ε, and/or are not accessible because of topological constraints.

Footprinting studies of the nuclear factors bound to the ε germline promoter *in vivo* and analyses of protein/protein interactions involving BSAP are required to test the validity of this model. However, the ability of BSAP to act in concert with other nuclear factors to activate or repress target genes is well established. Repression of the $3'\alpha$ enhancer (hs1,2) or activation of the $3'\alpha$ enhancer-hs4 by BSAP involves the combined efforts of a common set of factors, such as octamer binding proteins, NF-κB-like complexes, and in the case of the $3'\alpha$ enhancer (hs1,2), a novel G-rich DNA binding protein (53, 54). The choice between activation or repression seems to be strictly dependent on the topology of the binding sites for these factors, and may result from direct occlusion of their activation domains, or from the recruitment of other factor(s) that mediate repression or activation (55).

Additionally and/or alternatively, BSAP may contribute to coupling germline transcription and switching to cell proliferation. Switch recombination to $\gamma 1$ and expression of $\gamma 1$ and ε germline transcripts was severely reduced after incubation of activated murine B cells with DNA synthesis inhibitors (56). BSAP activity is known to be upregulated by stimulation of murine B cells with mitogens or CD40L, and downregulated by cross-linking of OX40 ligand (57). Antisense-mediated downregulation of BSAP resulted in a dramatic decrease in cell proliferation, and in the inhibition of class switching to IgG1 induced by IL-4 + LPS (58). A clue to the mechanisms underlying the link between BSAP and B-cell proliferation has been offered by recent results demonstrating that BSAP represses transcription of the tumor suppressor gene p53 (59). p53 appears to control the cell cycle by activating downstream target genes that arrest cells in late G1 phase, and furthermore mediates apoptosis in a variety of cell types. BSAP expression in the early stages of B-cell differentiation would inhibit p53 expression, leading to rapid growth and partial differentiation, while preventing cellular decisions concerning apoptosis. Once BSAP expression is reduced, p53 expression would become substantial, and the final stages of differentiation could occur (59).

REFERENCES

1. Coffman RL, Lebman DA and Rothman P (1993) The mechanism and regulation of immunoglobulin isotype switching. *Adv Immunol* **54**:229–269.

2. Stavnezer J (1996) Immunoglobulin class switching. *Curr Opin Immunol* **8**:199–205.
3. Iwasato T, Shimizu A, Honjo T and Yamagishi H (1990) Circular DNA is excised by immunoglobulin class switch recombination. *Cell* **62**:143–149.
4. Zhang K, Mills FC and Saxon A (1994) Switch circles from IL-4-directed ε class switching from human B lymphocytes – evidence for direct, sequential and multiple step sequential switch from μ to ε Ig heavy chain gene. *J Immunol* **152**:3427–3435.
5. Jung S, Rajewsky K and Radbruch A (1993) Shutdown of class switch recombination by deletion of a switch region control element. *Science* **259**:984–987.
6. Zhang J, Bottaro A, Li S, Stewart V and Alt FW (1993) Targeted mutation in the Ig2b exon results in a selective Iγ2b deficiency in mice. *EMBO J* **12**:3529–3537.
7. Lorenz M, Jung S and Radbruch A (1995) Switch transcripts in immunoglobulin class switching. *Science* **267**:1825–1828.
8. Liu YJ, Malisan F, de Bouteiller O *et al* (1996) Within germinal centers, isotype switching of immunoglobulin genes occurs after the onset of somatic mutation. *Immunity* **4**:241–250.
9. Arpin C, Déchanet J, Van Kooten C *et al* (1995) Generation of memory B cells and plasma cells *in vitro*. *Science* **265**:720–722.
10. Toellner K-M, Gulbranson-Judge A, Taylor DR, Sze DM-Y and MacLennan ICM (1996) Immunoglobulin switch transcript production *in vivo* related to the site and time of antigen-specific B cell activation. *J Exp Med* **183**:2303–2312.
11. Punnonen J, Cocks BG and de Vries JE (1995) IL-4 induces germ-line IgE heavy chain gene transcription in human fetal pre-B cells. Evidence for differential expression of functional IL-4 and IL-13 receptors during B cell ontogeny. *J Immunol* **155**:4248–4254.
12. Hodgkin PD, Lee J-H and Lyons AB (1996) B cell differentiation and isotype switching is related to division cycle number. *J Exp Med* **184**:277–281.
13. Kühn R, Rajewsky KR and Müller W (1991) Generation and analysis of interleukin-4 deficient mice. *Science* **254**:707–710.
14. Kopf M, Le Gros G, Bachmann M, Lamers MC, Bluethmann H and Köhler G (1993) Disruption of the murine IL-4 gene blocks Th2 cytokine responses. *Nature* **362**:245–248.
15. Morawetz RA, Gabriele L, Rizzo LV *et al* (1996) Interleukin-4-independent immunoglobulin class switch to immunoglobulin E in the mouse. *J Exp Med* **184**:1651–1661.
16. Noben-Trauth N, Kropf P and Müller I (1996) Susceptibility to *Leishmania major* infection in interleukin-4-deficient mice. *Science* **271**:987–990.
17. Hjulström S, Landin A, Jansson L, Holmdahl R and Heyman B (1995) No role of interleukin-4 in CD23/IgE-mediated enhancement of the murine antibody response *in vivo*. *Eur J Immunol* **25**:1469–1472.
18. von der Weid T, Kopf M, Köhler G and Langhorne J (1994) The immune response to *Plasmodium chabaudi* malaria in interleukin-4-deficient mice. *Eur J Immunol* **24**:2285–2293.
19. Warren WD and Berton MT (1995) Induction of germ-line γ1 and ε Ig gene expression in murine B cells. IL-4 and the CD40 ligand-CD40 interaction provide distinct but synergistic signals. *J Immunol* **155**:5637–5646.
20. Hou J, Schindler U, Henzel WJ, Ho TC, Brasseur M and McKnight SL (1994) An interleukin-4-induced transcription factor: IL-4 Stat. *Science* **265**:1701–1706.
21. Quelle FW, Shimoda K, Thierfelder W *et al* (1995) Cloning of murine and human Stat6, Stat proteins that are tyrosine phosphorylated in response to IL-4 and IL-3 but are not required for mitogenesis. *Mol Cell Biol* **15**:3336–3343.
22. Ihle JN and Kerr IM (1995) Jaks and Stats in signaling by the cytokine receptor superfamily. *Trends Genet* **11**:69–74.
23. Ivashkiv LB (1995) Cytokines and STATs: How can signals achieve specificity? *Immunity* **3**:1–4.

24. Schindler U, Wu P, Rothe M, Brasseur M and McKnight SL (1995) Components of a Stat recognition code: evidence for two layers of molecular selectivity. *Immunity* **2**:689–697.

25. Kotanides H and Reich NC (1993) Requirement of tyrosine phosphorylation for rapid activation of a DNA binding factor by IL-4. *Science* **262**:1265–1267.

26. Albrecht B, Peiritsch S and Woisetschläger M (1994) A bifunctional control element in the human IgE germline promoter involved in repression and IL-4 activation. *Int Immunol* **6**:1143–1151.

27. Delphin S and Stavnezer J (1995) Characterization of an IL-4 responsive region in the immunoglobulin heavy chain germline ε promoter: regulation by NF-IL-4, a C/EBP family member, and NF-κB/p50. *J Exp Med* **181**:181–192.

28. Köhler I and Rieber EP (1993) Allergy-associated Iε and Fcε receptor II (CD23b) genes activated via binding of an interleukin-4-induced transcription factor to a novel responsive element. *Eur J Immunol* **23**:3066–3071.

29. Wang D-Z, Cherrington A, Famakin-Mosuro B and Boothby M (1996) Independent pathways for de-repression of the mouse immunoglobulin heavy chain germ-line ε promoter: an IL-4 NAF/NF-IL4 site as a context-dependent negative element. *Int Immunol* **8**:977–989.

30. Shimoda K, van Deursen J, Sangster MY *et al* (1996) Lack of IL-4-induced Th2 response and IgE class switching in mice with disrupted Stat6 gene. *Nature* **380**:630–633.

31. Kaplan MH, Schindler U, Smiley ST and Grusby MJ (1996) Stat6 is required for mediating responses to IL-4 and for the development of Th2 cells. *Immunity* **4**:313–319.

32. Takeda K, Tanaka T, Shi W *et al* (1996) Essential role of Stat6 in IL-4 signalling. *Nature* **380**:627–630.

33. Kim J, Reeves R, Rothman P and Boothby M (1995) The non-histone chromosomal protein HMG-I(Y) contributes to repression of the immunoglobulin heavy chain germ-line ε RNA promoter. *Eur J Immunol* **25**:798–807.

34. Jung S, Siebenkotten G and Radbruch A (1994) Frequency of immunoglobulin E class switching is autonomously determined and independent of prior switching to other classes. *J Exp Med* **179**:2023–2026.

35. Sha WC, Liou H-C, Tuomanen EI and Baltimore D (1995) Targeted disruption of the p50 subunit of NF-κB leads to multifocal defects in immune responses. *Cell* **80**:321–330.

36. Snapper CM, Zelazowski P, Rosas FR *et al* (1996) B cells from p50/NF-κB knockout mice have selective defects in proliferation, differentiation, germ line C$_H$ transcription, and Ig class switching. *J Immunol* **156**:183–191.

37. Snapper CM, Rosas FR, Zelazowski P *et al* (1996) B cells lacking RelB are defective in proliferative responses, but undergo normal B cell maturation to Ig secretion and Ig class switching. *J Exp Med* **184**:1537–1541.

38. Liao F, Birshtein BK, Busslinger M and Rothman P (1994) The transcription factor BSAP (NF-HB) is essential for immunoglobulin germ-line ε transcription. *J Immunol* **152**:2904–2911.

39. Adams B, Dörfler P, Aguzzi A *et al* (1992) Pax-5 encodes the transcription factor BSAP and is expressed in B lymphocytes, the developing CNS, and adult testis. *Genes Dev* **6**:1589–1607.

40. Urbanék P, Wang Z-Q, Fetka I, Wagner EF and Busslinger M (1994) Complete block of early B cell differentiation and altered patterning of the posterior midbrain in mice lacking Pax5/BSAP. *Cell* **79**:901–912.

41. Kozmik Z, Wang S, Dörfler P, Adams B and Busslinger M (1992) The promoter of the CD19 gene is a target for the B-cell-specific transcription factor BSAP. *Mol Cell Biol* **12**:2662–2672.

42. Okabe T, Watanabe T and Kudo A (1992) A pre-B and B cell-specific DNA binding protein, EBB-1, which binds to the promoter of the V_{preB1} gene. *Eur J Immunol* **22**:37.

43. Reimold AM, Ponath PD, Li Y-S *et al* (1996) Transcription factor B cell lineage-specific activator protein regulates the gene for human X-box binding protein 1. *J Exp Med* **183**:393–401.

44. Zwollo P and Desiderio S (1994) Specific recognition of the blk promoter by the B-lymphoid transcription factor B-cell-specific activator protein. *J Biol Chem* **269**:15310–15317.

45. Singh M and Birshtein BK (1993) NF-HB (BSAP) is a repressor of the murine immunoglobulin heavy-chain 3′α enhancer at early stages of B-cell differentiation. *Mol Cell Biol* **13**:3611–3622.

46. Neurath MF, Strober W and Wakatsuki Y (1994) The murine Ig 3′ α enhancer is a target site with repressor function for the B cell lineage-specific transcription factor BSAP (NF-HB, Sα-BP). *J Immunol* **153**:730–742.

47. Busslinger M, Klix N, Pfeffer P, Graninger PG and Kozmik Z (1996) Deregulation of *PAX-5* by translocation of the Eµ enhancer of the Ig H locus adjacent to two alternative *PAX-5* promoters in a diffuse large-cell lymphoma. *Proc Natl Acad Sci USA* **93**:6129–6134.

48. Thienes CP, De Monte L, Monticelli S, Busslinger M, Gould HJ and Vercelli D (1997) The transcription factor BSAP enhances in both IL-4- and CD40-mediated activation of the human ε germline promoter. *J Immunol* **158**:5874–5882.

49. Albrecht B, Peiritsch S, Messner B and Woisetschläger M (1996) The transcription factor B cell-specific activator protein is not involved in the IL-4-induced activation of the human IgE germline promoter. *J Immunol* **157**:1538–1543.

50. Czerny T and Busslinger M (1995) DNA-binding and transactivation properties of Pax-6: three amino acids in the paired domain are responsible for the different sequence recognition of Pax-6 and BSAP (Pax-5). *Mol Cell Biol* **15**:2858–2871.

51. Lin Y-CA and Stavnezer J (1992) Regulation of transcription of the germ-line Igα constant region gene by an ATF element and by novel transforming growth factor-$\beta 1$-responsive elements. *J Immunol* **149**:2914–2925.

52. Xu M and Stavnezer J (1992) Regulation of transcription of immunoglobulin germ-line γ1 RNA: analysis of the promoter/enhancer. *EMBO J* **11**:145–155.

53. Michaelson JS, Singh M, Snapper CM, Sha WC, Baltimore D and Birshtein BK (1996) Regulation of 3′ IgH enhancers by a common set of factors, including κB-binding proteins. *J Immunol* **156**:2828–2839.

54. Singh M and Birshtein BK (1996) Concerted repression of an immunoglobulin heavy-chain enhancer, 3′αE (hs1,2). *Proc Natl Acad Sci USA* **93**:4392–4397.

55. Michaelson JS, Singh M and Birshtein BK (1996) B cell lineage-specific activator protein (BSAP) a player at multiple stages of B cell development. *J Immunol* **156**:2349–2351.

56. Lundgren M, Ström L, Bergquist L-O *et al* (1995) Cell cycle regulation of immunoglobulin class switch recombination and germ-line transcription: potential role of Ets family members. *Eur J Immunol* **25**:2042–2051.

57. Stüber E, Neurath M, Calderhead D, Perry Fell H and Strober W (1995) Cross-linking of OX40 ligand, a member of the TNF/NGF cytokine family, induces proliferation and differentiation in murine splenic B cells. *Immunity* **2**:507–521.

58. Wakatsuki Y, Neurath MF, Max EE and Strober W (1994) The B cell-specific transcription factor BSAP regulates B cell proliferation. *J Exp Med* **179**:1099–1108.

59. Stuart ET, Haffner R, Oren M and Gruss P (1995) Loss of p53 function through PAX-mediated transcriptional repression. *EMBO J* **14**:5638–5645.

11 Isotype Switching from μ to ε Immunoglobulin Heavy Chain Gene in Human B Cells as Determined by Switch Circle Analysis

KE ZHANG and ANDREW SAXON
The Hart and Louise Lyon Laboratory, UCLA School of Medicine, Los Angeles CA, USA

Immunoglobulin (Ig) isotype switching is a critical process in the immune system whereby B cells generate different types of effector antibody molecules without changing antigen specificity (1, 2). As B lymphocytes differentiate into memory or plasma cells, μ heavy chain gene expression changes to expression of other isotypes (2, 3). DNA rearrangement between two different isotype switch (S) regions is the major mechanism for isotype switching. This deletional rearrangement, so called S–S recombination, joins the Sμ region with a downstream S region to create a new transcriptional unit encompassing VDJ sequences (originally expressed with Cμ) and the targeted downstream C_H gene (3). This is accomplished by non-homologous recombination. Such deletional recombination is accompanied by excision of the intervening DNA between the involved upstream and downstream S regions. According to the proposed mechanism for deletional recombination, intervening DNA between two recombining S regions should loop out and ligate through its ends to form an extra-chromosomal circular DNA molecule, or Ig switch circle (4, 5). A polymerase chain reaction (PCR)-based system has been developed to analyze the switch circles excised from human B cells involved in isotype switching from μ to ε, μ to γ and μ to α genes (6, 7) so as to determine whether switch circular DNAs are excised via looping out and deletional recombination in human B cells and to provide an insight into the intermediate processes of isotype switching from μ to ε, γ and α genes in humans. In this chapter we will discuss the methodology and application of the switch circle analysis in understanding the isotype switch process from μ to ε heavy chain gene in humans. These studies revealed that isotype switch from the μ to the ε locus can be achieved by a variety of switching pathways; including direct switching from μ to ε, sequential switching from μ to ε via γ and triple step sequential switching from μ to ε via an α and γ gene. Furthermore, once switched, we demonstrate that isotype stabilization can occur by a process of secondary S region deletion.

IgE Regulation: Molecular Mechanisms. Edited by D. Vercelli. © 1997 John Wiley & Sons Ltd.

11.1 THE RATIONALE OF A PCR STRATEGY FOR
DETECTION OF SWITCH CIRCULAR DNA

During deletional recombination, the 5' part of the upstream S region sequence and 3' part of the targeted downstream S region sequence join together on the chromosome to form a hybrid S region. The 3' portion of the upstream S region sequence, the 5' sequences of the targeted S region and all the intervening sequence should be looped out in those B lymphocytes undergoing isotype switch. Based on these facts, a PCR based-strategy to assay the switch circles from human B cells was developed. As depicted in Figure 11.1a, the deleted DNA forms a circular structure by joining the 5' switch section of a downstream isotype to 3' switch sequences of a more proximal isotype. Thus the orientation of the designed PCR primer pair 2 (antisense sequences) and 5 (sense sequences) allows amplification of switch circle sequences formed by $S\mu$ to $S\varepsilon$ direct switching. Primer pair 1 and 6 were used as 'nested' primers for second-round PCR to increase the sensitivity and specificity of first-round PCR. Switch circular DNA formed by μ to ε sequential switch via any intervening Ig C_H would not be amplified by this set of primers. This follows because the 3' part of $S\mu$ sequences, where primer 2 and 1 are located, would be part of a switch circle containing the 5' S region of the intervening isotype (rather than ε) to which μ had initially switched (see Figure 11.1a, top switch circle).

Similarly, primer set 4 and 5, with primer set 3 and 6 used for second-round amplification, are designed to detect only switch circles representing γ to ε switch events (Figure 11.1b). The γ primers detect all four human γ genes ($\gamma3$, $\gamma1$, $\gamma2$, and $\gamma4$) as they are greater than 97% homologous to each other in the regions (8). Therefore it is likely that γ–ε switch circles derived from any of the four γ genes would be amplified by these primer sets. Primer pairs 4–5 and 3–6 would not detect μ to ε direct switching, because the 3' part of $S\mu$ would have been looped out and deleted during the prior switch recombination between $S\mu$ and $S\gamma$.

The orientation of the primers ensures that the amplified switch fragments are from the excised circular DNA and not from the rearranged genomic DNA. Thus, these approaches are able to test in humans the hypothesis that deleted intervening DNA indeed forms switch circular DNA, and to test whether both direct and sequential switch mechanisms are involved in μ to ε switching. Proper selection of primers based on their predicted orientation in switch circular DNA allows one to identify and study in a sensitive manner those specific switch events of interest (i.e. μ to γ, μ to α etc.) without being hindered by other types of switch circles or the S sequences in the retained genomic DNA. Indeed, such a system has now been adapted to study Ig isotype switching from μ to γ subclasses and to α in human B cells (7 and unpublished data).

This system provided a novel approach for the study of isotype switching, and particularly for analysis of low-frequency switch events such as those occurring in polyclonal or antigen-activated fresh human B cells, where the physical isolation and characterization of circular DNA will not give satisfactory results. Importantly, switch circle analysis provides conclusive direct data about actual switching events, information which may not be directly obtained by the analysis of the retained switch junctions in chromosomal DNA as secondary deletion of isotype switched B cells (9) or sequential switching create new recombination breakpoints on the rearranged chromosome. The breakpoints defined from switch circles represent the original recombination sites, a situation not necessarily reflected in breakpoints on switched chromosomes. Excised switch circles are believed not to further undergo replication (10, 11) making the chance of secondary deletion occurring in switch circles unlikely compared to the known occurrence of secondary deletions in retained switched loci on the active chromosome. Thus, breakpoints defined from switch circles more closely resemble the original recombination sites than breakpoints from the switched chromosomes.

11.1.1 PCR and Cloning Protocol

PCR was performed in a 25 μl volume/reaction with 10% dimethyl sulfoxide (DMSO), 50 mM KCl, 20 mM Tris–HCl (pH 8.4), 2.5 mM MgCl$_2$, 0.5 μM primers and 2.5 U of Taq polymerase. Circular DNA was specially prepared by the methods described previously (6). An amount of 'circular fraction DNA' derived from 1×10^6 cultured cells was used as the DNA template for each reaction. The first cycle of PCR was carried out at 94 °C for 10 min (without Taq polymerase) for complete DNA denaturation, 65 °C for 10 min for annealing (Taq polymerase was added to the tube at this step), and 72 °C for 10 min for extension. PCR was continued at 94 °C for 1 min, 65 °C for 1 min and 72 °C for 5 min for 40 cycles, with 15 min extension in the final cycle.

A second round of PCR using nested primers was run on the DNA templates derived from the first PCR reaction with the same conditions as the first round PCR, except for the changes in the primers. The first round PCR products from primer set 2 and 5 (μ and ε) were re-amplified by primer set 1 and 6 and the products from primer set 4 and 5 (γ and ε) were reamplified by primer set 3 and 6 (see Figure 11.1). A second round of amplifications was carried out at 94 °C for 1 min, 68 °C for 1 min and 72 °C for 3 min for 40 cycles, with a 15 min extension time for the final cycle. The primer sequences are shown in the following list:

(1) 5'-ATTGGCCCAGTGCCATGTCCTCCAGTTCAT-3', complementary to position 3738–3710 of Sμ
(2) 5'-CCATCTATGTCCAACAAGATCATGA-3', complementary to position 3766–3742 of Sμ
(3) 5'-CTCTGGCCATCGGTGCCACCTCA-3', complementary to position 4620–4598 of Sγ4
(4) 5'AGTCAGCACAGTCCAGGGCCTCTA3', complementary to position 4656–4633 of Sγ4
(5) 5'-AGGCTCCACTGCCCGGCACAGAAAT-3', corresponding to position 542–566 of Sε
(6) 5'-TGTCCCTTAGAGGACAGGTGGCCAAG-3', corresponding to position 1156–1181 of Sε (12).

194

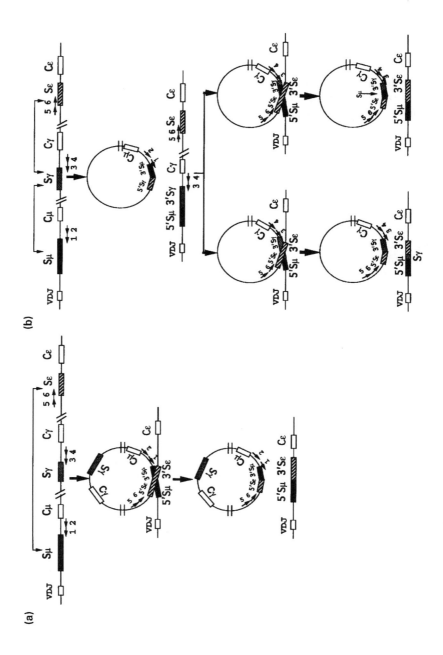

Figure 11.1. Schematic diagram showing the formation of switch circular DNA (switch circles) and the PCR strategy used for the detection of switch fragments contained within such switch circles. (a) Diagram of the occurrence and detection of μ to ε direct switch. A map of disrupted human Ig C_H chain genes that relate to this study is shown at the top. The S regions are indicated by shaded boxes and the constant regions are shown as an open box. The numbered arrows indicate the position and the orientation of the PCR primers; the arrows above the gene map are sense sequences and those below the map are antisense sequences. For μ to ε direct switching, after looping-out and deletion, a hybrid S–S region with $5'S\mu$–$3'S\varepsilon$ would be generated on the chromosome, as shown in the linear diagram at the bottom. The excised DNA should join their two ends to form a switch circular DNA with a $5'S\varepsilon$–$3'S\mu$ sequence, as shown in the circle. Primers 2 and 5 would amplify the switch fragments from switch circles if the deleted S–S regions are joined to form circular DNA. Primers 1 and 6 were used for the second round of PCR reactions to increase the sensitivity and specificity of the procedure. (b) Diagram of the occurrence and detection of μ to ε sequential switch via γ. Primers 4 and 5 were used for the first-round PCR, and primers 3 and 6 were used for second-round PCR in order to amplify γ to ε switching. The μ to γ switch would generate an $S\mu$–$S\gamma$ switch circle as shown, and a $5'S\mu$–$3'S\gamma$ sequence would be generated on the chromosome, as shown in the linear diagram. Subsequent γ to ε switch could generate two types of switch circles, depending on where the recombination sites occur. A switch circle that has $5'S\varepsilon$ directly joined to $3'S\gamma$ would be generated when the switch takes place between the $S\gamma$ part of the hybrid $5'S\mu$–$3'S\gamma$ region and $S\varepsilon$, as shown in the left hand side of (b). The chromosome would retain some $S\gamma$ sequences. A second type of switch circle, with $S\mu$ sequences interposed between the $5'S\varepsilon$ and the $3'S\gamma$ sequences, would result when switch recombination occurs between the remaining $5'S\mu$ part of the hybrid $5'S\mu$–$3'S\gamma$ region and $S\varepsilon$. This is shown on the right hand side of (b). In this case, the retained chromosomal S–S region will have $5'S\mu$ joined to $3'S\varepsilon$ (adapted from Ref. 6 (*J Immunol*), with permission)

The final PCR products were cloned by the TA cloning method (5). The clones that contained inserts were selected for mini-preparation and digested with EcoRI. After electrophoresis, the DNA was transferred to nylon membrane and screened by hybridization with a PCR-generated 257 bp probe that is specific for 5′ Sε sequences

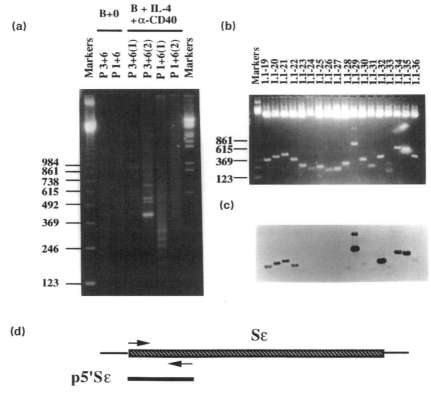

Figure 11.2. Detection and cloning of PCR-amplified recombinant S regions from switch circles containing Sε sequences. (a) Gel electrophoresis of switch fragments from switch circles PCR-amplified using μ–ε primers (P1 + 6) or γ–ε primers (P3 + 6). Multiple DNA bands of different sizes can be seen in stimulated cells. DNA from control (B + 0) and IL-4 plus anti-CD40 mAb-stimulated B cells (B + Stimuli) served as template for amplification of switch fragments by different primer sets (P). Two independent amplifications (indicated by the numbers in parenthesis) were performed with induced B cells with each set of primers. (b) Subcloning of the PCR products. Five microliters of the second-round PCR products (shown in (a)) were ligated into the TA cloning vector. Clones with inserts were randomly picked for mini-prep analysis. Inserts of different sizes derived from these clones are shown. (c) Southern blot analysis of the isolated subclones detecting those that contain 5′Sε sequences. The subclones from (b) were hybridized with a 257 bp PCR-generated probe representing 5′Sε sequences, as shown in (d). The clones that hybridized were subjected to sequence analysis, as they were likely to be derived from switch circles of interest. (d) Diagram for the PCR-generated probe P5′Sε that was used for Southern blot in (c). A 257 bp fragment was amplified by PCR and sequenced (from Ref. 6 (*J Immunol*), with permission)

(P5'Sε). The clones that hybridized with P5'Sε were subjected to DNA sequencing. An example of DNA 'switch circle fragments' amplification from IL-4 plus anti-CD40 monoclonal antibody (mAb)-stimulated B cells is shown in Figure 11.2. Multiple bands are visualized when amplified with the primer set for μ to ε direct switch (labeled p1 + 6) and the primer set for γ to ε sequential switch (labeled p3 + 6). No PCR bands are seen with unstimulated B cells (B + 0). The multiple bands are consistent with the prediction that breakpoints for switch recombination would be scattered over both S regions involved in the joining (10). An example of cloning of the PCR products is shown in Figure 11.2b, where 17 randomly selected individual subclones from the mini-preparation are shown. Hybridization with the 5' Sε specific probe (P5'Sε), as in Figure 11.2c indicated that these subclones contained Sε sequences of interest. The various sizes of the inserts imply that the subclones represent switch sequences from different switch circles.

11.2 DIRECT SWITCH FROM μ TO ε

Sequence analysis revealed that the clones reactive with P5'Sε and derived from primer pair 1 + 6 (specific for detection of μ–ε direct switching) had 5'Sε sequences directly joined to 3'Sμ sequences in a 5'–3' orientation. The amplified products of 'switch circle fragment' were expected to be 5'Sε–3'Sμ, as they are the reciprocal pieces to the switch fragment 5'Sμ–3'Sε in the rearranged chromosome. An example of such a clone is presented in Figure 11.3a, where the recombination breakpoint for

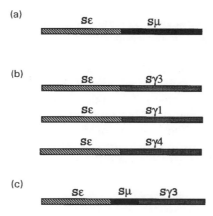

Figure 11.3. Schematic diagram of the structure of the amplified fragments derived from switch circular DNA. (a) Diagram of the structure of the circular DNA fragment with 5'Sε directly joined to 3'Sμ, reflecting μ to ε direct switching. (b) Diagram of the structure of the circular DNA fragment with 5'Sε directly joined to 3'Sγ3, Sγ1 and Sγ4, reflecting μ to ε indirect (sequential) switching through multiple γ genes. (c) Diagram of the structure of the circular DNA fragment with 5'Sε indirectly joined to 3'Sγ3, with Sμ sequences interposed between them, reflecting μ to ε indirect (sequential) switching through the γ3 gene

the clone is defined by alignment of the 'switch circle fragments' with the published germline $S\varepsilon$ and $S\mu$ region sequences. The direct $5'S\varepsilon–3'S\mu$ junctions in the switch circles conclusively demonstrate that switching from μ to downstream isotypes such as ε can be achieved by direct switching in stimulated primary human B cells, and does not require passing through an intermediary isotype. This conclusion with human B cells is consistent with subsequent experiments with $S\gamma 1$ (the equivalent of human $\gamma 4$) control region knock-out mice in which the switch frequency to the ε locus was not affected, even though $\gamma 1$ switch was completely blocked (13). Such results disprove the proposal that class switching to C_H genes distal to $C\mu$, such as $C\varepsilon$ and $C\alpha$, proceeds by obligate switch recombination via an $S\gamma$ intermediate. Sequential switching to ε via γ genes also occurs (see below), but it is not an obligatory step.

11.3 SEQUENTIAL SWITCH FROM μ TO ε VIA VARIOUS γ GENES

As mentioned earlier, we used a pair of primer sets to analyze γ to ε isotype switching. Nucleotide sequencing of clones resulting from amplification with primer set $3 + 6$ (Figure 11.1b) (that specifically detects γ to ε switching and reacts with P5'Sε) revealed that these clones representing switch circular DNA had $5'$ $S\varepsilon$ directly joined to $3'$ $S\gamma$ sequences in $5'–3'$ orientation, as predicted. An example of such a clone is presented in Figure 11.3b. Similarly, the recombination breakpoints for these clones were defined by alignment of the 'switch circle fragments' with published germline $S\varepsilon$ and $S\gamma$ region sequences.

Even though all the four human $S\gamma$ regions share high homology (8), there are γ subclass-specific characteristic nucleotides located in the amplified regions. Therefore the $S\gamma$ sequences from these clones were subjected to special scrutiny for 'diagnostic nucleotides' so as to provide sufficient data to determine from which of the four $S\gamma$ ($\gamma 1–4$) regions the clones were derived. Such diagnostic nucleotide analysis revealed that the γ sequences from the clones were derived from $\gamma 3$, $\gamma 1$ and $\gamma 4$, indicating that sequential switching from μ to ε could occur through various γ genes in human B cells. The detection of direct γ to ε switch was indirect but compelling evidence for μ-γ-ε switch, because all B cells start at μ. However, we were able to isolate a clone with residual $S\mu$ sequences interposed between $5'$ $S\varepsilon$ and $3'$ $S\gamma$ in the switch circle (Figure 11.3c). The existence of such clones is direct evidence for μ to ε sequential switch via γ genes, as shown in Figure 11.1b.

11.4 TRIPLE STEP SEQUENTIAL SWITCH TO ε VIA α AND γ

Multiple step sequential switching from μ to ε through more than one intermediate gene was also defined by using switch circle analysis. One switch circle clone contained an $S\alpha 1$ fragment interposed between $5'$ $S\varepsilon$ and $3'$ $S\gamma$ sequences (Figure

11.4a). The placement of Sα1 sequence between 5' Sε and 3' Sγ segments is evidence for previous recombination between Sμ and Sα1 prior to switching to γ4 or γ2. Thus, at a minimum, a triple step sequential switch model needs to be invoked to explain the generation of the switch circle that gave rise to this clone, which is schematically diagrammed in Figure 11.4b. The initial switch [1)] between Sμ and Sα1 generated a hybrid S region with a 5'Sμ–3'Sα1 chromosomal junction. The second switch [2)] occurred between the Sα1 portion of the hybrid 5'Sμ–3'Sα1 region and Sγ4 or Sγ2, leading to formation of a complex 5'Sμ–3'Sα1–(Sγ4 or Sγ2) chromosomal S region. A final switch event [3)] must have then taken place between the Sα1 sequences in the complex Sμ–Sα1–(Sγ4 or Sγ2) region, and Sε. This led us

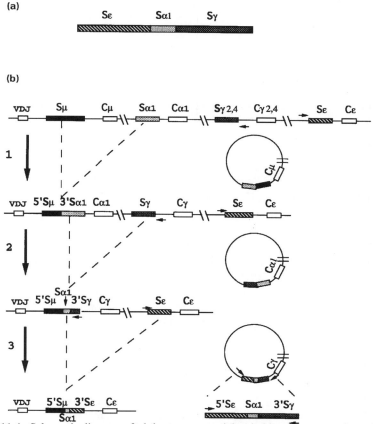

Figure 11.4. Schematic diagram of triple-step sequential switching from μ to ε through the α1 and γ genes. (a) Diagram of the structure of the circular DNA fragment with 5'Sε indirectly joined to 3'Sγ, with Sα1 sequences interposed between them, reflecting μ to ε indirect (sequential) switching through multiple α1 and a γ (γ2 or γ4) gene. (b) Delineation of the switching pathway for triple-step sequential switching (modified from Ref. 6 (*J Immunol*), with permission)

to detect an excised switch circle containing $5'S\varepsilon–S\alpha1–3'(S\gamma4$ or $S\gamma2)$ sequences, as shown in the circle at the bottom right. Reciprocally, this final switching step would create a chromosomal S region containing $5'S\mu–S\alpha1–3'S\varepsilon$ (bottom left) that allows for ε gene expression.

Whether such multi-step sequential switching represents an unusual path among the routes to ε switching is uncertain, as the chance of detecting the complex type of switch circles is much lower than the chance of detecting direct or two-step sequential switching. This would be true even if the frequency of three-step sequential switching were the same as direct or two-step switching. Switch circles reflecting multi-step sequential switching would be detected only in those cases where a portion of the second S region (i.e. $S\alpha1$) is retained in the chromosome during the next switch recombination (i.e. to $S\gamma4$ or $S\gamma2$), and then both downstream S sequences ($S\alpha1$, and $S\gamma4$ or $S\gamma2$) are excised as part of a subsequent switch circle. There are many opportunities for recombinations in multi-step sequential switching to remove the switch remnants of earlier S-S joining so that a later switch circle will not contain the elements of earlier switches, even though multi-step sequential switching has occurred (Figure 11.4b). Interestingly, the notion of switching from μ to ε via $\alpha1$ is in agreement with the report that ε switching could be frequently induced from IgA1 positive B cells by interleukin (IL)-4 stimulation (14).

11.5 SECONDARY DELETIONAL RECOMBINATION AS A MECHANISM FOR ISOTYPE STABILIZATION

Analysis of the Ig S region structure from many stable isotype switched B cells reveals that the majority of the ultimate switch recombination sites are located at the $5'$ end or even upstream of $S\mu$ (15). These findings are in contrast with results from switch circle analysis which reveal that the primary switch recombination sites are preferentially distributed in the middle or $3'$ end of the $S\mu$ region. Secondary deletion within recombined chimeric S regions has been proposed as a mechanism to account for these differences (1, 15). Such a hypothesis has been directly tested by a modified switch circle analysis approach in human B cells, as shown in Figure 11.5. Circular DNAs representing secondary deletion events were isolated and characterized by using a PCR specially designed to detect such events as secondary deletion circles (16). The results revealed that cells do undergo secondary deletions of S regions, often deleting the vast majority of S sequences as secondary deletion circles. These results definitively demonstrate that secondary deletion/recombination of chimeric S regions of human isotype switched B cells does occur. Such secondary deletion/recombination events can be potentially responsible for isotype stabilization of switched B cells, as the active Ig gene may have an insufficient amount of retained chimeric switch sequence to serve as a substrate for further S–S recombination (Figure 11.6).

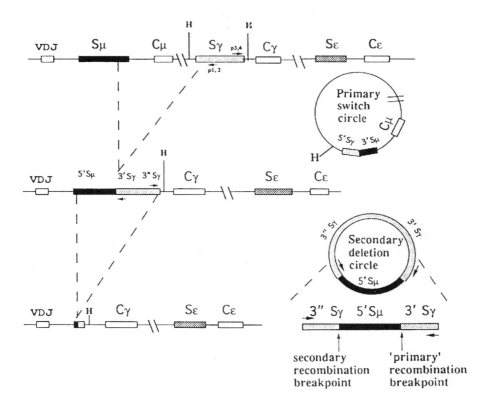

Figure 11.5. Schematic diagram demonstrating the formation of circular DNA representing primary and secondary recombination/deletion and the PCR strategy for detection of secondary deletion circles. A map of disrupted human Ig C_H chain gene region related to this study is shown at the top. The typical S regions with repetitive sequences are indicated by shaded boxes and the constant regions are shown as an open box. The numbered arrows indicate the position and the orientation of the PCR primers; the arrows above the gene map are sense sequences, and those below the map are antisense sequences. For initial μ to γ switching (primary switch), the 5′ $S\mu$ portion and 3′ $S\gamma$ portion would join on the chromosome to generate a hybrid $S\mu$–$S\gamma$ region. The intervening DNA excised from the chromosome forms a primary switch circle as shown. The hybrid $S\mu$–$S\gamma$ region, when undergoing a secondary deletion as predicted, would rearrange its most 3′ end (indicated as 3″$S\gamma$) to the 5′ end of the tandemly repeated sequences of the $S\mu$ region. This would leave a very abbreviated retained S region with minimal chromosomal tandem S region sequences, while excising circular DNA (secondary deletion circle) with a part of the initial hybrid S region joined directly to itself. Such a secondary deletion circle would be amplified by PCR using primers p2 and p3 (followed by p1 and p4 for second-round PCR) to give a unique $S\gamma$–$S\mu$–$S\gamma$ structure, as shown in the bottom part of the figure (from Ref. 9 (*J Immunol*), with permission)

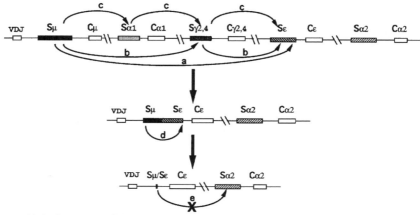

Figure 11.6. Summary of the switch pattern from the μ to the ε locus in human B cells, as defined by analysis of switch circles. Isotype switching from μ to ε can be achieved, at a minimum, by (i) direct switching from μ to ε (a: shown beneath the upper diagram of the Ig loci); (ii) sequential switching from μ to ε via one of the γ genes (b,b: shown beneath the upper diagram of the Ig loci), or (iii) triple-step sequential switching from μ to ε via $\alpha 1$ and γ genes ($\gamma 2$ or $\gamma 4$) (c,c,c: shown above the upper diagram of the Ig loci). The recombined chimeric switch regions resulting from isotype switching (d: μ to ε in this case) can undergo further secondary deletional recombination from the very 3' end to the 5' end of the chimeric S region (e), to eliminate the vast majority of the chimeric S region. Such a process therefore blocks the ability to undergo subsequent switching to a downstream isotype ($\alpha 2$ isotype in this case). Although the figure shows the secondary deletion for ε, this process occurs for the other isotypes as well

11.6 CONCLUSIONS

In this chapter we describe the application of switch circle analysis in approaching ε switching and secondary deletional recombination in human B cells. A highly sensitive and specific PCR-based assay has been developed to study the mechanism involved in the isotype switch from Ig Hμ to Ig Hε. By analysis of the generation of switch circles, an array of pathways to achieve isotype switch from μ to ε has been delineated. Isotype switching to the ε gene can be achieved by: (i) direct switching from μ to ε; (ii) sequential switching from μ to ε via multiple γ genes; and (iii) multi-step sequential switching from μ to ε via α and γ. While this approach provides an array of pathways that can be used in switching to ε, due to technical considerations it does not provide quantitative data as to the preferred use of specific pathways. The frequency of switching to ε via the available routes remains to be determined. Switch circle analysis also allowed us to conclude that looping out and deletional recombination is the mechanism for isotype switching in human B cells. The same principle of analysis of deleted switch circular DNA has subsequently been adapted to provide insights into the ability of various stimuli to drive isotype switching to γ subclasses and α genes. Circular DNA analysis also provided the first direct proof of secondary deletion within chimeric S regions of active Ig genes and strongly supports the idea that secondary deletional recombination is one mechanism for isotype stabilization.

ACKNOWLEDGMENTS

We want to acknowledge the scientific input and willingness to share unpublished data of Drs Ed E. Max and Fred Mills of CBER, FDA. We also want to acknowledge the excellent technical assistance of Hai-Kit Cheah. This work was supported by USPHS grants AI-15251, CA-12800 and the UCLA Asthma, Allergy and Immunologic Disease Center (AI-34567 funded by the NIAID and the NIEHS).

REFERENCES

1. Wang AC, Wilson SK, Hooper JE, Fudenberg HH and Nisonoff A (1970) Evidence for control of synthesis of the variable regions of heavy chains of immunoglobulin chains G and M by the same gene. *Proc Natl Acad Sci USA* **66**:337–343.
2. Pernis B, Forni L and Luzzati AL (1977) Synthesis of multiple immunoglobulin classes by single lymphocytes. *Cold Spring Harbor Symp Quant Biol* **41**:175–183.
3. Lutzker S and Alt FW (1989) Immunoglobulin heavy-chain class switching. In: *Mobile DNA*, Berg DE and Howe MM (Eds) pp. 693–714. American Society for Microbiology, Washington DC.
4. Honjo T and Kataoka T (1978) Organization of immunoglobulin heavy chain genes and allelic deletion model. *Proc Natl Acad Sci USA* **75**:2140–2144.
5. Jack HM, McDowell M, Steinberg CM and Wabl M (1988) Looping out and deletion mechanism for the immunoglobulin heavy-chain class switch. *Proc Natl Acad Sci USA* **85**:1581–1585.
6. Zhang K, Mills FC and Saxon A (1994) Switch circles from IL-4-directed ε class switching from human B lymphocytes: Evidence for direct, sequential, and multiple step sequential switch from μ to ε Ig heavy chain gene. *J Immunol* **152**:3427–3436.
7. Fujieda S, Zhang K and Saxon A (1995) IL-4 plus CD40 monoclonal antibody induces human B cells γ subclass specific isotype switching: Switching to $\gamma1$, $\gamma3$, and $\gamma4$, but not $\gamma2$. *J Immunol* **155**:2318–2329.
8. Mills FC, Mitchell MP, Harindranath N and Max EE (1995) Human Ig Sγ regions and their participation in sequential switching to IgE. *J Immunol* **155**:3021–3036.
9. Zhang K, Cheah H-K and Saxon A (1995) Secondary deletional recombination of rearranged switch region in Ig isotype switched B cells: a mechanism for isotype stabilization. *J Immunol* **154**:2237–2247.
10. Von Schwedler U, Jack HM and Wabl M (1990) Circular DNA is a product of the immunoglobulin class switch rearrangement. *Nature* **345**:452–456.
11. Iwasato T, Arakawa H, Shimizu A, Honjo T and Yamagishi H (1992) Biased distribution of recombination sites within S regions upon immunoglobulin class switch recombination induced by transforming growth factor β and lipopolysaccharide. *J Exp Med* **175**:1539–1546.
12. Mills FC, Brooker JS and Camerini-Otero RD (1990) Sequences of human immunoglobulin switch regions: Implications for recombination and transcription. *Nucleic Acids Res* **18**:7305–7316.

13. Jung S, Siebenkotten G and Radbruch A (1994) Frequency of immunoglobulin E class switching is autonomously determined and independent of prior switching to other classes. *J Exp Med* **179:**2023–2026.

14. Zhang X, Werner-Favre C, Tang H, Brouwers N, Bonnefoy J-Y and Zubler RH (1991) IL-4 dependent IgE switch in membrane IgA-positive human B cells. *J Immunol* **147:**3001–3007.

15. Matsuoka M, Yoshida K, Maeda T, Usuda S and Sakano H (1990) Formation of switch circular DNA in cytokine treated mouse splenocytes: Evidence for intramolecular DNA deletion in immunoglobulin class switch. *Cell* **62:**135–142.

12 Production of a Family of IgE Proteins by Alternative Splicing of the 3' End ε RNA

KE ZHANG and ANDREW SAXON
Division of Clinical Immunology and Allergy, University of California Los Angeles School of Medicine, Los Angeles CA, USA

Immunoglobulin E (IgE) was identified as the antibody mediating immediate allergic reactions some 30 years ago (1). Although the mechanism for IgE production and regulation has been extensively studied for many years, many aspects remain to be fully elucidated. The structural–functional heterogeneity of human IgE molecules, for example, is one of those unsolved questions. It has been observed for some time that human polyclonal IgE exhibits a heterogeneity of protein bands around the size of the classic secreted ε protein (2). Functional studies of human IgE also provide evidence for heterogeneity, because sera from only half of the atopic patients contain IgE that can passively sensitize basophils from normal individuals and trigger histamine release (3, 4). Galactin 3, an IgE binding protein, also shows differential binding to IgE (5, 6). Yet humans have only one functional ε heavy chain gene encoding the ε chain of IgE (7). Thus, once switch to ε is accomplished, the ε gene would be expected to code for a single membrane and a single secreted IgE protein, as is found for all other immunoglobulins. This expectation was challenged by the observation of three bands in Northern blot analysis of human ε mRNA (8), suggesting that the active ε gene might use alternative 3' RNA splicing to produce ε mRNAs encoding novel IgE protein(s). In this chapter we will discuss the structure of a family of ε-specific mRNA variants that encode novel ε protein isoforms as a basis to understanding the heterogeneity of IgE molecules and the possible linkage of these novel IgE isoforms with allergic diseases.

IgE Regulation: Molecular Mechanisms. Edited by D. Vercelli. © 1997 John Wiley & Sons Ltd.

12.1 ALTERNATIVE RNA SPLICING OF HUMAN ε MEMBRANE REGION EXONS GENERATES MULTIPLE SPECIES OF ε mRNA THAT ENCODE A FAMILY OF IGE PROTEINS

12.1.1 Identification of Putative ε Membrane Region Exons for the Human ε Heavy Chain Gene

As a basis for dissecting possible alternative ε RNA species involving human ε membrane exon sequences, the nucleotide sequence of human germline genomic DNA containing these exons was initially determined. This analysis identified a DNA segment, located about 1.8 kb downstream from the 3′ end of the ε CH4 domain, that showed strong sequence similarity to the ε membrane exons previously described in murine DNA at a similar location (Figure 12.1) (9–11). Of the 72 amino acid residues encoded in the two murine exons M1 and M2, 33 (46%) are conserved in the homologous human sequence. In particular, the hydrophobic residues in M1 that are thought to play a critical role in anchoring the protein to the lipid membrane of the B lymphocyte are well conserved. These include the LFLLSV segment found in most murine Ig H membrane regions and the C-terminal alanine residue. Although deletion/insertion differences are scattered in the intron sequences, in the exons they occur in only two places, with no alteration in the reading frame: two compensating deletions between nucleotides 220 and 230, and a 9 bp deletion between nucleotides 180 and 190. The latter probably resulted from an event involving repeated GACCT sequences that in the mouse are separated by nine base pairs. An additional 8 bp deletion just upstream, between nucleotides 177 and 178, may also be related to repeated sequences (CCCA). This deletion may play a critical role in generating the membrane forms of IgE in humans that differ from those found in mice (see below).

12.1.2 Splicing of CH4 to Two Distinct Splicing Acceptor Sites in the M1 Region Generates Two Species of RNA Encoding Two Membrane Forms of IgE

Based on the genomic DNA sequence of putative human ε membrane exons, we used reverse transcription (RT)–polymerase chain reaction (PCR) to fully elucidate the alternative splicing of ε mRNAs containing membrane exon sequences. Two species of mRNAs encoding membrane IgE were detected and identified by the presence of a hydrophobic transmembrane coding domain. One species, named CH4–M1′–M2, was generated by splicing from CH4 to a novel splicing acceptor site 156 nucleotides upstream of the M1 exon, to produce a membrane form of IgE with 52 extra amino acids in the extracellular portion between the CH4 and the M1 exon. The other mRNA form for membrane IgE, named CH4–M1–M2, was spliced from CH4 to the predicted splicing acceptor site of the M1 exon for other human immunoglobulins, and for murine immunoglobulins. Hydrophilicity analysis

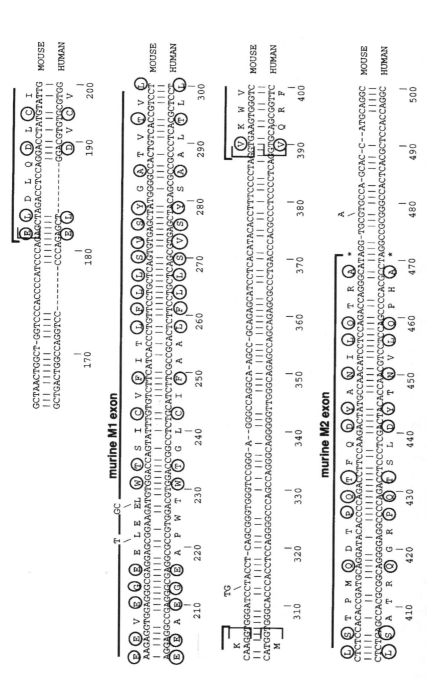

Figure 12.1. Nucleotide sequence of the human genomic fragment containing the ε membrane exons. A portion of the human sequence obtained in the present investigation is compared with the previously published murine sequence (23), in which exons M1 and M2 were identified on the basis of homology to the membrane exons of other isotypes. The amino acid translation (one letter code) is given, with conserved residues circled. From Ref. 10 (*J Exp Med*), with permission

revealed that the hydrophobic transmembrane domain is located in the M1 exon (9–11). A schematic model for two types of membrane-bound IgE is presented in Figure 12.2a. Semiquantitative PCR revealed that the CH4–M1–M2 product was present in less than 1% of the concentration of the species containing the longer M1' exon, indicating that the mRNA for the CH4–M1'–M2 form was largely dominant in IgE-producing B cells. Therefore, this form of RNA is the major type of membrane-bound IgE in humans. Indeed, such a longer membrane-bound IgE protein was detected on the surface of IgE-secreting cell lines by a specific anti-peptide anti-serum against the extracellular 52 amino acid domain (9).

Immunoglobulins exist in two forms, membrane bound or secreted, depending on alternative splicing and polyadenylation patterns of primary RNA transcripts. Indeed, alternative splicing of the μ heavy chain (12) was one of the early examples of this mechanism by which two proteins can be encoded by a single gene. For secreted immunoglobulins, the carboxy-terminal amino acids of the heavy chain are encoded contiguously with the terminal Ig H domain. For the membrane immuno-globulin form, RNA splicing eliminates the C-terminal residues of the secreted form and joins the remaining part of the last domain exon to one or two exons that encode amino acids characteristic of membrane immunoglobulins. The features of these membrane peptide segments are shown in Figure 12.3, which includes the sequences of human and murine immunoglobulin membrane segments published to date. The most characteristic feature is a segment of uncharged, mostly hydrophobic amino acids that presumably anchors the protein to the cell membrane lipids. With respect to this transmembrane segment, the human ε membrane sequence was found to be typical, including most of the consensus amino acid residues found in other isotypes, as well as a typical number of hydroxyl amino acids and a single cysteine. Some of these residues may play a role in interactions with other membrane-bound proteins that form part of the antigen receptor signal transduction machinery on the cell surface. Despite conservation of these features of the transmembrane region, it is clear that the degree of human–murine sequence similarity is lower for the ε membrane exons, as compared with the membrane exons of all other available isotypes (the relatively poor sequence conservation between human and mouse is also seen in the immunoglobulin domains of Cε). On the C-terminal cytoplasmic side of the transmembrane region, all sequences show at least one positively charged residue that is presumably important for establishing the orientation of the protein in the membrane (13) and which may also play a role in directing the protein to the appropriate post-translational processing pathways (14). The length of the cyto-plasmic domain of the human ε sequence is identical to that of the murine homolog and to all of the published γ membrane forms of both species (27 residues, counting from the conserved valine just beyond the transmembrane segment). On the extra-cellular side, near the transmembrane segment, the human ε sequence is typical in having a high density of negatively charged residues. These are also thought to play a role in orienting the protein with respect to membrane topology.

However, the human ε membrane sequence is unique among all the currently described murine and human membrane immunoglobulins in the length of the

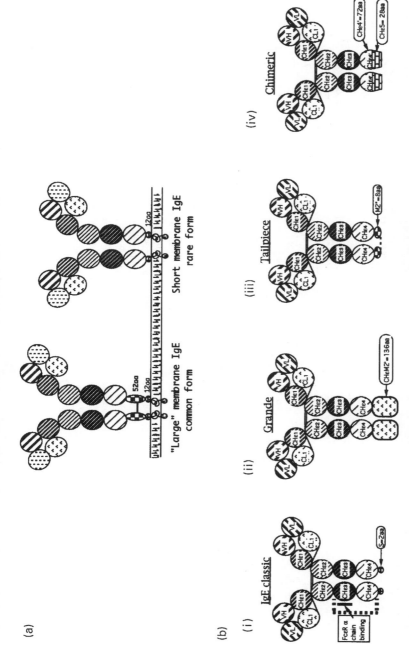

Figure 12.2. Cartoon of the IgE molecules derived from alternative splicing. (a) Diagram of the two forms of human membrane IgE. On the left is the common form of membrane IgE, which contains a novel 52 amino acid 'spacer' following the last constant region domain. The rare smaller membrane IgE is shown on the right. This protein is similar to the membrane IgE expressed in rodents. (b) Diagram of four isoforms of human secreted IgE. (i) represents the classic secreted IgE derived from read-through of the last constant region and the contiguous secreted terminus. The other three (ii, iii, iv) represent the novel secreted IgE resulting from alternative splicing

210

```
                (-)                           -----TRANSMEMBRANE-----        (+)                      Ref

 μ  Human                    EGEVSADEE  GFENLWATASTFIVLFLLSLFYSTTVTLFKVK                                a
    Mouse                    --N-E--    -----T--                                                       b
 δ  Human   LAMTPLIPQSKDENSDDYTFDDV  GSLWTTLSTFVALFILTLLYSGIVTFIKVK                                    c
    Mouse   IVN-IQHSCIM-Q--S-MDLEEE  NG--P-MC----L----F------                                          d
 γ  Human:1 ELQLEESCAEAQDG  ELDGLWTTITIFITLFLLSVCYSATVTFFKVKWIFSSVVDLKQTIIPDYRNMIGQGA                   e
         3  -------------------------L---                                                              f
         ψ  --------------------------------------------------------------------V----                 e
    Mouse:1 G---D-T---  --------S------A-L---  -----E---LV-E-K----AP                                    g
        2a  G-DDV---    --------S------S-L---  -----E---S---                                            g
        2b  --E-NGT---  --------S------S-L---  -----E--K-S--G---                                        g
         3  --E-NGT---  --------S------S-L---  -----QV---A---                                           g
 α  Human:α1 gscsvaDWQMPPPYVVLDLPQETLEEETPGANLWPTTTFPLTLFLLSLFYSTALTVTVSVRGPSGNREGPQY                   f,h
        α2  ---c---  ----------------------------K---                                                  f,h
    Mouse   ER-E-LS-L--QS-D-----A---S-----V------  ---T---F-SK-V--                                      i
 ε  Human   GLAGGSAQSQRAPDRVLCHSGQQQ  DVCVEEAEGEAPWT  WTGLCICIFAALFLLSVSYSAALTLLMVQRFLSATRQGRPQTSLDYTNVLQPHA   j
    Mouse   GLPRAAGGSVPHPRCHCGAGRADWPG PPEL  --DLQ-L-I--V---ELEEL--SI-V-IT----G-TG-V-K-KWV--TPM-DT---FQ--A-I--TR-   k

    CONSENSUS                         LW  F LELL  YS T  V
```

Figure 12.3. Amino acid sequences encoded by membrane exons. The available human and murine sequences are aligned to highlight conserved features, including the hydrophobic transmembrane region, flanked by acidic (extracellular) residues and basic (intracellular) residues. Within each isotype a human sequence was chosen as prototype, and other human and murine sequences are shown below by listing the residues that differ from the prototype. The six residues of human α that are listed in lower case letters represent the translation from an alternative RNA splice acceptor site. Consensus residues listed include those that appear in all aligned sequences (underlined) or all except one sequence (not underlined). References for the sequences are as follows: (a) Rabbitts *et al*, *Nucleic Acids Res* **9:**4509 (1981); (b) Early *et al*, *Cell* **20:**313 (1980); (c) White *et al*, *Science* **228:**733 (1985); (e) Cheng *et al*, *Nature* **296:**410 (1982); (f) Bensmana and Lefranc, *Immunogenetics* **32:**321 (1990) and Yamawaki-Kataoka *et al*, *Proc Natl Acad Sci USA* **79:**2623 (1982); (h) Yu *et al*, *J Immunol* **145:**3932 (1990); (i) Word *et al*, *EMBO J* **2:**887 (1983); (j) Zhang *et al*, *J Exp Med* **176:**233 (1992); (k) Ishida *et al* *EMBO J* **1:**1117 (1986). From Ref. 10 (*J Exp Med*), with permission

peptide segment between the membrane and the nearest extracellular immunoglobulin domain. The number of residues in this proximal extracellular region is characteristic for each isotype and well conserved between species, ranging from a minimum of 14 in μ (counting from the end of the last CH domain to the conserved tryptophan with which the transmembrane segment begins) to 33 in the long form of human α1 and α2 heavy chains (a shorter 27 residue form of the human α isotypes is also produced by an alternative splice (15), and the latter form matches the length of the murine homolog).

In contrast to the 20 residue length of this region in murine ε, the corresponding human ε segment is 68 amino acids long and quite proline rich. The sequence similarity between the human and mouse regions upstream of the murine M1 exon (Figure 12.1) suggests that the longer M1' sequence in humans was derived from the conversion of intron to exon sequence as a consequence of mutations affecting splice acceptor sites. As a possible example of such a mechanism, the 9 bp deletion in the human sequence between nucleotide 177 and 178 (Figure 12.1) and the A at position 172 may combine to 'weaken' the splice acceptor activity of the AG dinucleotide at position 181–2, because these sequence differences with the murine gene bring another AG dinucleotide (positions 172–3) too close for the optimum sequence configuration of a splice acceptor site (16). As a result, the more upstream splice acceptor site at position 28 (Figure 12.1) would be used preferentially. Alternatively, it is possible that a long exon in the common ancestor of mouse and man was shortened in the mouse line by a converse mechanism.

Though the biological function of the unique human ε extracellular segment remains to be determined, it is tempting to speculate that such a longer extracellular domain may play an important role in the signal transduction through membrane IgE by binding to specific ligand(s). Potentially, such an antigenically unique extracellular structure could be targeted to manipulate IgE production and expression, by eliminating membrane IgE-bearing IgE-producing B cells, but not the B cells that passively acquired IgE through the low affinity receptor for IgE (CD23).

12.1.3 Splicing of CH4 to Two Different Splicing Acceptor Sites of the M2 Exon Codes for Two Secreted IgE Isoforms

Studies employing RT–PCR also defined two novel species of ε mRNA derived from alternative splicing to the M2 exon region. One species, designated CH4–M2', represents a novel ε RNA species that results from splicing of CH4 directly to the M2 exon. Such ε RNA, designated M2' exon, encodes 136 amino acids in contrast to the 27 residues of M2 (Figure 12.2b), as a result of a frame shift. The conserved hydrophobic transmembrane region encoded by M1' (or M1) is absent from this mRNA, which therefore encodes a secreted protein. This protein is 134 amino acids longer than the classic ε heavy chain and its molecular weight is expected to be about 20 kDa larger than a classic secreted ε heavy chain protein. Another species of ε

RNA, designated CH4–M2″, is generated by splicing of CH4 to a novel splicing acceptor site in the terminal portion of the M2′ exon. This CH4–M2″ RNA also has a one-nucleotide reading frame shift compared with the CH4–M2′ form (2). The new CH4–M2″ mRNA encodes a secreted protein, as it also lacks the transmembrane domain. It differs from the classic secreted ε protein in the eight terminal amino acids, and is only six amino acids larger, so that it would not be distinguishable by size. A cartoon model for these secreted IgE isoforms is presented in Figure 12.2b.

To investigate whether the IgE protein isoforms encoded by CH4–M2′ and CH4–M2″ RNA exist and are secreted in the serum, polyclonal and monoclonal antibodies were generated against the CH4–M2′ and CH4–M2″ isoforms. The anti-M2′ antiserum raised against the C-terminal last 10 amino acids of the M2′ exon was specifically reactive with the 97 kDa ε protein in Western blots. While multiple bands were detected by the anti-human IgE heavy chain-specific monoclonal antibody (mAb), only the 97 kDa species of ε specifically reacted with the anti-M2′ antiserum (17). Such larger species of ε protein were detected by the anti-M2′ antiserum also in the serum of allergic patients. These results were confirmed by using an enzyme-linked immunosorbent assay (ELISA) that specifically detects the CH4–M2′ IgE isoform. These results indicate that CH4–M2′ mRNA encodes an IgE isoform that is present in human serum.

For detection of the CH4–M2″-encoded IgE isoform, two mAbs against the last eight amino acids of the C-terminal sequence of M2″ were used. These two mAbs were shown to specifically react with a genetically engineered, eukaryotically expressed CH4–M2″ isoform, but not with an expressed classic secreted ε protein. The existence of a secreted CH4–M2″-encoded IgE isoform in the sera of allergic patients was demonstrated by Western blot and ELISA (unpublished data).

Both the novel CH4–M2′ and CH4–M2″ secreted IgE protein isoforms show some notable features distinct from those of classic secreted IgE. Whether these remarkable differences in structure result in differences in biological function remains to be determined. With an extra 134 amino acid domain at the C-terminus, the function of CH4-M2′ may be expected to differ from that of classic secreted IgE. Such a domain may interfere with FcεR binding by disturbing the interchain CH4–CH4 interactions that maintain the CH2–CH3–CH4 structure or by directly blocking the CH3 binding site for FcεRI or FcεRII. Even though the M2″ exon encodes a peptide with only eight amino acids, it contains a cysteine residue at its COOH-terminal end. The consequences of this cysteine are of interest since cysteine residues located at the COOH-terminal end of heavy chains are usually associated with the J chain that is involved in the formation of the dimers or polymers of IgM and IgA1 (18). If the terminal cysteine in the M2″ exon plays the same role for IgE as does the terminal cysteine in the IgM and IgA1 polymers, then dimers or polymers of the IgE isoform encoded by the CH4–M2″ splicing product may exist. If such IgE forms exist, they may be expected to differ biologically from the classic secreted IgE or the other monomeric IgE isoform so far described. With the expression of genetically engineered IgE isoforms representing all the secreted isoforms (21), definitive data about functional differences among them will be provided.

12.1.4 Three Novel ε RNA Transcripts That Define a New ε Exon: CH5

The determination of the alternative splicing products of the human ε gene also led to define a novel exon, named CH5, that contains 106 nucleotides and is located in the intron between the CH4 and M1′ exons. The ε RNA containing this exon is produced by using a novel splicing donor site inside the CH4 exon (referred to as CH4′) that splices to an acceptor site for CH5 by a mutually exclusive splicing mechanism. The CH4′–CH5 structure then splices to three different splicing acceptor sites for M1′, M2′ and M2″ to generate three species of ε mRNA: CH4′–CH5–M1′–M2, CH4′–CH5–M2′ and CH4′–CH5–M2″. However, these three mRNA species encode the same IgE protein isoform, 10 amino acids smaller than the classic secreted ε protein, because translation of all the three mRNA species stops at a termination codon (TAA) within CH5 (Figure 12.2b). Replacement of the COOH-terminal 37 amino acid residues of the CH4 sequence with the 27 amino acids encoded by CH5 creates a domain that has one cysteine residue in a position different from the highly conserved cysteine that forms the immunoglobulin interchain disulfide bond (2). The presence of such a domain with a cysteine in an altered position may well affect the immunoglobulin domain folding (see below). ε RNA containing the CH5 exon, as well as the species of ε mRNAs mentioned above

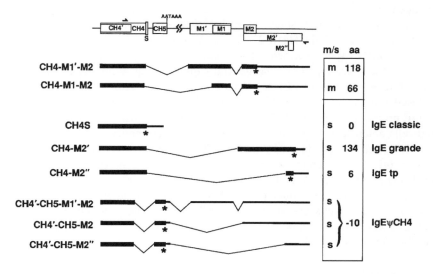

Figure 12.4. Diagrammatic summary of 3′-ends of various ε mRNA species generated by alternative splicing. A genomic DNA map of CH4 and the ε membrane exon region is shown at the top. All the sequence-conformed splice products are diagrammed, with their names to the left. Thick horizontal lines represent coding sequence; asterisks show the positions of in-frame termination codons. The table to the right indicates which RNA forms encoded membrane (m) or secreted (s) protein, and shows the number of amino acids by which the encoded proteins differ in size from the classic secreted ε protein (CH4S). Modified from Ref. 2 (*J Biol Chem*), with permission

(CH4–M2′ and CH4–M2″), were defined in all the IgE-secreting cell lines tested, in interleukin (IL)-4 plus anti-CD40 mAb-induced B cells, and in fresh B cells from hyper-IgE immunodeficiency syndrome patients (2), indicating that these alternative splicing pathways that generate secreted IgE isoform mRNA are common to all the IgE-producing B cells. The splicing- and alternative splicing-generated ε mRNA species are summarized in Figure 12.4.

12.2 EXPRESSION OF ε MRNA ISOFORMS IS DIFFERENTIALLY REGULATED AND DISEASE ASSOCIATED

12.2.1 The Pattern of ε mRNA Production in T-cell Dependent and T-cell 'Independent' IgE Synthesis

If the relative amounts of the different IgE isoform mRNA species could be altered, this would provide a mechanism for producing altered amounts of IgE isoforms under distinct biologic conditions. A reproducible relationship between the relative levels of ε mRNA species (splicing pattern) was first established using mRNA obtained from IL-4-stimulated peripheral blood mononuclear cells (PBMC), a T-cell dependent system. The mRNA for the ε variants could be detected in stimulated cells from all subjects. The most abundant mRNA species were the classic secreted (CH4-S) and the novel secreted CH4–M2″, followed closely by CH4–M2′. While the exact levels of ε mRNA species varied between individuals, the relative relationship of the levels (i.e. the splicing pattern) was generally quite similar. When IL-13 was used in place of IL-4, the pattern of ε mRNA variants was the same. The total ε mRNA produced was far less with IL-13-stimulated PBMC, which produced only 20% of the IgE protein induced by IL-4. This same pattern was detected in fresh unstimulated cells obtained from nasal lavage and in cell lines spontaneously secreting IgE (17). The ε mRNA produced by purified B cells under a variety of T-cell 'independent' IgE inducing conditions (e.g. using CD40, CD58 and hydrocortisone as the switch signal) revealed that under all these conditions the same ε mRNA pattern was observed, with the most abundant ε mRNA species being those for the classic secreted and the novel secreted IgE (CH4–M2″ form). Thus, the relative levels of ε mRNA observed with IL-4 or IL-13 (plus T cells) was taken as a 'normal' baseline state for ε isoform mRNA production (17).

12.2.2 The Production of ε mRNA Species is Differentially Regulated by Specific Stimuli

It was then determined whether specific stimuli which alter IgE production were also able to change the nature of the IgE produced (i.e. altering the relative amount of the ε mRNA species). B cells purified from non-atopic subjects were cultured with IL-4 and anti-CD40 mAb in the presence of specific stimuli, and changes in the production of total and specific ε mRNA variants were measured by quantitative RT–PCR. IL-10 increased the total amount of ε mRNA nearly 12-fold and showed a clear differential effect on the ε mRNA species. The production of the CH4–M2′ splice variant was preferentially increased, being 46 times more abundant in cultures with IL-10 than in cultures without it. The amounts of three other ε mRNA variants (CH4–M1′–M2, CH4–M2″ and CH4-S) increased by 10 to 12-fold. However, the CH4′–CH5 splice variant increased considerably less (two-fold). Accordingly, the ratio of CH4-S to CH4′–CH5 increased from 12:1 to 60:1 (Figure 12.5). Similarly, polyaromatic hydrocarbons extracted from diesel exhaust, compounds which enhance ongoing IgE production *in vitro*, led to a similar, but not identical, shift in IgE isoforms, with the most striking change being increased mRNA for CH4–M2′ and a far smaller increase in the levels of CH4–M2″ (19). In contrast, addition of IL-2, IL-13, or interferon (IFN)-γ did not alter the relative ratios of the ε mRNA variants. IL-6, while increasing total IgE and total ε mRNA, did not change the ε mRNA splicing pattern (Figure 12.5) (17). The ε mRNA splicing pattern could be modified by IL-10 after the pattern had already been established *in vitro* or in Epstein–Barr virus (EBV)-transformed, IgE-secreting cell lines (17).

It has been previously reported that the *in vitro* IgE response would be directly but only partially inhibited at the B cell level by specific antibodies directed against CD23/FcεRII (8). Extending this, we demonstrated that when purified B cells were stimulated with IL-4 plus anti-CD40 mAb in the presence of anti-CD23 mAb (25 μg/ml), ε mRNA decreased by over 60% and this was accompanied by a dramatic change in the ε mRNA pattern. There was a marked decrease in CH4–M2′ compared to all other variants such as to lead to the near obliteration of this mRNA in cells from some individuals. The finding that anti-CD23 mAb preferentially inhibits production of specific ε mRNA species demonstrates that production of ε mRNA can be differentially downregulated, and is consistent with the earlier observation that anti-CD23 mAb never fully inhibited IgE production (8).

12.2.3 A Distinct Pattern of ε mRNA Species is Observed *In Vivo* in Conditions with Altered IgE Production

To pursue *in vivo* the concept that ε RNA splicing was developmentally regulated, two approaches were used. First, because patients with high levels of IgE due to allergic or parasitic disease often have circulating B cells that spontaneously produce IgE, such cells were used to determine the pattern of ε mRNA produced *in vivo* in those conditions. These patients showed a pattern of ε mRNA analogous to the IL-10-driven pattern, as compared to the 'normal' IL-4 plus anti-CD40 mAb-driven pattern. CH4–M2′ mRNA was markedly increased, and CH4′–CH5 mRNA was barely discernible in the B cells from highly allergic patients, and often completely absent in the parasite-infected patients. This distinct ε mRNA pattern was unaltered when B cells from highly allergic patients were isolated and cultured with IL-4 plus anti-CD40 mAb for 14 days (i.e. the increased prominence of CH4–M2′ mRNA

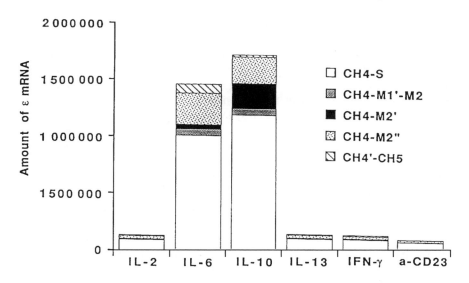

	IL-2	IL-6	IL-10	IL-13	IFN-γ	a-CD23
CH4'-CH5	5.2%	5.5%	1.2%	4.8%	4.5%	4.9%
CH4-M2"	16.5%	18.7%	13.4%	16.4%	16.8%	18.2%
CH4-M2'	3.4%	2.8%	12.9%	3.0%	4.0%	1.2%
CH4-M1'-M2	2.8%	3.9%	3.1%	3.6%	2.9%	3.8%
CH4-S	72.1%	69.1%	69.4%	72.2%	71.8%	71.9%

Figure 12.5. Effect of the post-switch signals on ε mRNA variant production. In the upper stack bar graph, the amount of each of the ε mRNA variants produced by B cells from non-atopic subjects under different conditions are shown. The cells were stimulated with IL-4 (100 U/ml) and anti-CD40 mAb (0.1 μg/ml) and cocultured with either IL-10 (500 U/ml), IL-6 (500 U/ml), IL-2 (500 U/ml), IFN-γ (500 U/ml) or anti-CD23 (25 μg/ml) for 14 days. The quantity of each variant was standardized for β-actin and the mean of experiments on seven subjects is shown as a stack diagram for each condition. The amount of ε mRNA was measured in densitometric units. In tabular form below the graph are the percentages of the total ε mRNA for each variant, for each experimental group. Addition of IL-6 and IL-10 increased the amount of total ε mRNA, while addition of CD23 mAb decreased total ε mRNA. However, as shown, only IL-10 and CD23 mAb altered the relative amounts of the variants produced. From Ref. 17 (*J Immunol*), with permission

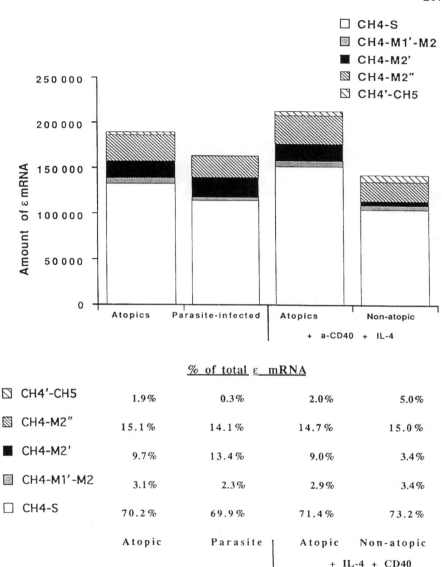

Figure 12.6. Different disease states produce different relative and absolute amounts of ε mRNA variants. In the upper graph, the amounts of the ε mRNA variants produced under different conditions are shown. The ε mRNA levels spontaneously produced by cells from subjects with high levels of serum IgE caused by severe atopy or parasitic infection are compared to those seen when B cells from the same severe atopic subjects or from non-atopic subjects were cultured for 14 days with IL-4 (100 U/ml) and anti-CD40 mAb (0.1 μg/ml). The stack bar graph demonstrates the mean amount of each variant (standardized for β-actin) from experiments with seven atopic, seven non-atopic and five parasite-infected subjects. The amount of ε mRNA was measured in densitometric units. In tabular form below the graph are the percentages of the total ε mRNA for each variant, for each experimental group. From Ref. 17 (*J Immunol*), with permission

persisted (Figure 12.6)). The ε mRNA patterns in B cells from a subset of patients with common variable immunodeficiency, who have primarily immature B cells in their circulation, were also examined (22). These patients make little immunoglobulins *in vivo* and though they make IgE in response to IL-4 plus anti-CD40 mAb stimulation, the amount of IgE is much less than normal. As predicted, the patients' cells did not make the 'normal' pattern of ε mRNA when stimulated by IL-4 plus anti-CD40 mAb. When IL-10 was added, the characteristic increase in CH4–M2′ mRNA was not observed, either (22 and data not shown).

The second approach was to determine the *in vivo* pattern of ε mRNA species expressed following *in vivo* nasal challenge. Challenges were performed with diesel exhaust particles (DEP), ragweed antigen or a combination of the two. Cells recovered from nasal lavage were assessed. DEP challenge resulted in a ≈ five-fold increase in lavage IgE protein, no increase in ragweed-specific IgE and a change in the relative levels of the ε mRNA species, with a minimal increase in CH4′–CH5 mRNA and a ≈ 20–30-fold increase in the other ε mRNA variants (20). Ragweed-challenge resulted in a similar pattern and a ≈ five-fold increase in ragweed-specific IgE. Notably, DEP plus ragweed challenge gave a ≈ 50-fold increase in ε mRNA for the secreted isoforms except for CH4′–CH5, which became even less abundant, while there was a ≈ 50-fold increase in ragweed-specific IgE.

The use of splice sites for human ε mRNA species is tightly regulated since the potential number of splice products far exceeds that which is actually produced (2). The studies also show that use of the ε alternative splices is regulated by a limited number of stimuli and the pattern of ε mRNA variant production follows a developmental, disease-related profile. While having found disease-related changes in the pattern of ε mRNA variants encoding distinct IgE isoforms, an analysis of the biologic activity of recombinant proteins and a measurement of their levels in disease conditions will be required to directly answer questions as to the biological relevance of the changes observed in ε mRNA splicing.

12.3 EXPRESSION OF THE NOVEL HUMAN SECRETED IgE ISOFORMS AS GENETICALLY ENGINEERED PROTEINS

As mentioned earlier, using polyclonal and monoclonal anti-peptide antibodies to M2′ and M2″ the protein products representing these novel IgE isoforms were detected in the supernatant and cytoplasm of IgE-secreting cell lines, in the serum from a patient with IgE myeloma, in the serum of some patients with very elevated IgE levels and in nasal secretions following *in vivo* challenges. However, the low levels of IgE present even in the serum of patients with markedly increased levels of IgE, and the similar molecular size of several isoforms argued against any attempt to purify the isoforms. Therefore, expression vectors were developed to produce genetically engineered secreted ε isoforms (Figure 12.7). The four human IgE isoforms predicted to be secreted proteins were expressed as human anti-dansyl antibodies in the murine myeloma cell line Sp2/0 (21). The IgE isoforms expressed are 'classic' (CH4-S), 'grandé' (CH4–M2′), 'tailpiece' (IgEtp protein) (CH4–M2″) and 'chimeric' (IgEψCH4 protein) (CH4′–CH5) (Figure 12.7). The expression vectors were transfected into an Sp2/0-derived cell line previously transfected with a chimeric light chain containing a murine anti-dansyl V_L domain and a human C_k domain.

Transfectomas expressing three of the isoforms (IgE classic, IgE grandé and IgEtp) produced a protein of 180–190 kDa which was reduced upon treatment with 2-mercaptoethanol to a heavy chain of ≈ 75 kDa and a light chain of ≈ 25 kDa, indicating that these isoforms were secreted as fully assembled H2L2 molecules. As expected, IgE classic and IgEtp migrated with identical mobility, while IgE grandé migrated more slowly (Figure 12.7). Transfectomas expressing chimeric IgE (IgEψCH4) secreted HL monomers which migrated as a broad 75–90 kDa band under non-reducing conditions (Figure 12.7). The diffuse migration of IgEψCH4 was due to heterogeneous glycosylation, as it was no longer evident when cells were cultured in the presence of tunicamycin. The incomplete assembly of IgEψCH4 is not entirely unexpected, given that H2 pairing is initially stabilized by non-covalent interactions between the heavy chain C-terminal domains. As discussed earlier, the C-terminal portion of Cε4 is replaced by sequences from CH5 in IgEψCH4. Among the residues replaced is a cysteine which is universally conserved in immunoglobulin domains, making it likely that the normal immunoglobulin domain structure is not present in the IgEψCH4 terminal domain (21).

Individual members of the human secreted IgE family are likely to differ in their ability to mediate IgE functions. While the contact residues for FcεRI and FcεRII are present in all the secreted IgE isoforms, the full CH4 domain is critical in constraining the three-dimensional 'donut' shape of the paired CH3–CH4 IgE regions that provide for the FcR binding ability of IgE. In this regard IgEψCH4 deserves special attention, because this isoform corresponds to secreted HL 'half molecules'. If IgEψCH4 binds to FcεRI as a half molecule, it would be at a marked disadvantage in cross-link receptors and may therefore be less able to arm mast cells and basophils for antigen-triggered release. Indeed, it may even function to inhibit such release.

12.4 CONCLUSIONS

In this chapter we have discussed the discovery that novel alternative splicing of the 3′ end of ε RNA generates a family of six isoforms of human IgE protein. This appears to result from an inability of humans to use the M1 splice acceptor. Alternatively spliced ε mRNA species encode four secreted human IgE isoforms. Of these, CH4-S encodes the prototype secreted IgE (IgE classic), the only secreted IgE found in rats and mice. The human CH4–M2′ mRNA encodes a secreted IgE isoform (IgE grandé) 134 amino acids larger than classic secreted IgE. The CH4–M2″ mRNA encodes a secreted IgE isoform (IgE tailpiece) six amino acids larger than classic secreted IgE, and containing a C-terminal cysteine. The ε mRNA splice from inside CH4 to the cryptic CH5 exon is unique among immunoglobulins and encodes

(a)

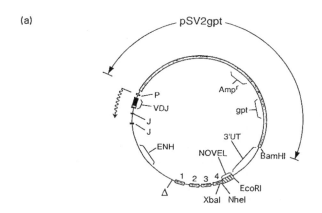

(b)

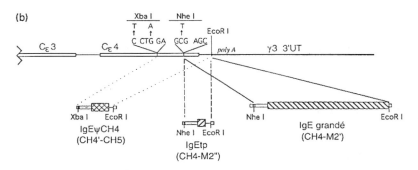

(c)

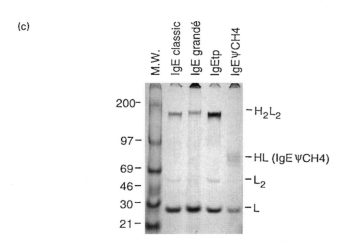

a single secreted IgE isoform (IgE chimeric, ψCH4) 10 amino acids smaller than classic secreted IgE. Expression of the full range of ε mRNA species is common to all the human IgE-producing cells examined. Compared to the 'normal' pattern, the ε RNA variants for secreted IgE are expressed in different relative amounts in allergic patients, in patients with parasitic infection, and in immunodeficient patients. Importantly, *in vivo* challenges with DEP and ragweed antigen also shift the ε RNA splicing pattern. Similarly, the relative amounts of ε mRNA species were shown to be differentially regulated *in vitro* by IL-10, CD23 ligation and polyaromatic hydrocarbons derived from DEP.

Together with classic IgE, two of the three novel secreted IgE isoforms (IgE grandé and tailpiece) have been shown to be present in humans. Measurement of the absolute and relative amounts of IgE isoforms *in vivo* under different disease and treatment conditions will require the establishment of assays. All four secreted IgE isoforms (classic, grandé, tailpiece and chimeric) have recently been expressed, and functional assessment of these expressed IgE isoforms is now possible. It is likely that differential expression of the structurally heterogeneous IgE isoforms will be directly linked to functional heterogeneity and human immediate hypersensitivity disease expression.

Figure 12.7. The expression of novel secreted IgE isoforms. (a) A diagram of the pSV2gpt expression vector for IgE grandé, highlighting relevant features. The immunoglobulin is encoded by an anti-dansyl variable domain exon (VDJ), ε constant domain exons (1,2,3,4) and sequence encoding the novel carboxy terminus (NOVEL). Two orphan J segments are also present (J). Expression is driven by an immunoglobulin heavy chain promoter/leader sequence (P) and an immunoglobulin heavy chain enhancer element (ENH). The wavy arrow indicates the direction of transcription. 3′UT indicates the human γ3 untranslated region. Amp^r and gpt indicate the β-lactamase and xanthine–guanine phosphoribosyltransferase genes used for selection in prokaryotic and eukaryotic cells, respectively. The *Xba*I, *Nhe*I and *Eco*RI sites introduced by PCR mutagenesis are shown. Also shown is the *Bam*HI site used to subclone the different constructs into expressions vectors. The *Sal*I and *Xho*I sites used to subclone into expression vectors were destroyed in the ligation and are indicated by a Δ. (b) Strategy used to generate isoform-specific IgE constructs. The top portion of the figure depicts the third and fourth constant domain exons of the genomic human ε gene and a 3′ untranslated region, γ3 3′UT (not drawn to scale), from the human γ3 immunoglobulin heavy chain locus. The mutations used to generate the *Xba*I and *Nhe*I sites in Cε4 are shown above the Cε4 exon. The *Xba*I and *Nhe*I sites in the three RT–PCR clones (at the bottom of the figure) were introduced with the same mutations. None of the mutations introduced amino acid substitutions. The three RT–PCR clones were then fused to the genomic exons at the *Xba*I and *Eco*RI sites, or at the *Nhe*I and *Eco*RI sites. (c) Immunoprecipitation of ^{35}S-methionine labeled IgE isoforms. Cell lines producing IgE classic, IgE grandé, IgEtp or IgEψCH4 were labeled for 6–18 hours with ^{35}S-methionine, and IgE was precipitated from the secretions using rabbit anti-human Fab followed by *Staphylococcus aureus*. Samples were loaded on a 5% gel under denaturing, non-reducing conditions. IgE classic, IgE grandé and IgEtp are secreted as species of 190 kDa. IgEψCH4 is secreted primarily as a HL form which migrates at 75–90 kDa, and free light chain of 25 kDa. Adapted from Ref. 21

ACKNOWLEDGMENTS

Much of this work has been performed with our colleagues and collaborators, Dr David Diaz-Sanchez, Dr Sherie Morrison, and Dr Jeff Lyzcak of UCLA, and Dr Ed E. Max of CBER, FDA. We also want to acknowledge the excellent technical assistance of Hai-Kit Cheah. This work was supported by USPHS grants AI-15251, CA12800 and the UCLA Asthma, Allergy and Immunologic Disease Center (AI-34567 funded by the NIAID and the NIEHS).

REFERENCES

1. Ishizaka K, Ishizaka T and Hornbrook MM (1966) Physiochemical properties of human reagenic antibody. Presence of a unique immunoglobulin as carrier of reagenic activity. *J Immunol* **97**:75–87.
2. Zhang K, Max EE, Cheah HK and Saxon A (1994) Complex alternative RNA splicing of ε immunoglobulin transcripts produces mRNAs encoding four potential secreted protein isoforms. *J Biol Chem* **269**:456–462.
3. MacDonald SM, Langdon JM, Greenlee BM and Kagey-Sobotka A (1991) IgE-dependent histamine-releasing factors. *Int Arch Allergy Appl Immunol* **94**:144–147.
4. MacDonald SM, Rafnar T, Langdon J and Lichtenstein LM (1995) Molecular identification of an IgE-dependent histamine-releasing factor. *Science* **269**:688–690.
5. Hsu DK, Zuber RI and Liu FT (1992) Biochemical and biophysical characterization of human recombinant IgE-binding protein, an S-type animal lectin. *J Biol Chem* **267**:14167–14174.
6. Frigeri LG and Liu FT (1992) Surface expression of functional IgE binding protein, an endogenous lectin, on mast cells and macrophages. *J Immunol* **148**:861–867.
7. Max EE, Battey R, Ney R, Kirsch I and Leder P (1982) Duplication and deletion in the human immunoglobulin E genes. *Cell* **29**:691–699.
8. Saxon A, Behle K, Kurbe-Leamer M, Max EE and Zhang K (1991) Inhibition of human IgE production via FcεRII stimulation results from a decrease in the mRNA for secreted but not membrane ε heavy chains. *J Immunol* **147**:4000–4007.
9. Peng C, Davis FM, Sun LK, Liou RS, Kim Y and Chang TW (1992) A new isoform of human membrane-bound IgE. *J Immunol* **148**:129–136.
10. Zhang K, Saxon A and Max EE (1992) Two unusual forms of human immunoglobulin E encoded by alternative RNA splicing of ε heavy chain membrane exons. *J Exp Med* **176**:233–243.
11. Hellman L (1993) Characterization of four novel ε chain mRNA and a comparative analysis of genes for immunoglobulin E in rodents and man. *Eur J Immunol* **23**:159–167.
12. Early P, Rogers J, Davis M *et al* (1980) Two mRNA's can be produced from a single immunoglobulin μ gene by alternative RNA processing pathways. *Cell* **20**:313–319.
13. Boyd D and Beckwith J (1980) The role of charged amino acids in the localization of secreted and membrane proteins. *Cell* **62**:1031–1033.
14. Mitchell RN, Shaw AC, Weaver YK, Leder P and Abbas AK (1991) Cytoplasmic tail deletion converts membrane immunoglobulin to a phosphatidylinositol-linked form lacking signaling and efficient antigen internalization functions. *J Biol Chem* **266**:8856–8860.
15. Yu L, Peng C, Starnes SM, Liou RS and Chang TW (1990) Two isoforms of human membrane-bound α immunoglobulin resulting from alternative mRNA splicing in the membrane segment. *J Immunol* **145**:3932–3936.

16. Self I, Khoury G and Dhar R (1979) BKV splice sequences based on analysis of preferred donor and acceptor sites. *Nucleic Acids Res* **6**:3387–3398.
17. Diaz-Sanchez D, Zhang K, Nutman TB and Saxon A (1995) Differential regulation of alternative 3' splicing of ε messenger RNA variants. *J Immunol* **155**:1930–1941.
18. Hasemann CA and Capra JD (1989) Immunoglobulins: structure and function. In: Paul WE (Ed.) *Fundamental Immunology*, pp. 209–233. Raven Press, New York.
19. Takenaka H, Zhang K, Diaz-Sanchez D, Tsien A and Saxon A (1994) Enhanced human IgE results from exposure to the aromatic hydrocarbons in diesel exhaust: direct effects on B cells IgE production. *J Allergy Clin Immunol* **95**:103–109.
20. Diaz-Sanchez D, Dotson AR, Takenaka H and Saxon A (1994) Diesel exhaust particles induce local IgE production *in vivo* and alter the pattern of IgE messenger RNA isoform. *J Clin Invest* **94**:1417–1427.
21. Lyczak JB, Zhang K, Saxon A and Morrison SL (1996) Expression of novel secreted isoforms of human immunoglobulin E proteins. *J Biol Chem* **271**:3428–3346.
22. Saxon A, Keld B, Diaz-Sanchez D, Guo B-C and Sidell N (1995) B cells from a distinct subset of patients with common variable immunodeficiency have increased CD95 (Apo-1/fas) and diminished CD38 expression and undergo enhanced apoptosis: rescue by CD40 and IL-4. *Clin Exp Immunol* **102**:17–25.
23. Ishida Y, Ueda S, Hayashida H, Miyata T and Honjo T (1982) The nucleotide sequence of the mouse immunoglobulin epsilon gene: comparison with the human epsilon gene sequence. *EMBO J* **1**:1117–1123.

13 Antibody Recognition of Recombinant Allergens and Allergen Fragments: Evidence for a Predominantly Direct Class Switch to IgE in Allergic Patients

RUDOLF VALENTA and TANJA BALL

Institute of General and Experimental Pathology, University of Vienna, Vienna, Austria

13.1 INTRODUCTION

Production of IgE antibodies against water-soluble low molecular weight protein antigens represents the hallmark of atopic diseases. Although IgE antibodies are produced in extremely low concentrations, they are able to cause a cascade of allergic symptoms (allergic rhinoconjunctivitis, asthma, up to anaphylactic shock) by activating effector cells (mast cells, basophils) via binding to Fcε receptors. The cross-linking of effector cell-bound IgE by allergens then leads to cell activation and release of biologic mediators (e.g. histamine, leukotrienes). Formation of IgE antibodies with specificity and high affinity for certain allergens is thought to require at least two steps that affect the constant and variable immunoglobulin regions: immunoglobulin class switch from IgM precursors to IgE-producing B cells, and affinity maturation by somatic mutation (1–5). It is well established that IgE production is regulated by cytokines (interleukin (IL)-4, IL-13) which switch IgM-expressing antigen-specific B lymphocytes to IgE production (6–8); however, controversial information is available regarding the exact mechanisms of class switch leading to the production of allergen-specific IgE antibodies in allergic patients (9, 10).

The question whether switch to IgE production occurs directly from IgM to IgE (i.e. direct class switching) or proceeds from IgM via certain IgG subclasses to IgE (i.e. sequential class switching) has been addressed in murine models as well as using cultured human B lymphocytes. While on the one hand it was demonstrated in mice that B cells stimulated with lipopolysaccharide (LPS) and IL-4 preferentially switch from IgM via IgG1 to IgE production (11, 12), it was also shown that in mutant mice, in which sequential switching to IgE via IgG1 was blocked, the

IgE Regulation: Molecular Mechanisms. Edited by D. Vercelli. © 1997 John Wiley & Sons Ltd.

frequency of cells switching to IgE was not affected (13). Polymerase chain reaction (PCR)-amplified switch circles isolated from cultured human B cells which were stimulated by IL-4 provided evidence for direct μ to ε, as well as sequential μ–γ–ε switching (14–17). Moreover, the analysis of Sμ/Sε switch regions from freshly isolated B lymphocytes from atopic patients argued for a predominantly direct IgM to IgE class switch program (18) (see also Chapters 8 and 11).

The above described experimental models investigated class switch mechanisms in B cells without known specificity for certain allergens and, therefore, make it difficult to judge whether sequential or non-sequential class switch is predominantly responsible for the production of specific IgE antibodies in allergic patients. It has recently become possible to use defined (i.e. recombinant) allergens to analyze the humoral and cellular immune response of atopic patients (19). The aim of the present contribution was the analysis of data obtained by measuring the recognition of defined (i.e. recombinant) allergens and allergen fragments (epitopes) by IgE and IgG antibodies from atopic patients, non-allergic individuals as well as from allergic patients after hyposensitization therapy. Furthermore, we discuss results obtained by inducing IgE responses in mice (20) and rhesus monkeys (21) through injection of recombinant allergens with Al(OH)$_3$ as adjuvant, in the context of class switch mechanisms.

13.2 IgE AND IgG RECOGNITION OF RECOMBINANT PLANT ALLERGENS

Due to the availability of recombinant allergens it has become possible to measure IgE and IgG subclass responses against defined components. An analysis of 51 sera from birch pollen allergic patients and 10 sera from non-allergic control individuals in a skin prick test study evaluating the biological activity of the major birch pollen allergen Bet v 1 (22) (Table 13.1) showed that:

(1) Allergic patients displayed different IgE and IgG subclass reactivity against the major birch pollen allergen Bet v 1. Sera were identified with undetectable or low levels of Bet v 1-specific IgE (Table 13.1: sera # 2, 17, 18, 23, 37, 39, 42, 44, and 50) but containing significant titers of Bet v 1-specific IgG1, IgG2, IgG3 and IgG4 antibodies;
(2) The levels of Bet v 1-specific IgE were not associated with the titers of certain IgG subclasses and frequently no Bet v 1-specific antibodies could be detected in certain subclasses;
(3) Non-allergic individuals failed to produce Bet v 1-specific IgE but frequently showed significant IgG subclass reactivity against Bet v 1 (Table 13.1: sera # 52, 55 and 56).

Similar results were obtained by serological testing of sera from grass-pollen allergic individuals for reactivity with recombinant timothy grass pollen allergens (23, 24) and in another skin test study performed with recombinant Bet v 1 and Bet v

2 (25). Again, no association of IgE and IgG subclass reactivities to recombinant birch pollen and timothy grass pollen allergens (Table 13.2) was found. The results obtained with recombinant plant allergens were confirmed by a study performed with recombinant Der p 2, a major mite allergen (26). Also in this study, the titers of IgE, IgG4 and other IgG subclasses against Der p 2 differed markedly. In summary, the serological measurements of specific IgE and IgG subclass reactivities to defined recombinant allergens indicate that IgE and IgG subclass responses in allergic patients are not synchronized and it appears that a considerable proportion of allergen-specific IgG antibodies bind either to different epitopes, or with considerably lower affinity, as compared with IgE antibodies.

13.3 IgE AND IgG RECOGNITION OF ALLERGEN EPITOPES

Recently, cell lines were established from a birch-pollen allergic patient who underwent hyposensitization therapy and secreted IgG antibodies with specificity for the major birch pollen allergen, Bet v 1 (27). One of the human monoclonal antibodies, BAB 1, was able to inhibit binding of allergic patient's IgE to Bet v 1, some antibodies (BAB4 and BAB5) did not significantly inhibit IgE binding and another antibody, BAB2, remarkably enhanced IgE binding, most probably by causing a conformational change of the allergen. These results indicated that sera from allergic patients contain IgG antibodies which bind to the same as well as to different epitopes as do IgE antibodies. Similar results were obtained by epitope mapping studies performed by gene fragmentation to reveal the antibody binding sites of plant and mite allergens. In a study performed with recombinant fragments of the major mite allergen Der p 2, the authors found that there were significant differences in epitope recognition between IgE and IgG4 antibodies and that IgE antibodies recognized restricted parts of the Der p 2 allergen compared with IgG4 (28). Our own studies analyzing the antibody binding sites of the major timothy grass pollen allergens Phl p 1 (29, T Ball et al, unpublished data) and Phl p 2 (R Valenta et al, unpublished data) as well as birch profilin, Bet v 2 (30), revealed that:

(1) IgE and IgG4 antibodies of allergic patients bind to the same and different epitopes;
(2) Sera from allergic patients who were not treated by hyposensitization produced rather low levels of IgG4 antibodies against IgE epitopes;
(3) Hyposensitization treatment can induce significant levels of IgG4 antibodies against IgE epitopes;
(4) Both IgE and IgG4 antibodies bind to the recombinant allergen fragments under conditions of high stringency (i.e. high concentrations of Tween 20 (0.5%)), and therefore appear to have high and comparable affinities.

Figure 13.1 shows an example of the recognition of recombinant Phl p 1 fragments by IgE and IgG4 antibodies from two grass-pollen allergic patients. As

Table 13.1. Comparison of serological and skin testing results obtained in a group of birch pollen allergic patients (sera 1–51) and non-allergic control individuals (sera 52–59). Total IgE levels, birch-pollen specific RAST, Bet v 1-specific IgE and IgG, skin prick (SPT) and intradermal tests (IDT) with birch pollen extract (ALK) or recombinant Bet v 1 (rBet v 1) are shown.

Patient	Total IgE (kU/L)	RAST birch (kU/L)	SPT ALK	SPT rBet v I	IDT ALK	IDT rBet v I	ELISA rBet v I IgE	Immunoblot rBet v I IgE	Immunoblot rBet v II IgE	ELISA rBet v I IgG1	ELISA rBet v I IgG2	ELISA rBet v I IgG3	ELISA rBet v I IgG4
1	58.7	6.65	+	+	+	+	0.12	+	–	0.19	0.23	0.00	0.35
2	149	4.05	+	+	+	+	0.04	+	+	0.92	0.31	0.00	0.21
3	230	26.5	+	+	+	+	0.92	+	–	1.24	0.50	0.00	0.75
4	29.1	6.41	+	+	+	+	0.10	+	–	0.84	0.60	0.36	0.60
5	263	60.9	+	+	+	+	1.66	+	–	0.50	0.22	0.00	0.70
6	125	29.4	+	+	+	+	0.74	+	–	1.10	1.40	0.14	0.92
7	289	17.4	+	+	+	+	0.43	+	–	1.42	1.18	0.81	2.50
8	325	100	+	+	+	+	2.06	+	–	1.64	1.17	0.03	1.50
9	192	14.5	+	+	+	ND	0.17	+	–	0.57	0.13	2.18	0.24
10	36	6.16	+	+	+	–	0.07	+	–	1.19	0.77	0.00	0.02
11	689	14.5	+	–	+	+	0.49	+	–	0.72	0.42	0.01	1.06
12	842	36	+	+	+	+	0.27	+	+	0.86	0.12	0.02	0.12
13	186	26.8	+	+	+	+	0.16	+	–	0.53	0.26	0.08	1.61
14	359	83.4	+	+	+	+	1.86	+	–	1.52	1.77	0.07	2.50
15	87.2	14.9	+	+	+	+	0.14	+	–	0.47	0.10	0.00	0.36
16	1251	85.4	+	+	+	+	2.05	+	+	0.32	0.77	0.08	0.56
17	118	5.07	+	+	+	+	0.05	+	–	0.86	0.17	0.04	0.28
18	199	4.16	+	+	+	+	0.05	+	–	0.09	0.25	1.03	0.43
19	115	13	+	+	+	+	0.18	+	–	1.47	2.50	0.80	2.50
20	127	33.5	+	+	+	ND	0.46	+	–	1.15	1.71	0.40	2.50
21	556	73.2	+	+	+	+	2.27	+	–	1.23	0.44	0.00	1.26
22	475	100	+	+	+	+	2.50	+	–	1.39	0.70	0.00	2.16
23	1958	12.8	+	+	+	ND	0	–	+	0.03	0.31	0.00	0.01
24	1083	38.4	+	+	+	+	1.12	+	+	0.98	0.37	0.00	1.73
25	1500	100	+	+	+	ND	1.51	+	+	1.60	2.50	0.40	2.50

#													
26	987	37.2	+	+	+	+	0.45	+	−	0.20	0.02	0.25	0.00
27	197	25.8	+	+	+	+	0.42	+	+	0.58	0.14	0.08	0.10
28	193	4.95	+	+	+	+	0.09	+	−	1.28	0.13	0.00	0.10
29	275	6.61	+	+	+	+	0.06	+	−	0.61	0.13	0.00	0.29
30	91.3	6.64	+	+	+	+	0.09	+	−	0.08	0.34	0.00	0.47
31	88	7.3	+	+	+	+	0.15	+	−	0.36	0.29	0.00	0.86
32	646	8.55	+	+	+	ND	0.07	+	−	0.77	0.81	0.24	0.68
33	1037	53.6	+	+	+	+	1.65	+	+	0.98	0.58	0.00	1.67
34	14.5	3.5	+	−	+	+	0.03	+	−	0.12	0.11	0.00	0.01
35	181	35.5	+	+	+	ND	0.72	+	−	1.61	2.50	0.18	2.50
36	468	41.3	+	+	+	+	0.86	+	−	1.18	0.58	0.37	0.98
37	83.8	4.71	+	+	+	+	0.03	+	−	0.62	0.45	0.11	0.35
38	286	82.5	+	+	+	ND	1.54	+	−	0.94	1.02	0.06	1.75
39	33.4	3.6	+	+	+	ND	0.02	+	−	0.41	0.04	0.02	0.62
40	332	59.1	+	+	+	+	1.99	+	−	1.31	1.56	1.45	1.33
41	108	10.5	+	+	+	+	0.10	+	−	0.50	0.23	0.15	1.09
42	385	3.6	+	+	+	+	0.03	+	−	0.91	0.59	1.69	1.54
43	393	28.6	+	+	+	+	0.84	+	−	1.15	1.26	1.55	1.08
44	186	7.53	+	+	+	ND	0.05	+	−	0.32	0.36	0.11	2.02
45	337	47.7	+	+	+	+	0.57	+	−	0.71	0.23	0.20	0.52
46	291	51.1	+	+	+	+	1.31	+	+	0.42	0.08	0.00	0.88
47	332	100	+	+	+	+	2.41	+	−	0.90	0.84	0.50	2.50
48	1320	100	+	+	+	+	2.41	+	−	0.82	1.37	0.40	1.95
49	442	41.3	+	+	+	+	0.93	+	−	1.10	0.55	0.06	1.84
50	663	19.8	−	−	−	−	0	−	+	0.30	0.02	0.05	0.01
51	314	25.1	+	+	−	+	0.56	+	+	0.87	0.36	0.09	1.03
52	33.4	<0.35	−	−	−	−	0	−	−	0.04	0.33	0.00	0.00
53	2	<0.35	−	−	−	−	0	−	−	0.05	0.02	0.12	0.00
54	41.7	<0.35	−	−	−	−	0	−	−	0.01	0.01	0.00	0.00
55	33.4	<0.35	−	−	−	−	0	−	−	0.00	0.39	0.01	0.00
56	50.2	<0.35	−	−	−	−	0	−	−	0.00	0.03	0.39	0.04
57	18.5	<0.35	−	−	−	−	0	−	−	0.00	0.00	0.00	0.00
58	2	<0.35	−	−	−	−	0	−	−	0.00	0.00	0.02	0.00
59	59.5	<0.35	−	−	−	−	0	−	−	0.00	0.00	0.03	0.04

Table 13.2. IgE and IgG subclass responses of grass-pollen allergic patients to natural (E) and recombinant timothy grass pollen allergens (I: Phl p 1; II: Phl p 2; V: Phl p 5) determined by enzyme-linked immunosorbent assay. Extinctions over baselines determined with a group of non-allergic individuals are shown.

#	1	2	3	4	5	6	7	8	9	10	11	12	13	
E	0.16	2.26	0.18	0.40	0.44	0.05	0.36	0.34	0.88	0.22	0.78	0.16	0.24	
I	0.10	0.52	0.11	0.10	0.29	0.05	0.29	0.13	0.47	0.13	0.16	0.09	0.10	IgE
II	0.08	0.19	0.09	0.05	0.05	0.04	0.12	0.10	0.13	0.06	0.12	0.05	0.07	
V	0.17	1.54	0.14	0.43	0.34	0.05	0.06	0.32	1.33	0.18	0.99	0.16	0.24	
E	0.15	0.60	0.50	0.28	0.20	0.09	0.16	0.73	0.20	0.13	0.47	0.26	0.25	
I	0.08	0.28	0.27	0.11	0.10	0.10	0.12	0.58	0.18	0.11	0.10	0.16	0.20	IgG$_1$
II	1.09	0.25	0.31	0.09	0.07	0.12	0.38	0.38	0.10	0.15	0.08	0.19	0.13	
V	0.10	0.45	0.48	0.30	0.09	0.10	0.10	0.81	0.65	0.16	0.14	0.25	0.19	
E	0.23	0.63	1.19	0.51	0.34	0.14	0.20	1.77	0.50	0.21	1.18	0.28	0.14	
I	0.23	0.50	0.64	1.13	0.61	0.94	0.64	0.55	1.04	0.24	1.32	1.16	0.36	IgG$_2$
II	1.01	0.19	0.48	0.47	0.29	0.34	0.24	0.58	0.71	0.44	0.54	0.54	0.46	
V	0.14	0.20	0.66	0.25	0.21	0.12	0.14	1.25	0.83	0.18	0.37	0.47	0.13	
E	0.11	0.28	0.12	0.08	0.13	0.15	0.12	0.35	0.13	0.08	2.04	0.07	0.09	
I	0.06	0.05	0.05	0.05	0.06	0.13	0.09	0.08	0.09	0.05	0.08	0.05	0.07	IgG$_3$
II	0.09	0.05	0.06	0.06	0.11	0.06	0.04	0.05	0.70	0.37	0.11	0.05	0.05	
V	0.26	0.07	0.05	0.05	0.06	0.11	0.05	0.09	0.08	0.28	0.07	0.58	0.05	
E	0.27	1.95	> 2.5	2.15	0.22	0.06	0.28	> 2.5	0.29	0.75	0.42	0.13	0.14	
I	0.08	0.40	2.31	0.36	0.21	0.06	0.18	2.05	0.16	0.35	0.27	0.08	0.10	IgG$_4$
II	0.20	0.50	> 2.5	0.19	0.07	0.07	0.12	> 2.5	0.17	0.27	0.14	0.06	0.07	
V	0.14	0.58	> 2.5	1.10	0.20	0.05	0.06	> 2.5	0.33	0.54	0.48	0.10	0.15	

summarized above, IgE and IgG4 antibodies bound to the same, as well as to different epitopes.

Although it has to be stated that the mentioned epitope mapping studies were performed with relatively large allergen fragments (15 amino acid polypeptides—10 kDa fragments), and it is therefore possible that the described allergen fragments contained more than one antibody binding site, the data suggest significant differences in the IgE and IgG4 recognition of allergens.

13.4 ONSET OF IgE AND IgG RESPONSES IN MURINE AND PRIMATE MODELS OF TYPE I ALLERGY

Using recombinant birch pollen allergens and $Al(OH)_3$ as adjuvant, IgE responses were induced in mice and rhesus monkeys (20, 21). It could be shown that recombinant Bet v 1 induced IgE antibodies which cross-reacted with Bet v 1-homologous allergens from other tree pollen and plant food. Furthermore, different allergenicity was noted for a major allergen, Bet v 1, and a less frequently recognized allergen, Bet v 2, in mice as well as rhesus monkeys. Table 13.3 further shows

231

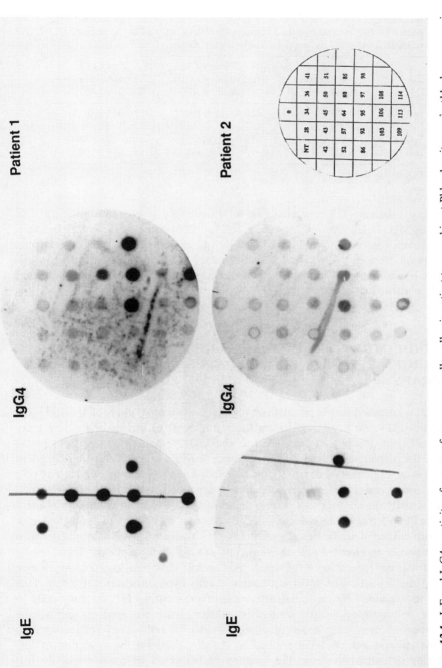

Figure 13.1. IgE and IgG4 reactivity of a serum from a grass-pollen allergic patient to recombinant Phl p 1 epitopes. λ gt11 phage expressing β-galactosidase (0) and Phl p 1 fragments (NT-114) were used to infect *E. coli* Y1090. Recombinant proteins were induced by overlay with nitrocellulose filters soaked in 10 mM isopropylthiogalactopyranoside (IPTG). Filters were incubated with serum and bound IgE was detected with ^{125}I-labeled anti-IgE antibodies (IgE) or mouse monoclonal anti-human IgG4 followed by a ^{125}I-labeled sheep anti-mouse antiserum (IgG4)

Table 13.3. Induction of IgE and IgG subclass responses against purified recombinant Bet v 1 in a group of seven immunized mice. The average time points of the first and maximal response in weeks, as well as the average OD (optical density) of the maximal response are shown.

	Time of first response (week $\pm$ SD)	Time of maximal response (week $\pm$ SD)	OD of maximal response ($\pm$ SD)
IgE	10.6 (± 4.08)	18.4 (± 8.16)	0.61 (± 0.15)
IgG1	15.4 (± 3.21)	27 (± 4.36)	2.5 (± 0)
IgG2a	20.9 (± 5.46)	35.9 (± 11.63)	1.6 (± 0.84)
IgG3	16.9 (± 1.07)	27 (± 8.19)	0.27 (± 0.05)

OD, optical density.

that Bet v 1-specific IgE production (at least under the given serum dilutions: i.e. IgE: 1:20; IgG1: 1:2000; IgG2a: 1:200; IgG3: 1:200) can be detected earlier than IgG subclass responses. While these data do not exclude the fact that the B cells which produced Bet v 1-specific IgE had switched to IgG production earlier on, the kinetics of the observed immune response argues against a preferential sequential μ–$\gamma 1$–ε class switch program.

13.5 INDUCTION OF IgE AND IgG4 RESPONSES AGAINST ALLERGEN EPITOPES DURING HYPOSENSITIZATION THERAPY

It is well established that hyposensitization treatment induces allergen-specific IgG4 antibodies (31). We have used recombinant fragments of the major timothy grass pollen allergen, Phl p 1, to measure IgE and IgG4 responses in sera from grass-pollen allergic patients before, during and after standard hyposensitization treatment (T Ball *et al*, unpublished data). Figure 13.2 shows the IgE and IgG4 reactivity of a serum from a grass-pollen allergic patient with recombinant Phl p 1 fragments. While initially the serum contained no detectable IgE and IgG4 antibodies reactive with the Phl p 1 fragments, induction of IgE responses was observed during and after the treatment. IgG4 antibodies against the Phl p 1 fragments were induced later than IgE antibodies and reacted with the same but also different fragments. These results suggest that the induction of IgE antibodies against defined allergen epitopes may precede the induction of IgG4 antibodies during hyposensitization therapy. This might be explained by an initial activation of pre-existing IgE memory cells to produce epitope-specific IgE antibodies, whereas later on—perhaps during the application of increasing doses of allergens—new B-cell clones are recruited to produce epitope-specific IgG4 antibodies. As discussed for the induction of IgE responses in animal systems, the kinetics of the onset of epitope-specific IgE and IgG antibodies and their partially different specificity seem to argue against

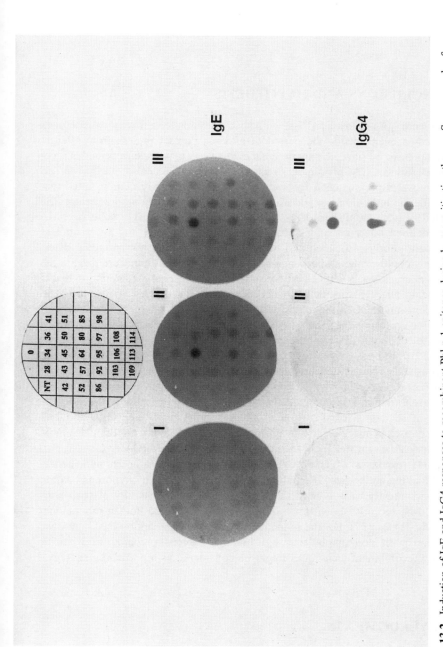

Figure 13.2. Induction of IgE and IgG4 responses to recombinant Phl p 1 epitopes during hyposensitization therapy. Serum samples from a grass pollen allergic patient were collected before (I), during (II) and after (III) hyposensitization treatment and tested for IgE (IgE) and IgG4 (IgG4) reactivity with recombinant phage clones expressing Phl p 1 fragments (NT-114) or β-galactosidase (0: negative control). Bound IgE and IgG4 antibodies were detected, as described in Figure 13.1

a sequential class switch program which proceeds from IgM via IgG4 to IgE production (see also Chapter 2).

13.6 CONCLUSIONS AND HYPOTHESIS

Although serum IgE is short lived, IgE with specificity for certain seasonal allergens can be detected even outside the period of allergen contact in sera from allergic patients. At present we have no experimental evidence as to whether repeated contact with allergen induces IgM precursors in allergic patients to switch from IgM to IgE or simply activates pre-switched IgE memory cells. It was early demonstrated that sera from allergic individuals in addition to IgE antibodies contain allergen-specific IgG (T Ball *et al*, unpublished data). Comparing the IgE and IgG subclass reactivities to defined allergens and epitopes, it appears that IgE and IgG subclass reactivities are poorly associated and directed in part to different antigenic determinants. This could explain why patients suffer from allergen exposure despite the presence of allergen-specific IgG antibodies. Given the reasonable assumption that B cells producing allergen-specific IgG subclasses were not deleted or inactivated in allergic patients and that, in the majority, allergen-specific IgG antibodies have high affinity for the corresponding allergen, comparable to IgE, the IgE and IgG subclass recognition of defined (i.e. recombinant) allergens and allergen epitopes as well as the kinetics of antibody responses observed in experimental animal models and during hyposensitization might be interpreted as a footprint of a preferentially not sequential (i.e. direct) class switch from IgM to IgE. However, these findings certainly represent rather indirect evidence and, in principle, do not exclude the occurrence of sequential class switch in allergic individuals. Since IgE and IgG subclass responses in allergic patients appear rather dissociated, it might be desirable to use hyposensitization treatment to induce allergen-specific IgG subclass (in particular, IgG4) responses which recognize preferentially IgE epitopes and, hence, represent blocking antibodies. The induction of IgG antibodies by hyposensitization treatment was already early noted (32, 33) and the blocking activity of such antibodies could be recently shown for a defined Bet v 1 specific human monoclonal IgG antibody, BAB1 (27). For the induction of such blocking antibodies, high dose immunization with non-anaphylactic IgE-binding haptens prepared from major allergens by recombinant techniques might be considered as a promising strategy.

ACKNOWLEDGMENTS

This work was supported by grant S06703 from the Austrian Science Foundation and by a grant from Pharmacia-Upjohn, Uppsala, Sweden.

REFERENCES

1. Radbruch A (1991) The molecular basis of immunoglobulin class switching: switch transcription versus switch recombination. *Immunol Res* **10**:381–385.
2. Alt FW, Oltz EM, Young F, Gorman J, Taccioli G and Chen J (1992) VDJ recombination. *Immunol Today* **13**:306–314.
3. Chen J and Alt FW (1993) Gene rearrangement and B cell development. *Curr Opin Immunol* **5**:194–200.
4. Harriman W, Volk H, Defranoux N and Wabl M (1993) Immunoglobulin class switch recombination. *Annu Rev Immunol* **11**:361–384.
5. Coffman RL, Lebman DA and Rothman P (1993) Mechanism and regulation of immunoglobulin isotype switching. *Adv Immunol* **54**:229–270.
6. Snapper CM and Paul WE (1987) Interferon-γ and B cell stimulatory factor-1 reciprocally regulate Ig isotype production. *Science* **236**:944–947.
7. Del Prete GF, Maggi E, Parronchi P *et al* (1988) IL-4 is an essential factor for the IgE synthesis induced *in vitro* by human T-cell clones and their supernatants. *J Immunol* **140**:4193–4198.
8. Punnonen J, Aversa G, Cocks BG *et al* (1993) Interleukin 13 induces interleukin-4-independent IgG4 and IgE synthesis and CD23 expression by human B cells. *Proc Natl Acad Sci USA* **90**:3730–3734.
9. Vercelli D and Geha RS (1992) Regulation of isoype switching. *Curr Opin Immunol* **4**:794–797.
10. Vercelli D (1993) Regulation of IgE synthesis. *Allergy Proc* **14**:413–416.
11. Mandler R, Finkelman FD, Levine AD and Snapper CM (1993) IL-4 induction of IgE class switching by lipopolysaccaride-activated murine B cells occurs predominantly through sequential switching. *J Immunol* **150**:407–418.
12. Siebenkotten G, Esser C, Wabl M and Radbruch A (1992) The murine IgG1/IgE class switch program. *Eur J Immunol* **22**:1827–1834.
13. Jung S, Siebenkotten G and Radbruch A (1994) Frequency of immunoglobulin E class switching is autonomously determined and independent of prior switching to other classes. *J Exp Med* **179**:2023–2026.
14. Mills FC, Thyphronitis G, Finkelman FD and Max EE (1992) Ig μ-ε isotype switch in IL-4-treated human B lymphoblastoid cells. Evidence for a sequential switch. *J Immunol* **149**:1075–1085.
15. Irsch J, Hendriks R, Tesch H, Schuurman R and Radbruch A (1993) Evidence for a human IgG1 class switch program. *Eur J Immunol* **23**:481–486.
16. Fujieda S, Zhang K and Saxon A (1995) IL-4 plus CD40 monoclonal antibody induces human B cells γ subclass-specific isotype switch: switching to γ1, γ3, γ4, but not γ2. *J Immunol* **155**:2318–2328.
17. Zhang K, Mills FC and Saxon A (1994) Switch circles from IL-4-directed ε class switching from human B lymphocytes. Evidence for direct, sequential, and multiple step sequential switch from μ to ε Ig heavy chain gene. *J Immunol* **152**:3427–3435.
18. van der Stoep N, Korver W and Logtenberg T (1994) *In vivo* and *in vitro* IgE isotype switching in human B lymphocytes: evidence for a predominantly direct IgM to IgE class switch program. *Eur J Immunol* **24**:1307–1311.
19. Valenta R and Kraft D (1995) Recombinant allergens for diagnosis and therapy of allergic diseases. *Curr Opin Immunol* **7**:751–756.
20. Vrtala S, Mayer P, Ferreira F *et al* (1996) Induction of IgE antibodies in mice and rhesus monkeys with recombinant birch pollen allergens; different allergenicity of Bet v 1 and Bet v 2. *J Allergy Clin Immunol* **98**:913–921.

21. Ferreira F, Mayer P, Sperr WR *et al* (1996) Induction of IgE antibodies with predefined specificity in rhesus monkeys with recombinant birch pollen allergens, Bet v 1 and Bet v 2. *J Allergy Clin Immunol* **97**:95–103.

22. Menz G, Dolecek C, Schönheit-Kenn U *et al* (1996) Serological and skin-test diagnosis of birch pollen allergy with recombinant Bet v 1, the major birch pollen allergen. *Clin Exp Allergy* **26**:50–60.

23. Vrtala S, Susani M, Sperr WR *et al* (1996) Immunologic characterization of purified recombinant timothy grass pollen (*Phleum pratense*) allergens (Phl p 1, Phl p 2, Phl p 5). *J Allergy Clin Immunol* **97**:781–787.

24. Laffer S, Spitzauer S, Susani M *et al* (1996) Comparison of recombinant timothy grass pollen allergens with natural extract for diagnosis of grass pollen allergy in different populations. *J Allergy Clin Immunol* **98**:652–658.

25. Pauli G, Oster JP, Deviller P *et al* (1996) Skin testing with recombinant allergens rBet v 1 and birch profilin, rBet v 2: diagnostic value for birch pollen and associated allergies. *J Allergy Clin Immunol* **97**:1100–1109.

26. Tame A, Sakiyama Y, Kobayashi I, Terai I and Kobayashi K (1996) Differences in titres of IgE, IgG4 and other IgG subclass anti-Der p 2 antibodies in allergic and non-allergic patients measured with recombinant allergen. *Clin Exp Allergy* **26**:43–49.

27. Visco V, Dolecek C, Denepoux S *et al* (1996) Human monoclonal antibodies that modulate the binding of specific IgE to birch pollen Bet v 1. *J Immunol* **157**:956–962.

28. Kobayashi I, Sakiyama Y, Tame A, Kobayashi K and Matsumoto S (1996) IgE and IgG4 antibodies from patients with mite allergy recognize different epitopes of *Dermatophagoides pteronyssinus* group II antigen (Der p 2). *J Allergy Clin Immunol* **97**:638–645.

29. Ball T, Vrtala S, Sperr WR *et al* (1994) Isolation of an immunodominant IgE hapten from an expression cDNA library. *J Biol Chem* **269**:28323–28328.

30. Fedorov AA, Ball T, Mahoney NM, Valenta R and Almo SC. (1997) Crystal structure and IgE-epitope mapping of birch pollen profilin: molecular basis for allergen cross-reactivity. *Structure* **5**:33–45.

31. Aalberse RC, Gaag R and Leeuwen J (1983) Serologic aspects of IgG4 antibodies. I. Prolonged immunization results in an IgG4-restricted response. *J Immunol* **130**:722–726.

32. Cooke RA, Bernhard JH, Hebald S and Stull A (1935) Serological evidence of immunity with co-existing sensitization in hay fever type of human allergy. *J Exp Med* **62**:733–750.

33. Loveless MH (1940) Immunological studies of pollinosis. I. The presence of 2 antibodies related to the same pollen-antigen in the serum of treated hay fever patients. *J Immunol* **38**:25–50.

Index

Index compiled by Liza Weinkove